Moderate and Deep Sedation in Clinical Practice

Moderate and Deep Sedation in Clinical Practice

Edited by

Richard D. Urman, MD, MBA
Harvard Medical School

Alan D. Kaye, MD, PhD
Louisiana State University School of Medicine

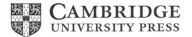

CAMBRIDGE UNIVERSITY PRESS

Cambridge, New York, Melbourne, Madrid, Cape Town,
Singapore, São Paulo, Delhi, Tokyo, Mexico City

Cambridge University Press
The Edinburgh Building, Cambridge CB2 8RU, UK

Published in the United States of America
by Cambridge University Press, New York

www.cambridge.org
Information on this title: www.cambridge.org/9781107400450

First published 2012

Printed in the United Kingdom at the University Press, Cambridge

A catalog record for this publication is available from the British Library

Library of Congress Cataloging-in-Publication Data

Moderate and deep sedation in clinical practice / edited by
Richard D. Urman, Alan D. Kaye.
    p. ; cm.
    Includes bibliographical references and index.
    ISBN 978-1-107-40045-0 (Paperback)
  1. Anesthesia–Handbooks, manuals, etc. 2. Conscious sedation–
Handbooks, manuals, etc. 3. Sedatives–Handbooks, manuals, etc.
I. Urman, Richard D. II. Kaye, Alan David.
    [DNLM: 1. Conscious Sedation. 2. Deep Sedation. WO 200]
    RD82.2.M63 2012
    617.9$'$6–dc23

                             2011023151

ISBN 978-1-107-40045-0 Paperback

To my patients, who are the ultimate beneficiaries of this work

To my colleagues from nursing, multiple medical specialties, and administration for their invaluable editorial input and collaboration

To my parents and my wife Zina Matlyuk-Urman, MD, for their encouragement and support

Richard D. Urman

To my mother Florence Feldman, who has never given up in her efforts to make a good life for her children and whose kindness and love I can never adequately repay

To my father Joel Kaye, for providing me with thousands of enlightening lessons in life and for helping to shape me into the man I am today

To my stepparents Gideon Feldman and Andrea Bennett-Kaye, who helped raise me, providing love, support, and wisdom over the last 30+ years

To my wife Kim Kaye, MD, and my children Aaron and Rachel Kaye, for making each day worth living

Alan D. Kaye

Contents

Contributors

Mary T. Antonelli, RN, MPH
Senior Director, Health Care Quality
and Patient Safety, New England Baptist
Hospital, Boston, MA, USA

Maria A. Antor, MD
Postdoctoral Researcher, Department of
Anesthesiology, Ohio State University,
Columbus, OH, USA

Alfredo R. Arribas, DOS, MS
Resident, Department of Oral and
Maxillofacial Surgery, Louisiana State
University, New Orleans, LA

Ron Banister, MD
Assistant Professor, Department of
Anesthesiology, Texas Tech University
Health Sciences Center, Lubbock, TX, USA

Donna Beitler, MS, RN
Nurse Educator, Johns Hopkins Hospital,
Baltimore, MD, USA

Ellen K. Bergeron, RN, MSN
Nursing Program Director, Center for
Nursing Excellence, Brigham and Women's
Hospital, Boston, MA, USA

Sergio D. Bergese, MD
Associate Professor, Department of
Anesthesiology, Ohio State University,
Columbus, OH, USA

Louise Caperelli-White, RN, MSN
Clinical Nurse Educator, Thoracic Surgical
ICU, Brigham and Women's Hospital,
Boston, MA, USA

Corey E. Collins, DO, FAAP
Director, Pediatric Anesthesia, Department
of Anesthesiology, Massachusetts Eye and
Ear Infirmary, Boston, MA, USA

Karen B. Domino, MD, MPH
Professor of Anesthesiology, Department
of Anesthesiology and Pain Medicine,
University of Washington School of
Medicine, Seattle, WA, USA

Charles Fox, MD
Vice Chair of Anesthesiology, Department
of Anesthesiology, Tulane University
Medical Center, New Orleans, LA, USA

Mary Elise Fox
Summer Research Assistant, Department of
Anesthesiology, Tulane University Medical
Center, New Orleans, LA, USA

Julie Gayle, MD
Tulane Avenue, New Orleans,
LA, USA

Kristi Dorn Hare, RN, MSN, CCRN, FNP.BC
Improvement Advisor, Sedation
and Analgesia Services, Performance
Improvement, University of California
Irvine Medical Center, Orange,
CA, USA

Eugenie S. Heitmiller, MD
Associate Professor of Anesthesiology and
Pediatrics, Department of Anesthesiology
and Critical Care Medicine, the Johns
Hopkins Hospital, Baltimore, MD, USA

Bommy Hong, MD
Resident, Department of Anesthesiology
and Critical Care Medicine, the Johns
Hopkins Hospital, Baltimore, MD, USA

Joseph C. Hung, MD
Chief Resident, Department of
Anesthesiology and Critical Care Medicine,
the Johns Hopkins Hospital, Baltimore,
MD, USA

Philip Kalarickal, MD, MPH
Assistant Professor of Anesthesiology,
Department of Anesthesiology, Tulane
University Medical Center, New Orleans,
LA, USA

Adam M. Kaye, PharmD
Department of Pharmacy Practice,
Thomas J. Long School of Pharmacy and
Health Sciences, University of the Pacific,
Stockton, CA, USA

Alan D. Kaye, MD, PhD
Professor and Chairman, Department of
Anesthesiology, Louisiana State University,
New Orleans, LA, USA

Jeffrey S. Kelly, MD, FACEP
Associate Professor, Department of
Anesthesiology and Critical Care Medicine,
Wake Forest University School of
Medicine, Winston-Salem, NC, USA

Eunhea Kim, MD
Resident in Anesthesiology, Department of
Anesthesiology, Perioperative and Pain
Medicine, Brigham and Women's Hospital,
Boston, MA, USA

Lyubov Kozmenko, RN
Acting Director of Simulation,
Nursing Skills and Technology Center,
Louisiana State University School of
Nursing, New Orleans, LA, USA

Valeriy Kozmenko, MD
Director of Simulation, Department of
Anesthesia, Louisiana State University
School of Medicine, New Orleans, LA, USA

Laura Kress, RN, MAS
Assistant Director of Nursing Practice, the
Johns Hopkins Hospital, Baltimore, MD, USA

Martin Kubin, MD
Resident Physician, Department of
Anesthesiology and Critical Care Medicine,
the Johns Hopkins Hospital, Baltimore,
MD, USA

Usman Latif, MD, MBA
Resident, Department of Anesthesiology
and Critical Care Medicine, the Johns
Hopkins Hospital, Baltimore, MD, USA

Henry Liu, MD
Associate Professor of Anesthesiology,
Department of Anesthesiology, Tulane
University Medical Center, New Orleans,
LA, USA

Todd Liu, MD
Resident, Department of Anesthesiology
and Critical Care Medicine, the Johns
Hopkins Hospital, Baltimore, MD, USA

Joyce C. Lo, MD
Department of Anesthesiology,
Perioperative and Pain Medicine,
Brigham and Women's Hospital, Boston,
MA, USA

Kai Matthes, MD, PhD
Lecturer in Anesthesia, Department of
Anesthesia, Perioperative and Pain
Medicine, Children's Hospital Boston,
Harvard Medical School, Boston,
MA, USA

Julia Metzner, MD
Professor of Anesthesiology,
Department of Anesthesiology and Pain
Medicine, University of Washington
School of Medicine, Seattle,
WA, USA

Rahul Mishra, DO
Resident, Department of Anesthesiology,
Texas Tech University Health Sciences
Center, Lubbock, TX, USA

Debra E. Morrison, MD
Director, Pediatric and Neonatal
Anesthesiology, Medical Director for
Sedation, Health Sciences Clinical
Professor, Department of Anesthesiology
and Perioperative Care, University of
California, Irvine Medical Center,
Orange, CA, USA

Arnab Mukherjee, MD
Resident in Anesthesia, the Johns Hopkins
Hospital, Baltimore, MD, USA

Heikki E. Nikkanen, MD
Instructor in Emergency Medicine, Brigham
and Women's Hospital, Boston, MA, USA

Erika G. Puente, MD
Research Scientist, Department of
Anesthesiology, Ohio State University,
Columbus, OH, USA

Benjamin R. Record, DDS
Clinical Director, Baton Rouge Clinic,
Program Director General Practice
Residency, Assistant Professor,
School of Dentistry, Louisiana State
University Health Science Center,
New Orleans, LA, USA

James Riopelle, MD
Clinical Professor, Department of
Anesthesia, Louisiana State University
School of Medicine, New Orleans, LA, USA

Brenda Schmitz, RN, MS
Clinical Practice Consultant, Department
of Radiology, Northwestern Memorial
Hospital, Chicago, IL, USA

David E. Seaver, RPh, JD
Risk Manager, Risk Management and
Clinical Compliance, Brigham and
Women's Hospital, Boston, MA, USA

Patricia M. Sequeira, MD
Clinical Assistant Professor, Department of
Anesthesiology, New York University
School of Medicine, New York, NY, USA

Theodore Strickland, MD
Assistant Professor of Anesthesiology,
Department of Anesthesiology, Tulane
University Medical Center, New Orleans,
LA, USA

Heather Trafton, MS, PA-C
Manager of PA Compliance and
Development, PA Services, Brigham
and Women's Hospital, Boston,
MA, USA

J. Gabriel Tsang, MBBS
Resident, Department of Anesthesiology
and Critical Care Medicine, the Johns
Hopkins Hospital, Baltimore,
MD, USA

Alberto Uribe, MD
Postdoctoral Researcher, Department of
Anesthesiology, Ohio State University,
Columbus, OH, USA

Richard D. Urman, MD, MBA
Assistant Professor of Anesthesia and
Director, Procedural Sedation Management
and Safety, Harvard Medical School/
Brigham and Women's Hospital, Boston,
MA, USA

Ghousia Wajida, MD
Critical Care Medicine Fellow,
Department of Anesthesiology and Critical
Care Medicine, Wake Forest University
School of Medicine, Winston-Salem,
NC, USA

Emmett E. Whitaker, MD
Senior Resident, Department of
Anesthesiology and Critical Care Medicine,
the Johns Hopkins Hospital, Baltimore,
MD, USA

Jamie Wingate, MD
Resident in Anesthesia, the Johns Hopkins
Hospital, Baltimore, MD, USA

Michael Yarborough, MD
Assistant Professor of Anesthesiology,
Department of Anesthesiology, Tulane
University Medical Center, New Orleans,
LA, USA

Foreword

In the last decade, the role of the healthcare provider has changed with the evolution of sedation practices. Today, sedation is being administered by a variety of caregivers in many different settings. An increasing number of procedures are being performed under moderate (formerly known as "conscious") and deep sedation in both the inpatient and outpatient arenas. For the healthcare practitioner, it is critical to have knowledge of pharmacology, monitoring, and regulatory requirements, as well as of local and national policies related to the administration of sedation. The healthcare practitioner must be able to provide sedation safely in the appropriate setting and for appropriately selected patients and procedures, in order to have the desired clinical outcomes and improved patient and proceduralist satisfaction. Today, a variety of healthcare professionals are involved in sedation: nurses, physician assistants, non-anesthesia physicians, and anesthesia professionals. This book is a must-have guide to help you understand your role and what is expected of you. As an administrator I highly recommend this book as an invaluable A-to-Z reference guide for setting up and running a successful sedation program. This book contains up-to-date information on education and credentialing, competency assessment, monitoring needs, pain management, and emergency resuscitation for a variety of sedation areas: radiology, endoscopy, cardiology, emergency department, intensive care, ambulatory centers and offices, among others. Since regulatory requirements and guidelines are constantly in flux, this book includes the latest expectations from The Joint Commission, and many general and specialty-specific guidelines that affect sedation practice are conveniently listed in the Guidelines and Standards chapter.

Drs. Urman and Kaye have done an amazing job, drawing upon their many years of anesthesia and sedation experience to provide the reader with the latest evidence-based, practical knowledge of the various aspects of sedation practice. The book starts by defining sedation levels and helping you select and evaluate patients. The editors have made it easy to understand the different components needed to provide sedation safely. Pharmacology, regulatory parameters, quality management, legal considerations, and documentation tips are discussed. Information is provided on all spectrums, from pediatric to geriatric, and covering emergency department, medical-surgical, intensive care, and outpatient settings.

Having worked in the healthcare industry for over 35 years in critical care and medical-surgical units, and as an administrator in hospital inpatient and outpatient settings, I believe this is the most complete resource available. This book has contributions from many nationally known individuals who are experts in their respective fields. I hope that their experience and commitment to our patients will make a difference in your practice, and that this book will help to bring the level of knowledge and competency of your staff to a higher level.

Martha G. Smith, RN, MN
Director of Patient Care Services,
Interim Louisiana State University Hospital,
Spirit of Charity Trauma Center, New Orleans, LA, USA

Preface

With the tremendous growth of procedures being performed under moderate (formerly known as "conscious") and deep sedation, it is essential for all physicians, nurses, physician assistants, and other healthcare providers and administrators to develop appropriate policies and educational programs to provide safe patient care. Because guidelines and regulations put forth by many professional societies, The Joint Commission (TJC), and the Centers for Medicare and Medicaid (CMS) are constantly evolving, it is important to stay current and well-informed.

Procedures performed under moderate and deep sedation are increasing in complexity and duration, and many patients present with significant existing medical problems. A vast majority of these procedures are performed outside of the operating room in both inpatient and outpatient settings. Consequently, non-anesthesia providers are becoming more involved in the supervision and administration of moderate and deep sedation.

Our intention was to compile a practical, comprehensive, up-to-date handbook that can be used to set up and maintain a safe moderate/deep sedation program in your healthcare facility. We cover all essential topics such as definitions of sedation levels, patient evaluation and recovery, pharmacology, monitoring and equipment, legal and patient safety issues, controversies, and emergency resuscitation. We discuss specific clinical and administrative aspects for the nursing and physician assistant staff. The handbook describes special considerations for unique patient populations such as pediatrics, the elderly, and patients with significant medical problems. Finally, we cover topics related to the procedures performed in the endoscopy, cardiology, and radiology suites, the intensive care unit, the emergency department, the dental practice, and the infertility clinic. Our chapter contributors constitute many national experts in their respective fields.

We hope that you find this handbook an invaluable resource, whether you are a clinician or an administrator.

Richard D. Urman, MD, MBA
Alan D. Kaye, MD, PhD

Guidelines and standards

Richard D. Urman

American Academy of Pediatrics (AAP) and American Academy of Pediatric Dentistry (AAPD)

Guidelines for monitoring and management of pediatric patients during and after sedation for diagnostic and therapeutic procedures: an update (2006). *Pediatrics* 2006; **118**: 2587–602. Available online at www.aapd.org/media/Policies_Guidelines/G_Sedation.pdf.

American Association of Critical-Care Nurses (AACN)

Position statement on the role of the RN in the management of patients receiving IV moderate sedation for short-term therapeutic, diagnostic, or surgical procedures (2002). Available online at www.aacn.org/WD/Practice/Docs/Sedation.doc.

American Association of Nurse Anesthetists (AANA)

Position statement on the qualified providers of sedation and analgesia: considerations for policy guidelines for registered nurses engaged in the administration of sedation and analgesia (2003). Available from AANA (www.aana.com).

Latex allergy protocol (1993). *AANA J* 1993; **61**: 223–4. Available online at www.aana.com/aanajournalonline.aspx.

American Association of Oral and Maxillofacial Surgeons (AAOMS)

Statement by the American Association of Oral and Maxillofacial Surgeons concerning the management of selected clinical conditions and associated clinical procedures: the control of pain and anxiety (2010). Available online at www.aaoms.org/docs/practice_mgmt/condition_statements/control_of_pain_and_anxiety.pdf.

Anesthesia in outpatient facilities (2007). In *AAOMS Parameters of Care: Clinical Practice Guidelines*, 4th edn (*AAOMS ParCare 07*). 55.PC07-CD. Available from AAOMS (www.aaomsstore.com).

American College of Cardiology (ACC) and American Heart Association (AHA)

ACC/AHA guidelines on perioperative cardiovascular evaluation and care for noncardiac surgery (2007). *J Am Coll Cardiol* 2007; **50**: 159–242. Available online at content.online-jacc.org/cgi/content/short/50/17/e159.

American College of Emergency Physicians (ACEP)

ACEP policy statement: sedation in the emergency department (2011 revision). Available online at www.acep.org/policystatements.

Clinical policy: procedural sedation and analgesia in the emergency department (2005). *Ann Emerg Med* 2005; **45**: 177–96. Available online at www.acep.org/clinicalpolicies.

Policy statement: delivery of agents for procedural sedation and analgesia by emergency nurses (2005). *Ann Emerg Med* 2005; **46**: 368. Available online at www.acep.org/policystatements.

American College of Radiology (ACR) and Society of Interventional Radiology (SIR)

ACR–SIR practice guideline for sedation and analgesia (Res. 45, 2010). Available online at www.acr.org/guidelines.

American Dental Association (ADA)

Guidelines for teaching pain control and sedation to dentists and dental students (2007). Available online at www.ada.org/sections/about/pdfs/anxiety_guidelines.pdf.
Guidelines for the use of sedation and general anesthesia by dentists (2007). Available online at www.ada.org/sections/about/pdfs/anesthesia_guidelines.pdf.

American Nurses Association (ANA)

Procedural sedation consensus statement (2008). Available online at www.nursingworld.org/NursingPractice.

American Society for Gastrointestinal Endoscopy (ASGE)

Position statement: nonanesthesiologist administration of propofol for GI endoscopy (2009). *Gastrointest Endosc* 2009; **70**: 1053–9.
Sedation and anesthesia in GI endoscopy (2008). *Gastrointest Endosc* 2008; **68**: 815–26.
Guidelines for conscious sedation and monitoring during gastrointestinal endoscopy (2003). *Gastrointest Endosc* 2003; **58**: 317–22.

American Society of Anesthesiologists (ASA)

Standards for basic anesthetic monitoring (2011). Available online at www.asahq.org/For-Healthcare-Professionals/Standards-Guidelines-and-Statements.aspx.
Statement on anesthetic care during interventional pain procedures for adults (2010). Available online at www.asahq.org/For-Healthcare-Professionals/Standards-Guidelines-and-Statements.aspx.
Statement on granting privileges for deep sedation to non-anesthesiologist sedation practitioners (2010). Further information from ASA (www.asahq.org).
Continuum of depth of sedation: definition of general anesthesia and levels of sedation/analgesia (2009). Available online at www.asahq.org/For-Healthcare-Professionals/Standards-Guidelines-and-Statements.aspx.
Distinguishing monitored anesthesia care ("MAC") from moderate sedation/analgesia (conscious sedation) (2009). Available online at www.asahq.org/For-Healthcare-Professionals/Standards-Guidelines-and-Statements.aspx.
Guidelines for office-based anesthesia (2009). Available online at www.asahq.org/For-Healthcare-Professionals/Standards-Guidelines-and-Statements.aspx.
Standards for postanesthesia care (2009). Available online at www.asahq.org/ For-Healthcare-Professionals/Standards-Guidelines-and-Statements.aspx.

Statement on qualifications of anesthesia providers in the office-based setting (2009). Available online at www.asahq.org/For-Healthcare-Professionals/Standards-Guidelines-and-Statements.aspx.

Statement on safe use of propofol (2009). Available online at www.asahq.org/For-Healthcare-Professionals/Standards-Guidelines-and-Statements.aspx.

Statement on nonoperating room anesthetizing locations (2008). Available online at www.asahq.org/For-Healthcare-Professionals/Standards-Guidelines-and-Statements.aspx.

Guidelines for ambulatory anesthesia and surgery (2008). Available online at www.asahq.org/For-Healthcare-Professionals/Standards-Guidelines-and-Statements.aspx.

Statement on granting privileges for administration of moderate sedation to practitioners who are not anesthesia professionals (2006). Available online at www.asahq.org/For-Healthcare-Professionals/Standards-Guidelines-and-Statements.aspx.

Statement on granting privileges to nonanesthesiologist practitioners for personally administering deep sedation or supervising deep sedation by individuals who are not anesthesia professionals (2006). Available online at www.asahq.org/For-Healthcare-Professionals/Standards-Guidelines-and-Statements.aspx.

Practice guidelines for sedation and analgesia by non-anesthesiologists (2002). *Anesthesiology* 2002; **96**: 1004–17. Available online at www.asahq.org/For-Healthcare-Professionals/Education-and-Events/Guidelines-for-Sedation-and-Analgesia-by-non-anesthesiologists.aspx.

Practice advisory for preanesthesia evaluation (2002). *Anesthesiology* 2002; **96**: 485–96.

Association of periOperative Registered Nurses (AORN)

Position statement on allied health care providers and support personnel in the perioperative practice setting (2011). Available online at www.aorn.org/PracticeResources/AORNPositionStatements/Position_HealthCareProvidersAndSupportPersonnel.

Position statement on creating a practice environment of safety (2011). Available online at www.aorn.org/PracticeResources/AORNPositionStatements/Position_CreatingaPatientSafetyCulture.

Perioperative standards and recommended practices (2011). Available from AORN (www.aornbookstore.org).

Position statement on one perioperative registered nurse circulator dedicated to every patient undergoing a surgical or other invasive procedure (2007). Available online at www.aorn.org/PracticeResources/AORNPositionStatements/Position_RegisteredNurseCirculator.

Recommended practices for managing the patient receiving moderate sedation/analgesia (2002). *AORN J.* 2002; **75**: 642–6, 649–52.

Centers for Medicare and Medicaid Services (CMS)

CMS interpretive guidelines for anesthesia and sedation (summary). Available online at www.asahq.org/For-Members/Practice-Management/Interpretive-Guidelines-Templates.aspx and www.asahq.org/For-Members/Advocacy/Federal-Legislative-and-Regulatory-Activities/Interpretive-Guidelines.aspx (accessed June 2011).

Emergency medicine and CMS interpretive guidelines. Available online at www.acep.org/Content.aspx?id=75563 (accessed June 2011).

Society of Critical Care Medicine (SCCM)

Clinical practice guidelines for the sustained use of sedatives and analgesics in the critically ill adult (2002). *Crit Care Med* 2002; **30**: 119–41.

The Joint Commission

Accreditation handbook for office-based surgery: what you need to know about obtaining accreditation (2011). Available online at www.jointcommission.org/assets/1/18/2011_OBS_Hdbk.pdf.

Comprehensive accreditation manual for hospitals (CAMH): the official handbook (2011 update). Available online at www.jcrinc.com/Joint-Commission-Requirements/Hospitals.

University HealthSystem Consortium (UHC)

Moderate sedation best practice recommendations (2005). Available from University Health-System Consortium, 2001 Spring Road, Suite 700, Oak Brook, Illinois 60523, USA (www.uhc.edu).

Position statement on the role of the RN in moderate sedation best practice recommendations (2001). Available from UHC (www.uhc.edu).

Deep sedation best practice recommendations (2001). Available from UHC (www.uhc.edu).

Chapter

1

Introduction to moderate and deep sedation

Emmett E. Whitaker, Arnab Mukherjee, Todd Liu,
Bommy Hong, and Eugenie Heitmiller

History of sedation

Some have argued that the development of sedation and analgesia may be one of the preeminent advances in both medical science and human technology. The power to manipulate and alter human consciousness and perception of pain has opened the door to extraordinary possibilities for medical practice. However, the origins of these advances reach far back to the limits of written history. Ancient Greeks recognized that naturally occurring substances such as mandrake root and alcohol could alter consciousness and be used during surgical manipulations [1,2]. Inca shamans used coca leaves to assist in trephination operations in which burr holes drilled into the skull were thought to cure illnesses [1]. And surgeons in the Middle Ages used ice and so-called "refrigeration anesthesia" to dull pain sensation prior to incision [2,3].

The modern practice of sedation is the end result of a process of evolution in alteration of consciousness, likely starting with the discovery of the analgesic properties of ether [1,4]. A medical student from Rochester, New York, named William Clarke used ether during a tooth extraction in January 1842. Many believe that this procedure may have been the first successful use of ether. Sedative technique using ether was further developed by Crawford Long during a neck tumor excision [1,4,5]. Later in 1842, Horace Wells would be the first to give a public demonstration at Massachusetts General Hospital. Unfortunately, when the patient cried out in pain, he was ridiculed and the use of ether was called "humbug" [1,4,5]. William Morton later would return to the same "Ether Dome" at Massachusetts General Hospital to successfully demonstrate the use of ether [1,5,6].

Over the years, the practice of sedation/analgesia has evolved significantly. Some patients prefer sedation to general anesthesia, and they often feel less anxious about receiving the former. Indeed, many healthcare practitioners prefer sedation because it offers a rapid return to pre-sedation condition and because of other patient, provider, and procedure-related factors.

Moderate and Deep Sedation in Clinical Practice, ed. Richard D. Urman and Alan D. Kaye.
Published by Cambridge University Press. © Cambridge University Press 2012.

Table 1.1. Procedures performed under sedation administered by non-anesthesia-trained professionals

Head and neck	Superficial thoracic	Extremity procedures	Gastrointestinal/ abdominal	Vascular	Gynecologic/ urologic	Emergency department/ radiology
Dental extractions	Breast augmentation	Carpal tunnel release	Endoscopic retrograde cholangiopancreatography	Hemodialysis access placement	Dilatation and curettage	Reduction of dislocation or fracture
Blepharoplasty	Breast biopsy	Trigger finger release	Colonoscopy	Pacemaker insertion	Fulguration of vaginal lesions	Complex suturing
Rhytidoplasty	Bronchoscopy	Removal of pins/wires/ screws	Endoscopic ultrasound	Angiography	Fulguration of anal lesions	Insertion of elective chest tube
Rhinoplasty	Chest tube insertion	Closed reduction	Gastroscopy	Cardiac catheterization	Cystoscopy	MRI
Laceration repair				Radiofrequency ablation	Incision and drainage of Bartholin's cyst	Arteriograms
Cataract extraction				Electrophysiologic testing	Vasectomy	Liver biopsy

Recently, the definitions of "general anesthesia" and "sedation" have undergone a period of development, leading to further characterization of the two techniques as distinct. It should be recognized that practitioners of early dental and oral maxillofacial surgery were at the forefront of developing the practice of sedation [6]. By the 1980s, most sedation of healthy patients for such dental procedures was administered by a registered nurse (RN), supervised by the physician, using benzodiazepine with an opioid [4].

One of the central questions surrounding the practice of sedation relates to who should administer it. Many agree that the individuals most trained in the administration of sedative/ hypnotic drugs, airway management, and patient resuscitation should administer sedation. Unfortunately, the demand for such providers is significantly greater than the supply. Therefore, many different providers, from physicians to registered nurses to physician assistants, provide sedation in today's healthcare milieu. Additionally, a broad spectrum of procedures have been carried out under sedation administered by non-anesthesia-trained registered nurses (Table 1.1) [7].

As the technology and practice of sedation and monitoring have evolved, the scope of practice of many providers has expanded. With time, sedative techniques have transitioned out of the operating room and into more diverse locations. Procedures have become shorter and less invasive, and technology and medical science have advanced. Furthermore, persons administering and managing sedation for a patient have diversified in tandem. Procedural sedation has been administered by anesthesiologists, certified registered nurse anesthetists (CRNAs), registered nurses, medical technicians, physician assistants, dentists, surgeons, and even by patients themselves (with supervision). Sedation is more attractive than general anesthesia to many stakeholders because it offers a potentially shorter recovery time, requires limited airway management, requires fewer personnel, is often more cost-effective, and may result in better patient satisfaction [8,9,10].

Recent technological advances have drastically changed the practice of sedation. One of the most significant was certainly the development of pulse oximetry during World War II by Glen Millikan [11]. Using optics to monitor the hemoglobin oxygen saturation provides a wealth of information to the clinician. This development has revolutionized the safety of sedation.

Another critical milestone has been the evolution of sedative medications. Early sedative drugs generally had a slower onset and longer duration of action than many modern drugs, as well as many undesirable side effects. Over time, new agents were discovered or developed that reduced these limitations. One of the most common sedative medications is midazolam [12]. The popularity of this drug is likely due to its quick onset, short duration of action, and favorable safety profile. It lacks analgesic properties but can cause desirable amnesia. Propofol can be used to induce general anesthesia, but subhypnotic doses have benefits of titratable sedation with rapid onset/offset. Its antiemetic properties are especially beneficial in the ambulatory setting, but it should be noted that it lacks analgesic effects [7,12]. Currently, the opioid of choice for sedation analgesia for many practitioners is fentanyl. Again, this popularity is likely related to its potency and short duration of action, such that it can be administered quite safely by an experienced practitioner [7,12,13].

Definitions of sedation

In 2002, the American Society of Anesthesiologists (ASA) appointed a task force to update practice guidelines for non-anesthesiologists administering sedation and analgesia. Levels

Table 1.2. Continuum of depth of sedation: definitions of general anesthesia and levels of sedation/analgesia

	Minimal sedation	Moderate sedation/analgesia ("conscious sedation")	Deep sedation/analgesia	General anesthesia
Responsiveness	Normal	Purposeful[a] response to verbal or tactile stimulation	Purposeful[a] response after repeated or painful stimulation	Unarousable even with painful stimulus
Airway	Unaffected	No intervention required	Intervention may be required	Intervention often required
Spontaneous ventilation	Unaffected	Adequate	May be inadequate	Frequently inadequate
Cardiovascular function	Unaffected	Usually maintained	Usually maintained	May be impaired

Source: American Society of Anesthesiologists Task Force on Sedation and Analgesia by Non-Anesthesiologists [14].
[a] Reflex withdrawal from a painful stimulus is not considered a purposeful response.

of sedation/anesthesia were defined according to responsiveness, airway, spontaneous ventilation, and cardiovascular function, as shown in Table 1.2 [14].

The levels of sedation presented in Table 1.2 are useful only if there are agreed-upon definitions of the different levels of consciousness. The ASA defines these levels as follows [14]:

(1) **Minimal sedation (anxiolysis)** – a drug-induced state during which patients respond normally to verbal commands. Although cognitive function and coordination may be impaired, ventilatory and cardiovascular functions are unaffected.

(2) **Moderate sedation/analgesia (conscious sedation)** – a drug-induced depression of consciousness during which patients respond purposefully to verbal commands, either alone or accompanied by light tactile stimulation. No interventions are required to maintain a patent airway, and spontaneous ventilation is adequate. Cardiovascular function is usually maintained.

(3) **Deep sedation/analgesia** – a drug-induced depression of consciousness during which patients cannot be easily aroused but respond purposefully following repeated or painful stimulation. The ability to independently maintain ventilatory function may be impaired. Patients may require assistance in maintaining a patent airway, and spontaneous ventilation may be inadequate. Cardiovascular function is usually maintained.

(4) **General anesthesia** – a drug-induced loss of consciousness during which patients are not arousable, even by painful stimulation. The ability to independently maintain ventilatory function is often impaired. Patients often require assistance in maintaining a patent airway, and positive pressure ventilation may be required because of depressed spontaneous ventilation or drug-induced depression of neuromuscular function. Cardiovascular function may be impaired.

The ASA further states that it is not always possible to predict how an individual patient will respond to a particular sedation plan. If a patient's level of sedation progresses to a stage that is deeper than originally planned, the practitioner should be able to rescue the patient from the deeper level of sedation. For example, individuals who administer *moderate sedation/analgesia (formerly known as "conscious sedation")* should be able to rescue patients who enter a state of *deep sedation/analgesia,* and those administering *deep sedation/analgesia* should be able to rescue patients who enter a state of *general anesthesia* [14]. It is important to emphasize that general anesthesia does not necessitate endotracheal intubation: one can administer general anesthesia, as defined by the ASA, without any airway device in place. Finally, there is a distinction between moderate sedation/analgesia and monitored anesthesia care (MAC). Specifically, the ASA defines MAC as "the anesthesia assessment and management of a patient's actual or anticipated physiological derangements" that may occur during the procedure. Furthermore, the provider of MAC must be qualified to convert to general anesthesia and rescue the patient's airway, and must be trained in all aspects of anesthesia care [15].

With the tremendous growth in the number and complexity of procedures, sedation has expanded in practice to many non-anesthesia and non-physician practitioners. Many professional organizations have established their own practice guidelines and standards (see *Guidelines and Standards, XIV*). For example, the ASA guidelines specify recommendations in the following areas [14]:

(1) patient evaluation
(2) pre-procedure preparation
(3) monitoring in regard to level of consciousness, pulmonary ventilation, oxygenation, and hemodynamics
(4) recording of monitored parameters
(5) availability of an individual responsible for monitoring
(6) training of personnel
(7) availability of emergency equipment
(8) use of supplemental oxygen
(9) combinations of sedative–analgesic agents
(10) titration of agents
(11) anesthetic induction agents used for sedation/analgesia (propofol, ketamine)
(12) intravenous access
(13) reversal agents
(14) recovery care

Involvement and regulation of nurses practicing sedation

In the USA, there is little in the way of federal regulation with regard to scope of practice issues for registered nurses practicing sedation, so many look to state boards of nursing for regulation. Thus, there is much variability in the limitations placed on nurses practicing sedation across the United States. Nevertheless, the Association of periOperative Registered Nurses (AORN) has produced guidelines for what every registered nurse should know about "conscious sedation." These published recommended practices provide guidelines for who manage the care of patients during sedation/analgesia [16].

According to the AORN, moderate sedation/analgesia is "produced by the administration of amnesic, analgesic, and sedative pharmacologic agents." Furthermore, "moderate sedation/analgesia produces a condition in which the patient exhibits a depressed level of consciousness and an altered perception of pain but retains the ability to respond appropriately to verbal and/or tactile stimulation and maintains protective reflexes" [16].

The desire to lend safety to the practice of non-anesthesia RNs has led many state nursing boards to develop acceptable practices for such providers. In turn, each individual institution will use these guidelines to produce its own sedation protocols in accordance with state law. All nurses participating in the administration of sedation and analgesia should periodically review most recent policies and procedures in their respective state and institution.

Outside of state law, there are a number of nonlegal organizations that develop position statements and practice guidelines. These are frequently used in concert with state law to develop individual sedation policies. Position statements are developed by a panel of experts and, in the absence of clinical evidence, are based largely on expert opinion. Practice guidelines are systematically developed and evidence-based, and are designed to assist the practitioner in making clinical decisions on a day-to-day basis. Such guidelines should be clear and free of bias. Finally, "recommended practices" represent an organization's official position on an issue and, in this case, are considered "statements of optimum performance criteria on various aspects of technical and professional perioperative nursing practice" [15].

Knowledge of these regulatory issues is important. In the case of malpractice proceedings, all of the above-mentioned guidelines are used to develop a standard of care, which is considered to be what a reasonable, equivalent practitioner would do in a given situation. In order to be convicted of malpractice, one must not have met the standard of care. Thus, all practitioners should be familiar with guidelines relevant to their practice.

With the ever-widening scope of sedation, practitioners must recognize the importance of standardizing practice. Organizing bodies such as the ASA, the AORN, the American Association of Nurse Anesthetists, the Society for Gastrointestinal Nurses and Associates, the American Society of PeriAnesthesia Nurses, the Emergency Nurses Association, and the American Association of Critical Care Nurses are constantly updating and releasing practice guidelines for those who practice sedation (see *Guidelines and Standards, XIV*). Furthermore, in the United States, most state governments use these guidelines to regulate practice through legislation. The Joint Commission also surveys all healthcare organizations to ensure that professional standards are maintained and protocols are followed in regard to administering sedation to patients [13,14,17]. Patient safety must be the number one priority for practitioners who administer sedation.

Summary
The practice of sedation has evolved significantly over the past 30 years. Once mainly the task of anesthesiology personnel, the demand for sedation services has outstripped the supply. The result has been the expansion of the scope of practice of other professionals. With continued attention to a high standard of safety, many different professionals are able to provide sedation services to those patients who need them.

References
1. Sabatowski R, Schafer D, Kasper SM, Brunsch H, Radbruch L. Pain treatment: a historical overview. *Curr Pharm Des* 2004; **10**: 701–16.

2. Houghton IT. Some observations on early military anaesthesia. *Anaesth Intensive Care* 2006; **34** (Suppl 1): 6–15.

3. Furnas DW. Topical refrigeration and frost anesthesia. *Anesthesiology* 1965; **26**: 344–7.

4. Finder RL. The art and science of office-based anesthesia in dentistry: a 150-year history. *Int Anesthesiol Clin* 2003; **41**: 1–12.

5. Hammonds WD, Steinhaus JE. Crawford W. Long: pioneer physician in anesthesia. *J Clin Anesth* 1993; **5**: 163–7.

6. Ash HL. Anesthesia's dental heritage (William Thomas Green Morton). *Anesth Prog* 1985; **32**: 25–9.

7. Watson DS, Odom-Forren J. *Practical Guide to Moderate Sedation/Analgesia*, 2nd edn. New York, NY: Mosby, 2005.

8. Weaver JM. Two notable pioneers in conscious sedation pass their gifts of pain-free dentistry to another generation. *Anesth Prog* 2000; **47**: 27–8.

9. Meredith JR, O'Keefe KP, Galwanker S. Pediatric procedural sedation and analgesia. *J Emerg Trauma Shock* 2008; **1**: 88–96.

10. Blake DR. Office-based anesthesia: dispelling common myths. *Aesthet Surg J* 2008; **28**: 564–70.

11. Severinghaus JW, Astrup PB. History of blood gas analysis. VI. Oximetry. *J Clin Monit* 1986; **2**: 270–88.

12. American Association of Nurses. *Policy Statement on Conscious Sedation*. Washington, DC: AAN, 1991.

13. Cravero JP, Blike GT. Review of pediatric sedation. *Anesth Analg* 2004; **99**: 1355–64.

14. American Society of Anesthesiologists Task Force on Sedation and Analgesia by Non-Anesthesiologists. Practice guidelines for sedation and analgesia by non-anesthesiologists. *Anesthesiology* 2002; **96**: 1004–17.

15. American Society of Anesthesiologists (ASA). Distinguishing monitored anesthesia care ("MAC") from moderate sedation/analgesia (conscious sedation). Park Ridge, IL: ASA, 2009. Available online at www.asahq.org/For-Healthcare-Professionals/Standards-Guidelines-and-Statements.aspx (accessed June 2011).

16. Association of periOperative Registered Nurses (AORN). Recommended practices for managing the patient receiving moderate sedation/analgesia. *AORN J* 2002; **75**: 642–6, 649–52.

17. Hung CT, Chow YF, Fung CF, Koo CH, Lui KC, Larn A. Safety and comfort during sedation for diagnostic or therapeutic procedures. *Hong Kong Med J* 2002; **8**: 114–22.

Chapter 2

Pharmacology principles

Alan D. Kaye, Julie Gayle, and Adam M. Kaye

Introduction

An increasing number of procedures requiring moderate and deep sedation are being performed outside the surgical suite. As a result, qualified non-anesthesia providers are administering moderate and deep sedation to patients for a variety of diagnostic, therapeutic, and/or surgical procedures. Practitioners should aim to provide patients with the benefits of sedation and/or analgesia while minimizing the associated risks. In order to do so, individuals responsible for patients receiving sedation and/or analgesia should understand the pharmacology of the agents being administered as well as the role of pharmacologic antagonists for opioids and benzodiazepines. Furthermore, combinations of sedative and analgesics should be administered as appropriate for the procedure being performed and the condition of the patient. Policies and standards regarding administration of sedation and analgesia by non-anesthesia providers are addressed elsewhere in the book. The following chapter focuses on the pharmacology of the drugs most commonly used to provide moderate and deep sedation and their available reversal agents.

Pharmacology basics

A drug that activates a receptor by binding to that receptor is called an **agonist**. An **antagonist** is a drug that binds to the receptor without activating the receptor and simultaneously prevents the agonist from stimulating the receptor. **Synergism** is when the effect of two drugs exceeds their algebraic sum. This is commonly seen with benzodiazepines

Moderate and Deep Sedation in Clinical Practice, ed. Richard D. Urman and Alan D. Kaye.
Published by Cambridge University Press. © Cambridge University Press 2012.

Table 2.1. Causes of variability of individual responses
to a drug

1. Drug interactions	
2. Pharmacokinetics	Age
	Renal function
	Hepatic function
	Cardiac function
	Bioavailability
	Body composition
3. Pharmacodynamics	Genetic differences
	Enzyme activity

and opioids when they are used in combination. **Pharmacokinetic** properties of a drug determine its onset of action and duration of drug effect. More specifically, pharmacokinetics describes the absorption, distribution, metabolism, and excretion of a drug (i.e., what the body does to the drug.) **Pharmacodynamics** describes the responsiveness of receptors to a drug and the mechanism by which these effects occur (i.e., what the drug does to the body). Individuals respond differently to the same drug, and often these different responses reflect the pharmacokinetics and/or pharmacodynamics among patients (Table 2.1).

Pharmacokinetics (determines onset of action and duration of drug effect) is affected by route of administration, absorption, and volume of distribution. **Volume of distribution** is influenced by characteristics of the drug including lipid solubility, binding to plasma proteins, and molecular size. Pharmacodynamics and pharmacologic drug effects are described in terms of dose–response curves, which depict the relationship between the dose of a drug administered and the resulting pharmacologic effect. Dose–response curves predict the effect of the drug on the patient with increasing dose. Titration of a drug should proceed based on expected pharmacodynamics of the drug given. Key considerations during titration of medications include appropriate choice for the patient's condition (e.g., renal failure, liver failure, previous drug exposure), appropriate choice of incremental dosing (i.e., time and quantity), and periodic monitoring. Preexisting disease processes also effect elimination half-time, which is an important consideration when administering sedation. **Elimination half-time** is the time necessary for plasma concentration of a drug to decrease to 50% during the elimination phase. Because elimination half-time is directly proportional to volume of distribution and inversely proportional to its clearance, renal and hepatic disease (altered volume of distribution and/or clearance) affect elimination half-time. It is important to understand that elimination half-time does not reflect time to recovery from drug effects. Elimination half-time allows for an estimation of the time it will take to reduce the drug concentration in the plasma by half. After about five elimination half-times, a drug is nearly totally eliminated from the body. Therefore, drug accumulation is likely if dosing intervals are less than this period of time.

Context-sensitive half-time

Elimination half-time does not always explain duration of action of many drugs used in sedation, especially if multiple boluses or infusions are used. Context-sensitive half-time (CSHT) is defined as the time taken for blood plasma concentration of a drug to decline by 50% after a drug infusion has been stopped. The "context" refers to the duration of the

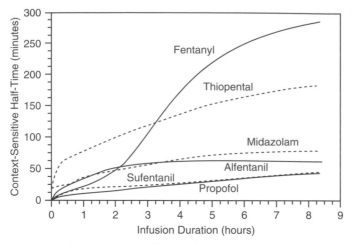

Figure 2.1. Context-sensitive half-times of drugs used in sedation.

infusion of the drug. Figure 2.1 shows examples of several classes of drugs (benzodiazepines, opioids, barbiturates, propofol) with their CSHT (minutes) plotted against duration of infusion (hours). As depicted in this representative graph, several hours of continued infusion or multiple repeated boluses given at close intervals can result in significant accumulation of the active drug in the patient. This can lead to exaggerated side effects (sedation, respiratory depression) and delayed recovery. Therefore, it is prudent to take CSHT of the drug into consideration, especially during longer (> 2 hour) procedures, and also to keep track of the total amount of drug(s) given by adding up all the boluses and/or infusions.

Synergy effects

Drugs used in sedation can have synergistic (i.e., additive) effects. This presents both advantages and disadvantages for the practitioner. The advantage is that one can achieve the desired level of sedation by using several agents while minimizing the total amount of each. For example, fentanyl has analgesic properties while midazolam is more useful as a sedative and an anxiolytic drug. On the other hand, when these drugs are administered together, it can lead to exaggerated sedation and respiratory effects. Therefore, titration to effect and close monitoring are needed. Table 2.2 shows commonly used drug classes and their relative effects on sedation, anxiety, and pain, and on the cardiovascular and respiratory systems.

Routes of administration

Routes of administration include parenteral (intravenous, intramuscular, inhalational) and enteral (oral, rectal, nasal). For the purposes of moderate and deep sedation, intravenous administration is perhaps most useful. Drugs administered by the intravenous (IV) route generally have a more rapid onset than those administered by the intramuscular (IM) route. Intravenous sedative/analgesic drugs should be given in small, incremental doses titrated to desired end points of sedation and analgesia, with adequate time allowed between doses to achieve those effects. Ideally, each component should be administered individually to

Table 2.2. Drug classes commonly used in sedation and their effects

Drug class	Effects				
	Sedation	Anxiolysis	Pain	Cardiovascular system	Respiratory system
Local anesthetic	−	−	++	$+^a$	−
Benzodiazepine	++	++	−	+	$+^a$
Opioid	+	+	++	+	++
Propofol	++	+	−	++	++
Barbiturate	++	+	−	++	++
Ketamine	++	+	++	+	$+^a$
Dexmedetomidine	++	+	+	+	−

−, no effect; +, moderate effect; ++, significant effect.
^{a} significant effect if overdosed

assess the need for additional analgesia to relieve pain or additional sedation to decrease anxiety or awareness.

Preemptive analgesia

Transmission of pain processes from tissue damage leads to sensitization of both peripheral and central pain pathways. Specifically, injury to nociceptive nerve fibers induces neural and behavioral changes that persist long after the injury has healed or the offending stimulus has been removed. This post-injury pain hypersensitivity can be due to posttraumatic changes in either the peripheral nervous system or the central nervous system. The noxious stimulus-induced neuroplasticity can be preempted by administration of analgesics or by regional neural blockade. Providing agents prior to surgery to reduce postoperative pain is termed **preemptive analgesia**, and its aim is to prevent sensitization of nociceptors before surgical stimulus. Thus, preemptive analgesia is a treatment that is initiated before surgical procedure to reduce sensitization of pain pathways. When appropriate drug doses are administered just prior to surgery, local anesthetic infiltration, gabapentin, opioids, acetaminophen, NMDA-receptor antagonist, cyclooxygenase (COX) inhibitors, nerve block, subarachnoid block, and epidural block have all been shown to provide postoperative pain benefits.

Drug interactions

Potential drug interactions require the clinician providing sedation to be cognizant of potential drug–drug effects, which can lead to morbidity and to mortality. Synergistic effects of two or more sedatives are well described and may result in central nervous system (CNS) and respiratory depression. Anesthesia providers spend years studying and refining their craft, and this is not always the case for the non-anesthesia sedation provider. Therefore, it is strongly recommended that healthcare providers develop an excellent understanding of the side effects as well as potential drug interactions of the agents they are using in the clinical setting. This must include herbals, of which there are over

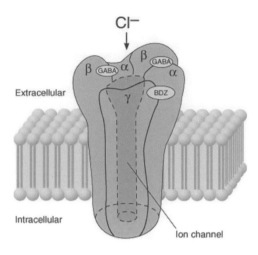

Figure 2.2. Schematic of benzodiazepine–GABA–chloride ion channel complex. BDZ, benzodiazepine.

29,000 available, and many of which can interact in unfavorable ways with conventional sedative medications. For example, St. John's wort can cause a lethal serotonergic crisis with meperidine, and kava-kava can potentiate CNS depression with any sedatives. Many of the "G" herbals – including ginger, garlic, ginseng, and ginkgo – can increase the risk of bleeding.

Benzodiazepines

Benzodiazepines are well suited for moderate and deep sedation because of their anxiolytic, amnesic, and sedative properties. At recommended doses and with careful titration, this drug class provides hypnosis (sedation) and anterograde amnesia with minimal effects on the cardiovascular and respiratory systems in healthy patients. Benzodiazepines do not provide analgesia. Commonly administered benzodiazepines include midazolam (Versed), diazepam (Valium), and lorazepam (Ativan).

Mechanism of action of the benzodiazepines is by facilitating the actions of gamma-aminobutyric acid (GABA) receptors in the brain. GABA is the principal inhibitory transmitter in the CNS. Benzodiazepines are highly lipid-soluble and rapidly enter the CNS, bind to GABA receptors in the brain and enhance opening of chloride channels (Figure 2.2). Increased chloride conductance produces hyperpolarization of the postsynaptic neuronal cell membrane and reduces excitability.

Desired clinical effects of the benzodiazepines used during moderate and deep sedation include anxiolysis, hypnosis (sedation), anterograde amnesia, anticonvulsant effects, and spinal-cord-mediated skeletal muscle relaxation. The different clinical effects of each benzodiazepine are due to binding of the GABA receptor at different sites. A large disparity exists between the level of sedation and the degree of amnesia. Patients may seem conscious, but they are amnesic to events and instructions. Benzodiazepines produce minimal changes in hemodynamic parameters (blood pressure, heart rate, cardiac output). However, dose-related effects of the benzodiazepines range from anxiolysis and amnesia to obtundation of airway reflexes and central respiratory depression. Recommended dose ranges of midazolam, diazepam, and lorazepam and other considerations are shown in Table 2.3.

Table 2.3. Commonly used benzodiazepines: dosing and other considerations

Drug (brand name)	Dosing (intravenous)		Onset	Duration	Considerations
	Pediatric	Adult			
All benzodiazepines					Major side effects are respiratory depression and hypotension. Reduce dose by one-third to one-half when used with other CNS-depressing drugs or in the elderly or debilitated.
Midazolam (Versed)	*Incremental bolus:* 0.05–0.1 mg/kg *Titrate:* 0.25 mg/kg every 5 min *Max:* 0.2 mg/kg	*Initial:* 0.5–2.5 mg **slowly** over 2 min *Titrate:* 0.5 mg increments *Max:* 5 mg	1–5 min	1–2.5 h	
Diazepam (Valium)	*Incremental bolus:* 0.1–0.3 mg/kg increments over minimum of 3 min *Max:* 0.6 mg/kg	*Initial:* 2.5–10 mg slowly *Titrate:* 2–5 mg every 5–10 min *Max:* 20 mg	30 s – 5 min	2–6 h	Diazepam is painful on injection. Should not be diluted.
Lorazepam (Ativan)	*Incremental bolus:* 0.05 mg/kg over 2 min May repeat ½ dose every 10–15 min *Max:* 2 mg	*Initial:* 0.02–0.05 mg/kg over 2 min; may repeat ½ dose every 10–15 min *Max:* 2 mg	5–10 min	4–6 h	Lorazepam is painful on injection. Prior to IV use, must be diluted with an equal amount of compatible diluent.

Midazolam (Versed)

Midazolam is a short-acting, water-soluble benzodiazepine possessing sedative, amnesic, anxiolytic, and anticonvulsant properties. Furthermore, midazolam has replaced diazepam for use in moderate and deep sedation. Midazolam is 2–3 times more potent than diazepam and is commonly used in procedural sedation. Midazolam's amnesic effects are more potent than its sedative effects. Like diazepam, midazolam is highly bound to plasma proteins. It is rapidly redistributed from the brain to other tissues and metabolized by the liver. Thus, it has a short duration of action. Metabolism in the liver is by hydroxylation, and midazolam is excreted by the kidneys after conjugation. Elimination half-time of midazolam is 1–4 hours, and shorter than diazepam. The elimination half-time may be doubled in the elderly as a result of age-related decreases in hepatic blood flow and possibly enzyme activity. Midazolam should be used with caution in the morbidly obese due to their increased volume of distribution and the prolonged half-life of the drug.

Diazepam (Valium)

Diazepam is a water-insoluble benzodiazepine also used in procedural sedation as well as in the treatment of anxiety and seizures. Like midazolam, it is classified as an anxiolytic, amnesic, anticonvulsant, and sedative. Diazepam is dissolved in propylene glycol and sodium benzoate and may cause pain on injection. Due to its high lipid solubility, diazepam is taken up rapidly into the brain. It is then redistributed extensively to other tissues. Because diazepam is highly protein-bound, diseases associated with decreased albumin concentration (e.g., malnutrition, liver disease, renal dysfunction, burns, and sepsis) may increase its effects. Diazepam is metabolized by the liver, producing two active metabolites: desmethyldiazepam and oxazepam. Desmethyldiazepam is metabolized more slowly and is slightly less potent than diazepam, but contributes to the sustained effects of the drug. In healthy individuals, elimination half-time is 21–37 hours. This range is markedly increased in those with cirrhosis of the liver and increased age, which is consistent with the increased sensitivity of these patients to the drug's sedative effects. Abrupt discontinuation of diazepam after prolonged administration may result in withdrawal symptoms. These symptoms include anxiety, hyperexcitability, and seizures.

Lorazepam (Ativan)

Lorazepam is a long-acting benzodiazepine with similar properties to midazolam and diazepam, but with more potent amnesic properties. Metabolized in the liver, its metabolites are inactive. Lorazepam has an elimination half-time of 10–20 hours, with urinary excretion accounting for greater than 80% of the dose given. It has a slower onset of action and much slower metabolic clearance compared to midazolam. Onset with IV administration is within 1–2 minutes and peak effect occurs at 20–30 minutes. Duration of lorazepam is 6–10 hours. Despite its slower onset of action, lorazepam is occasionally used for longer procedures requiring amnesia, sedation, and anxiolysis.

Adverse effects of benzodiazepines

Severe adverse effects may occur when benzodiazepines are administered with other drugs such as opioids. In combination with opioids, cardiovascular and hemodynamic perturbations become more significant. Respiratory depressant effects on spontaneous ventilation are enhanced dramatically when opioids are used in combination with benzodiazepines, and these are dose-dependent. These effects are also exaggerated in patients with chronic obstructive pulmonary disease. Furthermore, benzodiazepines exhibit a longer elimination half-time and greater sedative effect in elderly patients. Venoirritation may occur with diazepam and lorazepam.

Opioids

Opioids, also known as narcotics, are potent analgesics commonly used to provide pain relief during procedures. Opioids in combination with benzodiazepines provide adequate moderate and/or deep sedation and analgesia for many potentially painful procedures. Some of the more commonly used opioid agonists are morphine, fentanyl (Sublimaze), hydromorphone (Dilaudid) and meperidine (Demerol) (Table 2.4).

Mechanism of action of opioids describes the workings of all exogenous substances, natural or synthetic, that bind to opioid receptors and produce some agonist effects. Opioids act as agonists of opioid receptors at presynaptic and postsynaptic sites inside and outside the CNS. Occupancy of opioid receptors results in increased potassium conductance, calcium channel inactivation, or both, which produces an immediate decrease in neurotransmitter release. Opioid receptor activation results in mostly presynaptic inhibition of neurotransmitters (i.e., acetylcholine, dopamine, norepinephrine, and substance P). Opioid effects are dose-dependent and occur because of opioid binding at receptor sites. These receptor sites, located primarily in the CNS, include the mu, kappa, delta, and sigma receptors. The affinity of most opioid agonists for receptors correlates well with their analgesic potency. Desired clinical effects of opioids include analgesic, sedative, antitussive, and antishivering effects. Agonist action at the mu receptor is responsible for analgesia, euphoria, and sedation. Kappa receptor activation results in sedation and weak analgesia. Agonist action at the delta receptor also produces weak analgesia. The analgesic effect from systemic administration of opioids likely results from receptor activity at several different sites. These include sensory neurons in the peripheral nervous system, the dorsal horn of the spinal cord, the brainstem medulla, and the cortex of the brain. Each of the sites plays an important role in opioid-induced analgesia. The dorsal horn of the spinal cord provides analgesia by inhibiting transmission of nociceptive information. The medulla potentiates descending inhibitory pathways that modulate ascending pain signals. The cerebral cortex decreases the perception and emotional response to pain.

However, due to the widespread distribution of opioid receptors, many varied and unwanted effects may occur. Respiratory depression and physical dependence, pruritus and bradycardia result from agonist activity at the above receptor sites. Furthermore, agonism of the sigma receptor results in hypertension, tachycardia, delirium, and dysphoria. Other unwanted side effects of opioid agonists include orthostatic hypotension, skeletal muscle rigidity, nausea and vomiting, constipation and delayed gastric emptying, urinary retention, pupillary constriction, and sphincter of Oddi spasm.

Morphine

Morphine is the prototype opioid agonist with which all other opioids are compared. Morphine produces analgesia, euphoria, and sedation. The cause of pain persists, but even low doses morphine increase the pain threshold and modify the perception of pain. Continuous, dull pain is relieved by morphine more effectively than sharp, intermittent pain. Analgesia is most prominent when morphine is administered before the painful stimulus occurs. In the absence of pain, morphine may produce dysphoria rather than euphoria. When morphine is given IV, onset of the clinical effects occurs within a few minutes, and they peak within 15–30 minutes; elimination half-time is 2–4 hours. When administered IM, morphine is well absorbed, with an onset of effect in 15–30 minutes; peak effect occurs in 45–90 minutes, and the duration of action is 4 hours. Morphine

Table 2.4. Commonly used opioid agonists: dosing and other considerations

Drug (brand name)	Dosing (intravenous)		Onset	Duration	Considerations
	Pediatric	Adult			
All opioids					Reduce dose by one-third to one-half when given with other CNS-depressing drugs, or in the elderly or debilitated. May cause CNS and/or respiratory depression, nausea, vomiting, hypotension, dizziness.
Morphine	*Incremental bolus:* 0.05–0.15 mg/kg slowly *Titrate:* to desired effect *Max:* 3.0 mg single dose	*Initial:* 1–2 mg slowly *Titrate:* 1–2 mg slowly every 5–10 min *Max:* 15 mg	5–10 min	3–4 h	
Hydromorphone (Dilaudid)		*Initial:* 0.1–0.2 mg *Titrate:* 0.1–0.2 mg *Max:* 2.5 mg	3–5 min	2–3 h	
Fentanyl (Sublimaze)	Not recommended outside critical care areas in pediatrics	*Initial:* 0.05–2 µg/kg slowly over 3–5 min *Titrate:* 1 µg/kg at 30 min intervals *Max:* 4 µg/kg	30–60 s	30–60 min	Fentanyl and meperidine are contraindicated in patients who have received monoamine oxidase (MAO) inhibitors within last 14 days.
Meperidine (Demerol)	*Initial:* 1–1.5 mg/kg *Titrate:* 1 mg/kg increments *Max:* < 100 mg	*Initial:* 10 mg *Titrate:* 10 mg increments *Max:* 150 mg	1–5 min	1–3 h	

is metabolized by conjugation with glucuronic acid at both hepatic and extrahepatic sites, especially the kidney. Its active metabolite, morphine-6-glucuronide, produces analgesia and ventilatory depression by way of agonism of the mu receptors. Thus, elimination of morphine in patients with renal failure may be impaired, causing an accumulation of metabolites and unexpected depression of ventilation even with small doses of opioids.

Table 2.5. Equianalgesic opioid dosage table for a 70 kg adult

Drug	Duration	Oral	Parenteral	Half-life
Codeine	4–6 h	200 mg	120 mg IM	3 h
Morphine	3–6 h	30–60 mg	10 mg IM/IV	1.5–2 h
Hydromorphone	4–5 h	7.5 mg	1.5 mg IM/IV	2–3 h
Meperidine	2–4 h	300 mg	75 mg IM/IV	3–4 h
Fentanyl	1–2 h	N/A	0.1 mg IM/IV	1.5–6 h
Oxycodone	4–6 h	20 mg	N/A	N/A
Methadone	4–6 h	10–20 mg	10 mg IM/IV	15–40 h
Oxymorphone	3–6 h	N/A	1 mg IM/IV	
Levorphanol	6–8 h	4 mg	2 mg IM/IV	
Hydrocodone	3–4 h	30 mg	N/A	

Adapted from Urman and Vadivelu [1].

Hydromorphone (Dilaudid)

Hydromorphone is an opioid analgesic and is a semisynthetic derivative of morphine with 5–6 times the potency of morphine. Hydromorphone can be used to relieve moderate to severe pain, and can be administered via oral, intramuscular, or intravenous routes, among others. It has slightly faster onset of action and slightly shorter duration of action than morphine. Unlike morphine, it is metabolized to inactive compounds and results in less histamine release. Adverse side effects of hydromorphone are similar to those of other potent analgesics such as morphine and meperidine, but it may be a useful alternative in patients with contraindications or allergies to other opioids.

Fentanyl (Sublimaze)

Fentanyl is a phenylpiperdine-derivative synthetic opioid agonist structurally related to meperidine. Analgesic effects of fentanyl are 75–125 times more potent than those of morphine (Table 2.5). Fentanyl is often used as the analgesic component in moderate and deep sedation because of its rapid onset and minimal histamine release. A single dose of fentanyl IV has a more rapid and shorter duration of action than morphine. The greater lipid solubility of fentanyl compared to morphine explains its more rapid onset and greater potency. The short duration of a single dose of fentanyl associated with a rapid fall in plasma concentration reflects its rapid redistribution into inactive tissue sites such as skeletal muscle and fat. However, when multiple IV doses of fentanyl are administered, or with continuous infusion, progressive saturation of inactive tissues occurs. As a result, duration of analgesia and depression of ventilation may be prolonged when the plasma concentrations of the drug do not decrease rapidly. Metabolism of fentanyl occurs in the liver. IV fentanyl results in clinical effects within 30 seconds to 1 minute. Peak effects occur within 10 minutes and duration of action is 30–60 minutes following a single dose. Analgesic concentrations of fentanyl greatly potentiate the effects of midazolam and decrease the dose requirements of propofol. Synergism of opioids and benzodiazepines plays an important role in achieving hypnotic states for potentially painful procedures. However, the combination can easily result in ventilatory depression.

Meperidine (Demerol)

Meperidine is a synthetic opioid agonist, and like fentanyl it is a phenylpiperidine derivative. Meperidine is about one-tenth as potent as morphine. Meperidine is a shorter-acting opioid agonist than morphine with duration of action about 2–4 hours. Meperidine produces sedation and euphoria similar to that of morphine in equal analgesic doses. Metabolism is primarily hepatic. The principal metabolite, normeperidine, produces CNS stimulation in high concentrations. Urinary excretion is the principal elimination route. Elimination half-time of meperidine is 3–5 hours. Decreased renal function can predispose to accumulation of meperidine. Structurally, meperidine is similar to atropine and possesses atropine-like effects which may result in dry mouth, tachycardia, and pupillary dilatation. Myocardial depression can occur with meperidine at clinically relevant doses. Meperidine should not be used in patients on monoamine oxidase (MAO) inhibitors. In patients taking antidepressant drugs (MAO inhibitors, fluoxetine), meperidine may precipitate serotonin syndrome (autonomic instability with hypertension, tachycardia, diaphoresis, hyperthermia, agitation, and hyperreflexia) or potentiate side effects of serotonin reuptake inhibitors. In addition, meperidine may cause seizures in patients with renal insufficiency or a history of seizures, or when used in repeated or high doses. Normeperidine-induced seizures are more likely in patients who have received high chronic meperidine therapy, large doses of meperidine over a short period, and/or have an impaired ability to eliminate the metabolite. Elderly patients manifest decreased protein binding of meperidine, resulting in increased free drug in the plasma and an apparent increased sensitivity to the opioid. Because of its unique and extensive side-effect profile, meperidine is recommended as a second-line analgesic.

Adverse effects of opioids

Opioids have a direct effect on the respiratory center in the brain, resulting in a dose-dependent depression of the ventilatory response to carbon dioxide. Opioids also blunt the increase in ventilation resulting from hypoxia. They can produce generalized skeletal muscle rigidity. At clinically relevant doses, morphine and fentanyl do not cause significant myocardial depression. However, morphine and fentanyl can reduce cardiac output by causing a dose-dependent bradycardia. Other unwanted effects include nausea and vomiting, constipation, biliary spasm, and urinary retention.

Other drugs for deep sedation

Other drugs used for deep sedation include propofol (Diprivan), ketamine (Ketalar), dexmedetomidine (Precedex), and etomidate (Amidate) (Table 2.6).

Propofol (Diprivan)

Propofol is a substituted isopropylphenol with rapid, short-acting sedative hypnotic and antiemetic properties. Mechanism of action involves potentiation of the GABA receptor complex. Propofol is highly lipid-soluble, which explains the drug's rapid onset with bolus administration and makes it a readily titratable drug for intravenous sedation. The concentration of propofol decreases rapidly after intravenous bolus due to redistribution. Propofol

Table 2.6. Other drugs: dosing and considerations

Drug (brand name)	Dosing (intravenous)		Onset	Duration	Considerations
	Pediatric	Adult			
Propofol (Diprivan)	—	*Bolus:* 10–50 mg *Titrate:* 25–100 µg/kg/min	Within 30 s	2–4 min	Do not give to patients with egg or soybean oil allergy. Does not have any analgesic properties. Pain on injection may be reduced by lidocaine. May cause respiratory depression, hypotension, hiccoughs, wheezing, coughing.
Ketamine (Ketalar)	*Initial:* 1–2 mg/kg IV *IM dose:* 2 mg/kg	*Initial:* 10 mg, or 0.2–0.75 mg/kg	1 min	5–15 min	Consider concurrent midazolam. Contraindicated in patients with increased intracranial pressure. May cause hypertension, confusion, delirium, hallucinations, nystagmus, nausea, hypersecretions, respiratory depression, agitation upon awakening.
Dexmedetomidine (Precedex)	—	*Loading dose:* 1 µg/kg/h over 10–20 min *Titrate:* 0.2-0.7 to 1 µg/kg/h	10–15 min	2–4 h	Reduce loading dose by one-half for patients 65 years or older, and for those with impaired renal or hepatic function. May cause bradycardia, hypotension, and dry mouth. Concomitant use of other CNS depressants will result in increased levels of sedation.
Etomidate (Amidate)	0.2–0.3 mg/kg (ketamine preferred)	0.2 mg/kg over 30–60 s	< 1 min	3–5 min (up to 10 min)	Effects may be prolonged in liver failure. May cause nausea/vomiting, muscle twitching, respiratory depression.

is well suited for deep sedation because it allows for prompt recovery without residual sedation and a low incidence of nausea and vomiting. Typical dosing for minimal analgesia and amnesia effects is 25–100 µg/kg/min. Metabolism of propofol is both hepatic and nonhepatic (pulmonary uptake and first-pass elimination, renal excretion). Hepatic metabolism is rapid and extensive, resulting in metabolites that are excreted in the urine. Elimination half-time is 0.5–1.5 hours. Despite the rapid clearance of propofol by metabolism, there is no evidence of impaired elimination in patients with cirrhosis. Even at low doses, propofol can cause decreased oxygen levels and increased carbon dioxide levels, and inhibit airway reflexes. Because of its pronounced respiratory depressant effects and narrow therapeutic range, propofol should only be administered by individuals trained in airway management.

Propofol is a popular choice for sedation of mechanically ventilated patients in the intensive care unit. Propofol has been implicated in propofol infusion syndrome, in which critically ill patients requiring long-term (> 24 hours) sedation develop lactic acidosis, rhabdomyolysis, renal failure, and cardiac failure. Propofol can also cause pain and irritation upon IV injection. Mixing of propofol with any other drug is not recommended. Mixing of propofol with lidocaine to prevent pain with IV injection may result in coalescence of oil droplets, which may pose a risk of pulmonary embolism. The formulation of propofol containing soybean oil, glycerin, yolk lecithin, and sodium edentate has been implicated in episodes of bronchoconstriction following drug administration. Therefore, it should be avoided in patients with allergies to the above ingredients. Risk of infection and hypertriglyceridemia is also a concern. As supplied, it should be handled with aseptic technique and discarded once open for 6 hours.

Water-soluble preparations of propofol are available, including **fospropofol**, which is a prodrug that is metabolized to propofol, formaldehyde, and phosphate. Advantages of a water-soluble preparation include reduced pain at the site of intravenous administration and reduced chance for bacteremia and hyperlipidemia.The maximum recommended dose of fospropofol is 12.5 mg/kg, its peak levels are lower than for equipotent doses of propofol, and the drug has a longer-lasting effect.

Ketamine (Ketalar)

Ketamine, a phencyclidine derivative (PCP), is different from other hypnotic drugs in that it produces a cataleptic state in which a patient's eyes remain open with a slow nystagmic gaze. Ketamine is a CNS depressant resulting in dissociative state and analgesia. Hypertonus and purposeful skeletal muscle movements often occur with ketamine administration. The major effect of ketamine is thought to be produced through inhibition of the N-methyl-D-aspartate (NMDA) receptor complex. Ketamine also interacts with opioid, nicotinic, and muscarinic receptors. Ketamine's onset of action is rapid, reaching peak plasma concentrations within 1 minute after IV administration and 5 minutes after IM administration. Intense analgesia can be achieved with subanesthetic doses of ketamine at 0.2–0.5 mg/kg IV. Ketamine's clinical effects occur rapidly, with a return to consciousness within 15 minutes after a single dose.

Ketamine produces profound analgesia, stimulation of sympathetic nervous system, bronchodilation, and minimal respiratory depression. Ketamine is not significantly bound to plasma proteins and leaves the blood rapidly, to be distributed into the tissues. Ketamine is extremely lipid-soluble, which accounts for the rapid effects on the brain after administration. It is metabolized by hepatic microenzymes and has a large volume of distribution, resulting in an elimination half-time of 2–3 hours. Ketamine's active metabolite, norketamine, is one-third as potent as ketamine. Chronic administration of ketamine results in enzyme induction and tolerance to subsequent doses. Ketamine produces sympathetic nervous system stimulation with increases in blood pressure, heart rate, and cardiac output. It should be used with caution in patients with hypertension and coronary artery disease. Critically ill patients may experience the opposite effects, including hypotension and decreased cardiac output as a result of depletion of catecholamine stores and exhausted sympathetic nervous system compensatory mechanisms.

Ketamine does not cause significant ventilatory depression or affect airway tone. However, secretions are increased with ketamine administration and patients remain at risk for nausea and vomiting. Unpleasant emergence reactions limit the use of ketamine outside of the operating room. Combinations of ketamine and benzodiazepines limit these unwanted reactions and also increase amnesia.

Dexmedetomidine (Precedex)

Dexmedetomidine is a highly selective alpha-2-adrenergic agonist principally used for the short term sedation of intubated and ventilated patients in an intensive care setting. Hypnosis results from stimulation of the alpha-2 receptors in the locus ceruleus, and the analgesic effect originates at the level of the spinal cord. Dexmedetomidine as a single agent produces sedation, pain relief, anxiety reduction, stable respiratory rates, and predictable cardiovascular responses. Dexmedetomidine facilitates patient comfort, compliance, and comprehension by offering sedation with the ability to rouse patients. Dexmedetomidine produces sedative and analgesic effects without respiratory depression. Dexmedetomidine (0.2–0.7 mg/kg/h) is useful for postoperative critical care patients requiring mechanical ventilation. It does not result in clinically significant ventilatory depression, and sedation mimics natural sleep. The elimination half-time of dexmedetomidine is 2–3 hours. Dexmedetomidine is highly protein-bound and undergoes rapid and extensive metabolism in the liver. Its metabolites are excreted in the urine. Moderate decreases in heart rate may occur with dexmedetomidine infusion. Other adverse effects are probably due to unopposed vagal stimulation and include heart block, severe bradycardia, or asystole. Because of its sympatholytic actions, dexmedetomidine may also result in hypotension. Should it become necessary to reverse the sedative and cardiovascular effects of IV dexmedetomidine, atipamezole (Antisedan) is a specific and selective alpha-2-receptor antagonist that rapidly and effectively reverses these effects.

Etomidate (Amidate)

Etomidate is an intravenous agent with hypnotic but not analgesic properties. It produces minimal hemodynamic effects at clinically relevant doses. Etomidate is a carboxylated imidazole derivative of which one isomer possesses hypnotic qualities. Etomidate appears to have GABA-like effects; seemingly producing hypnosis through potentiation of GABA-mediated chloride currents. Etomidate is metabolized by hydrolysis via hepatic microsomal enzymes and plasma esterases. Etomidate is primarily cleared in the urine and has a short elimination half-time of 2–5 hours. Involuntary myoclonic movements are common with administration of etomidate. The frequency of the myoclonic-like activity can be attenuated by prior administration of an opioid. Awakening after a single injection of etomidate is rapid, typically without residual depressant effects. Etomidate has a high incidence of pain on injection and may result in venous irritation. Nausea and vomiting after administration may occur. The limiting factor on its use is the ability of etomidate to transiently depress adrenocortical function.

Adjunct medications
Diphenhydramine (Benadryl)

First-generation H_1 antihistamines cross the blood–brain barrier because of their lipophilic molecular structure, leading to sedation. It should be noted that adverse reactions may be due to their inhibition on muscarinic, serotoninergic and adrenergic receptors. Toxicity with overdose, whether intentional or accidental, has been reported. Antiemetic effects may be elicited, and clinically relevant uses can extend beyond the treatment of allergic symptoms to the treatment of vestibular disorders, as sedatives, as sleeping aids, and as antiemetics. In this regard, diphenhydramine, typically in a dose of 25–50 mg IV, can provide safe and effective sedation in most patients. Specific potential side effects include dry mouth, drowsiness, dizziness, nausea/vomiting, constipation, headaches, photosensitivity, and urinary retention.

Scopolamine

Scopolamaine is a muscarinic antagonist. It possesses sedative properties and is a treatment for nausea/vomiting and motion sickness. Historically, from the 1940s to the 1960s it was used to induce twilight sleep in laboring mothers to eliminate the memory of pain. In rare instances, this agent is utilized to provide amnesia and sedation in a variety of settings. Rare side effects include confusion, rambling speech, agitation, hallucinations, paranoid behaviors, and delusions. Preparations include oral, subcutaneous, IV, transdermal patch, and opthalmic.

Nonsteroidal anti-inflammatory drugs (NSAIDs)

Prostaglandins were first identified from semen, prostate, and seminal vesicles by Goldblatt and von Euler in the 1930s. The discovery of the cyclooxygenase reaction through which arachidonic acid is cyclized to yield prostaglandin, the identification of the cyclooxygenase enzyme, and the demonstration by Sir John Vane that aspirin, indomethacin, and NSAIDs were all inhibitors of cylooxygenase, all occurred in the early 1970s. Work by Habenicht in 1985 and later work by Needleman in 1990 ultimately demonstrated that an endogenous COX-1 and an inducible enzyme COX-2 existed.

It should not be surprising that NSAIDs have served as analgesics, anti-inflammatory, and antipyretic medicines since 1898 and are effective in mild to moderate surgical pain, with one benefit of this class of drugs being that they lack the adverse effects of opioids, including respiratory depression. Some common NSAIDs available include ibuprofen, naproxen, aspirin, indomethacin, and meloxicam. Surgical bleeding may be adversely affected by platelet dysfunction from NSAIDs.

Using structure activity relationships, pharmaceutical companies in the 1990s invested billions of dollars to develop more selective NSAIDs, namely COX-2 inhibitors (e.g., Celecoxib). These selective agents were introduced in 1999 and worked differently than older NSAIDs. Extensive research nearly 20 years ago identified the COX-2 site, as an inducible enzyme that is the location for the mediation of pain, inflammation, and fever pathways. All NSAIDs and aspirin inhibit active sites of COX-1 and COX-2. These agents typically bind with the side chain of Arg-120, forming a weak ionic bond. Many of the NSAIDs have a carboxylic acid or enolic acid portion that allows this bond formation. The COX-2 enzyme binding is in what is called a catalytic side pocket, and for aspirin this bonding is 10–100 times less efficient, thereby reducing its effectiveness at the COX-2 site.

These agents have many uses, including for mild to moderate pain relief and as a component for preemptive analgesia. Ketorolac (toradol) and ibuprofen (caldolor) are available as an intravenous preparation, and considerable research is ongoing to develop a COX-2 intravenous preparation in the near future. The use of NSAIDs can help reduce the amount of opioids administrated to the patient.

Acetaminophen

Acetaminophen (paracetamol) is widely used to reduce pain and fever. Intravenous acetaminophen can be found on more and more formularies, as its efficacy and safety profile have shown promise in recent literature. Double-blind clinical trials showed that IV acetaminophen reduced the need for opioid rescue medication. The pain medicine has been found to be well tolerated in recent clinical trials, having a tolerability profile similar to placebo. Furthermore, adverse reactions are extremely rare. An IV formulation of acetaminophen is available in Europe and is currently undergoing extensive clinical development for use in the United States. This IV formulation should have important implications for management of pain and fever for patients undergoing surgical procedures and interventions, as well in the intensive care unit.

Clonidine

Clonidine is a central alpha-2-receptor agonist, and is an antihypertensive medication. As a depletory of free and total catecholamine levels, it inhibits the release of norepinephrine. It has been used for many treatments beyond elevated blood pressure, including opioid withdrawal, other hyperarousal states, insomnia, and neuropathic pain, related to its sedative, anxiolytic, and analgesic properties. It is used in numerous preparations, including oral, transdermal, and epidural, to prolong the effects of analgesia when used together with local anesthetics. Since clonidine is a mild sedative, it can be used as a premedication before surgery or procedures. Prominent other side effects include lightheadedness, dry mouth, dizziness, and constipation.

Local anesthetics

Local anesthetics (LAs) prevent the generation and the conduction of the nerve impulse. Their primary site of action is the cell membrane, and the major mechanism of action of these drugs involves their interaction with one or more specific binding sites within the sodium (Na^+) channel. The degree of block produced by a given concentration of local anesthetic depends on how the nerve has been stimulated and on its resting membrane potential. Thus, a resting nerve is much less sensitive to a local anesthetic than one that is repetitively stimulated; higher frequency of stimulation and more positive membrane potential cause a greater degree of anesthetic block. These frequency- and voltage-dependent effects of local anesthetics occur because the local anesthetic molecule in its charged form gains access to its binding site within the pore only when the Na^+ channel is in an open state, and because the local anesthetic binds more tightly to and stabilizes the inactivated state of the Na^+ channel. As a general rule, small nerve fibers are more susceptible to the action of local anesthetics than are large fibers.

Local anesthetics, as unprotonated amines, tend to be only slightly soluble. Therefore, they are generally marketed as water-soluble salts, usually hydrochlorides. Inasmuch as the local anesthetics are weak bases (typical pK_a values range from 8 to 9), their hydrochloride salts are mildly acidic. This property increases the stability of the local anesthetic esters and any accompanying vasoconstrictor substance. Under usual conditions of administration, the pH of the local anesthetic solution rapidly equilibrates to that of the extracellular fluids. Although the unprotonated species of the local anesthetic is necessary for diffusion across cellular membranes, the cationic species interacts preferentially with Na^+ channels. Changes in pH of the injected local anesthetic solution can produce a shortening of onset time, with marked decreases paralleling major pH changes. The limiting factor for the pH adjustment is the solubility of the base form of the drug. For each local anesthetic, there is a pH at which the amount of base in solution is maximal (a saturated solution).

Another approach to shortening onset time for producing surgical anesthesia has been through the use of carbonated local anesthetic solutions. The local anesthetic salt is the carbonate, and the solution contains large amounts of carbon dioxide to maintain a high concentration of the carbonate anion. Combinations of local anesthetic with an opioid are increasingly used in situations where one desires sensory blockade without significant motor block, as in obstetrical anesthesia and pain management. The addition of epidural and intrathecal opioids allows use of lower concentrations of local anesthetic.

Plasma concentrations of local anesthetics are dependent on:

- the dose of the drug administered
- the absorption of the drug from the site injected, which depends on the vasoactivity of the drug, site vascularity, and whether a vasoconstrictor such as epinephrine has been added to the anesthetic solution
- biotransformation and elimination of the drug from the circulation

Peak local anesthetic blood levels that develop are directly related to the dose administered at any given site.

Undesired effects of local anesthetics

Table 2.7 shows the toxic dose of several local anesthetics.

Central nervous system

Following absorption, local anesthetics may cause stimulation of the CNS, producing restlessness and tremor that may proceed to clonic convulsions. In general, the more potent the anesthetic the more readily convulsions may be produced. Alterations of CNS activity are thus predictable from the local anesthetic agent in question and the blood concentration achieved. Central stimulation is followed by depression; death is usually caused by respiratory failure.

Cardiovascular system

Following systemic absorption, local anesthetics act on the cardiovascular system. The primary site of action is the myocardium, where decreases in electrical excitability, conduction rate,

Table 2.7. Local anesthetics: duration of action and toxic dose

Local anesthetic (brand name)	Concentrations (%)	Maxium total recommended dose	Volume of maximum total recommended dose	Average onset and duration of action
Procaine (Novocaine)	0.25–0.5%	350–600 mg	140–240 mL of 0.25% 70–120 mL of 0.5%	Onset: 2–5 min Duration: 15–60 min
Chloroprocaine (Nesacaine)	1–2%	≤ 800 mg	80 mL of 1% 40 mL of 2%	Onset: 6–12 min Duration: 30 min
Lidocaine, plain (Xylocaine)	1–2%	3–5 mg/kg; ≤ 300 mg	30 mL of 1% 15 mL of 2%	Onset: 1–2 min Duration: 30–60 min
Lidocaine, with epinephrine	1–2% lidocaine Epinephrine: 1 : 100,000 or 1 : 200,000	5–7 mg/kg; ≤500 mg	50 mL of 1% 25 mL of 2%	Onset: 1–2 min Duration: 60–240 min
Bupivacaine, plain (Marcaine, Sensorcaine)	0.25–0.5%	2.5 mg/kg; ≤ 175 mg	70 mL of 0.25% 35 mL of 0.5%	Onset: 5 min Duration: 120–240 min
Bupivacaine, with epinephrine	0.25–0.5% bupivacaine Epinephrine: 1 : 200,000	≤ 225 mg	90 mL of 0.25% 45 mL of 0.5%	Onset: 5 min Duration: 180–360 min
Mepivacaine (Polocaine)	1%	≤ 400 mg	40 mL of 1%	Onset: 3–5 min Duration: 45–90 min

Adapted from Windle [2].

and force of contraction occur. In addition, most local anesthetics cause arteriolar dilatation. The cardiovascular effects usually are seen only after high systemic concentrations are attained and effects on the CNS are produced. However, on rare occasions lower doses will cause cardiovascular collapse and death, due to either an action on the pacemaker or the sudden onset of ventricular fibrillation. However, it should be noted that ventricular tachycardia and fibrillation are relatively uncommon consequences of local anesthetics other than bupivacaine. Finally, it should be stressed that untoward cardiovascular effects of local anesthetic agents may result from their inadvertent intravascular administration, especially if epinephrine also is present.

Lidocaine

Lidocaine (Xylocaine), introduced in 1948, is currently the most commonly used local anesthetic.

Pharmacological actions

The pharmacological actions that lidocaine shares with other local anesthetic drugs have been described widely. Lidocaine produces faster, more intense, longer-lasting, and more extensive anesthesia than does an equal concentration of procaine. It is a good choice for individuals sensitive to ester-type local anesthetics.

Absorption, fate, and excretion

Lidocaine is absorbed rapidly after parenteral administration and from the gastrointestinal and respiratory tracts. Although it is effective when used without any vasoconstrictor, in the presence of epinephrine the rate of absorption and the toxicity are decreased, and the duration of action usually is prolonged. Lidocaine is dealkylated in the liver by mixed-function oxidases to monoethylglycine xylidide and glycine xylidide, which can be metabolized further to monoethylglycine and xylidide. Both monoethylglycine xylidide and glycine xylidide retain local anesthetic activity. In human beings, about 75% of xylidide is excreted in the urine as the further metabolite, 4-hydroxy-2,6-dimethylaniline [3].

Toxicity

The side effects of lidocaine seen with increasing dose include drowsiness, tinnitus, dysgeusia, dizziness, and twitching. As the dose increases, seizures, coma, and respiratory depression and arrest will occur. Clinically significant cardiovascular depression usually occurs at serum lidocaine levels that produce marked CNS effects. The metabolites monoethylglycine xylidide and glycine xylidide may contribute to some of these side effects.

Clinical uses

Lidocaine has a broad range of clinical uses as a local anesthetic. It has utility in almost any application where a local anesthetic of intermediate duration is needed. Lidocaine also is used as an antiarrhythmic agent.

Bupivacaine

Bupivacaine (Marcaine, Sensorcaine), introduced in 1963, is a commonly used amide local anesthetic. Its structure is similar to that of lidocaine, except that the amine-containing group is a butyl piperidine. It is a potent agent capable of producing prolonged anesthesia. Its long duration of action plus its tendency to provide more sensory than motor block has made it a popular drug for providing prolonged analgesia during labor or the postoperative period. By taking advantage of indwelling catheters and continuous infusions, bupivacaine can be used to provide several days of effective analgesia.

Bupivacaine was developed as a modification of mepivacaine. Its structural similarities with mepivacaine are readily apparent. Bupivacaine has a butyl (four-carbon substitution) group on the hydrophilic nitrogen.

Bupivacaine has made a contribution to regional anesthesia second in importance only to that of lidocaine. It is one of the first of the clinically used local anesthetic drugs that provides good separation of motor and sensory blockade after its administration. The onset of anesthesia and the duration of action are long and can be further prolonged by the addition of epinephrine in areas with a low fat content. Only small increases in duration are seen when bupivacaine is injected into areas with a high fat content. For example, a 50% increase in duration of brachial plexus blockade (an area of low fat content) follows the addition of epinephrine to bupivacaine solutions; in contrast, only a 10–15% increase in duration of epidural anesthesia results from the addition of epinephrine to bupivacaine solutions, since the epidural space has a high fat content.

Toxicity

Bupivacaine is more cardiotoxic than equieffective doses of lidocaine. Clinically, this is manifested by severe ventricular arrhythmias and myocardial depression after inadvertent intravascular administration of large doses of bupivacaine. The enhanced cardiotoxicity of bupivacaine probably is due to multiple factors. Lidocaine and bupivacaine both block cardiac Na^+ channels rapidly during systole. However, bupivacaine dissociates much more slowly than does lidocaine during diastole, so a significant fraction of Na^+ channels remains blocked at the end of diastole (at physiological heart rates) with bupivacaine [4]. Thus the block by bupivacaine is cumulative and substantially more than would be predicted by its local anesthetic potency. At least a portion of the cardiac toxicity of bupivacaine may be mediated centrally, as direct injection of small quantities of bupivacaine into the medulla can produce malignant ventricular arrhythmias [5]. Bupivacaine-induced cardiac toxicity can be very difficult to treat, and its severity is enhanced in the presence of acidosis, hypercarbia, and hypoxemia.

Clinical uses

In the United States, bupivacaine has been used mainly for obstetrical anesthesia and postoperative pain control when analgesia without significant motor blockade is highly desirable, as this is achievable with low bupivacaine concentrations. In contrast to lidocaine, however, when high blood levels occur with bupivacaine, a higher incidence of cardiotoxic effects is seen. Bupivacaine has a poorer therapeutic index than lidocaine in producing electrophysiological toxicity of the heart [6]. Although bupivacaine metabolism is slower in the fetus and newborn than in the adult, active biotransformation is accomplished by the fetus and newborn.

A second major role of bupivacaine is in subarachnoid anesthesia. It produces very reliable onset of anesthesia within 5 minutes, and the duration of anesthesia is approximately 3 hours. In many ways, it is similar to tetracaine; however, the dose of bupivacaine required is somewhat larger – specifically, 10 mg of tetracaine is approximately equal to 12–15 mg of bupivacaine. The onset of sympathetic blockade following spinal anesthesia appears to be more gradual with bupivacaine than with tetracaine. Also, the sensory blockade produced by bupivacaine lasts longer than the motor blockade, which is in contrast to what occurs with etidocaine and tetracaine. Bupivacaine can be used for subarachnoid anesthesia in either the glucose-containing hyperbaric solution (0.75%) or with the isobaric solution by using the drug packaged for epidural use as a 0.25% or a 0.5% concentration.

Ropivacaine

The cardiac toxicity of bupivacaine stimulated interest in developing a less toxic long-lasting local anesthetic. The result of that search was the development of a new amino ethylamine, ropivacaine, the S-enantiomer of 1-propyl-2′,6′-pipecolocylidide. The S-enantiomer, like most local anesthetics with a chiral center, was chosen because it has a lower toxicity than the R isomer. This is presumably due to slower uptake, resulting in lower blood levels for a given dose. Ropivacaine is slightly less potent than bupivacaine in producing anesthesia. In several animal models, it appears to be less cardiotoxic than equieffective doses of bupivacaine. In clinical studies, ropivacaine appears to be suitable for both epidural and regional anesthesia, with duration of action similar to that of bupivacaine. Interestingly, it seems to be even more motor-sparing than bupivacaine.

Clinical uses of local anesthetics

Local anesthesia is the loss of sensation in a body part without the loss of consciousness or the impairment of central control of vital functions. It offers two major advantages. The first is that the physiological perturbations associated with general anesthesia are avoided. The second is that neurophysiological responses to pain and stress can be modified beneficially, as described earlier in the chapter under the section on *Preemptive analgesia*. As discussed above, local anesthetics have the potential to produce deleterious side effects. The choice of a local anesthetic and care in its use are the primary determinants of such toxicity. There is a poor relationship between the amount of local anesthetic injected and peak plasma levels in adults. The serum level also depends on the area of injection. It is highest with interpleural or intercostal block and lowest with subcutaneous infiltration. Thus recommended doses serve only as general guidelines.

Treatment of local anesthetic systemic toxicity (LAST)

Symptoms of local anesthetic systemic toxicity (LAST) may include tinnitus, metallic taste in the mouth, lip numbness, lightheadedness, seizures, arrhythmias, and finally cardiovascular collapse. If suspicion for toxicity is high, prompt and effective airway management is crucial in preventing hypoxia and acidosis, which are known to potentiate LAST.

If seizures occur, they should be rapidly treated with benzodiazepines. Small doses of propofol or thiopental are also acceptable. Although propofol can stop seizures, large doses further depress cardiac function, and propofol should be avoided when there are signs of cardiovascular compromise.

If cardiac arrest occurs, initiate ACLS. Avoid calcium channel blockers and beta-adrenergic receptor blockers. If ventricular arrhythmias develop, amiodarone is the preferred treatment (lidocaine or procainamide are not recommended).

Lipid emulsion therapy can be initiated at the first signs of LAST, but after airway management. Dosing consists of a 1.5 mL/kg 20% lipid emulsion bolus, followed by an infusion of 0.25 mL/kg/min, continued for at least 10 minutes after circulatory stability is attained. If circulatory stability is not attained, consider giving another bolus and increasing infusion to 0.5 mL/kg/min. Approximately 10 mL/kg lipid emulsion over 30 minutes is recommended as the upper limit for initial dosing. Remember that propofol is not a substitute for lipid emulsion. Failure to respond to lipid emulsion and vasopressor therapy should prompt institution of cardiopulmonary bypass. Because there can be considerable lag in beginning cardiopulmonary bypass, it is reasonable to notify the closest facility capable of providing it when cardiovascular compromise is first identified during LAST. (Adapted from Weinberg [7].)

Reversal agents for benzodiazepines and opioids

The benzodiazepine and opioid antagonists are important drug classes to consider when administering moderate and/or deep sedation. Reversal agents provide a mechanism to quickly restore sensorium following short procedures. In addition, should abolition of

Table 2.8. Reversal agents

Drug (brand name)	Dosing (intravenous)		Onset	Duration	Considerations
	Pediatric	Adult			
Flumazenil (Romazicon)	0.005–0.1 mg/kg, with 0.01 mg/kg most used dose	0.2 mg over 15 s, repeat at 0.2 mg every 60 s to 1 mg max; may repeat at 20 min intervals *Max:* 3 mg in 30 min	30–60 s	< 60 min	Can precipitate seizures in those with history of seizures and tricyclic overdose. If seizures occur they may be refractory until flumazenil is metabolized. May cause visual disturbances, diaphoresis, arrhythmias.
Naloxone (Narcan)	Less than 5 years or 20 kg: 0.001–0.1 mg/kg, may repeat every 2–3 min *Max:* 2 mg Greater than 5 years or 20 kg: 2 mg dose, may repeat as needed	0.4 mg every 2–3 min *Max:* 10 mg	2 min	45 min	Can precipitate ventricular tachycardia and fibrillation in those with cardiovascular disease or receiving cardiotoxic drugs. May cause nausea and vomiting, sweating, tachycardia, hypertension, pulmonary edema.

airway reflexes and/or respiratory depression occur due to benzodiazepine and/or opioid administration, reversal agents are available (Table 2.8).

Flumazenil (Romazicon)

Flumazenil is a specific benzodiazepine-receptor antagonist that effectively reverses most of the CNS effects of benzodiazepines. Flumazenil is a competitive antagonist that prevents or reverses all agonist effects of benzodiazepines in a dose-dependent manner. It reverses the sedative-hypnotic effects of benzodiazepines as well as the depression of ventilation that can occur when benzodiazepines are combined with opioids. Titration of flumazenil to the desired level of consciousness is recommended (Table 2.8). Lower total doses of flumazenil, 0.3–0.6 mg IV, are generally adequate to decrease the degree of sedation, whereas doses of 0.5–1.0 mg IV abolish the therapeutic effects of benzodiazepines. Because the duration of action of the benzodiazepines is longer (up to 6 hours) than flumazenil's duration of action (30–60 minutes), supplemental doses may be necessary to maintain antagonist activity.

A continuous low-dose infusion of flumazenil of 0.1–0.4 mg/hour may be used rather than repeated doses to maintain wakefulness. Reversal of benzodiazepines is not without risk. In patients with a history of seizures, flumazenil can result in precipitation of withdrawal seizure activity. Therefore, flumazenil is not recommended for use in patients taking antiepileptic drugs for the control of seizure activity. Flumazenil antagonism of the benzodiazepine sedative effects generally does not cause acute anxiety, hypertension, or tachycardia. Also, the drug is not associated with alterations in coronary hemodynamics in patients with coronary artery disease. Presumably, flumazenil's weak intrinsic agonist activity attenuates effects of abrupt reversal of the benzodiazepines.

Naloxone (Narcan)

Naloxone is a nonselective antagonist at all three opioid receptors. It is a competitive opioid antagonist that promptly reverses opioid-induced analgesia and depression of ventilation. The short duration of action of naloxone (30–45 minutes) is thought to be due to its rapid removal from the brain. Return of opioid effects occurs unless supplemental doses of naloxone are administered. Alternatively, a continuous infusion of naloxone (3–5 µg/kg/h IV) may be used rather than additional IV boluses of the drug. Antagonism of opioid-induced ventilatory depression results in reversal of analgesia. Slow titration of naloxone may reverse the unwanted respiratory effects while allowing for partial agonism of opioid receptors and some analgesia. Naloxone is primarily metabolized in the liver. Adverse reactions may occur with reversal of opioid activity, including tachycardia, hypertension, dysrhythmias, nausea, vomiting, and diaphoresis. Nausea and vomiting appear to be closely related to the dose and speed of injection and may be attenuated by administration of the drug over 2–3 minutes. Cardiovascular stimulation after intravenous administration of naloxone is presumed to result from the sudden perception of pain and sympathetic nervous system stimulation. As a result, hypertension, tachycardia, cardiac dysrhythmias (including ventricular fibrillation), and pulmonary edema can occur. Furthermore, withdrawal symptoms may occur with reversal of both benzodiazepines and/or opioids in patients dependent on them.

Clinical pearls

- **Sedating to a desired effect.** To administer sedation safely requires an understanding of drug pharmacokinetics such as half-life, context-sensitive half-time, and common side effects. However, sedating to a desired effect is sometimes more of an art than a science. It also requires experience and understanding both of the procedure and of patient characteristics. If the patient has had sedation before, it is important to examine prior records for documentation of drugs given, total dosages used, and reported patient comfort.
- **Desired ideal characteristics of the drugs** used in moderate and deep sedation include: rapid onset; easily controlled depth of sedation and possibility for reversal, if needed; rapid recovery; minimal respiratory effects; amnesic and analgesic effects, cardiovascular stability; nonallergic and with no active metabolic byproducts. However, none of the drugs used in moderate or deep sedation has *all* of the desired characteristics outlined above. Therefore, a combination of drugs is often employed to achieve many of the desired effects while minimizing the unwanted side effects.

- **Common objectives of sedation include:**

  (1) *Decreasing patient anxiety.* This is best accomplished with benzodiazepines.

  (2) *Increasing pain threshold.* Pain can be preempted and treated with acetaminophen and/or nonsteroidal anti-inflammatory agents (NSAIDs) such as ibuprofen (PO, IV) and ketorolac (IV). Short- and long-acting opioid medications can provide more effective pain control, but can be associated with several side effects.

  (3) *Imposing some degree of amnesia.* Benzodiazepines are the most effective agents for this purpose.

  (4) *Maintaining minor variation of vital signs* such as blood pressure, heart rate, and oxygen saturation. Some of the medications used can lead to hypotension (propofol, opioids), bradycardia (dexmedetomidine, high-dose opioids), and decreased respiratory rate (propofol, opioids). Using a combination of drugs from different classes can help achieve desired sedation end points while resulting in fewer unwanted side effects.

- **Slowly titrate medication(s) to desired effect.** Many facilities will place limits on the total amount of particular medication that can be administered in a given time period. It is important to remember that each patient may respond differently to a given amount of medication, and that one may observe delayed side effects, such as respiratory depression. Slowly titrating to desired effects and setting limits on total dose that can be given can help prevent unintended oversedation (see ASA continuum of depth of sedation, Table 1.2 [8]).

- **Drug dosing modifications** may be necessary to account for the patient's body habitus (obesity can lead to increased drug volume of distribution), cardiac status (decreased cardiac output), nutritional status (drug protein binding), liver and/or kidney dysfunction (decreased drug metabolism and excretion), extremes of age, concurrent use of other drugs (a patient's regularly taken drugs can interact with the administered drugs and result in increased side effects), and allergies.

- **Have I given enough sedation and analgesia?** As mentioned above, slowly titrating to desired effect is most prudent. Administer drugs appropriate for the given level of stimulation during the procedure. Also, it is important to be familiar with the procedure and anticipate a more/less stimulating period before it actually occurs. Also, take the patient's comorbidities (e.g., chronic pain, liver or kidney disease, obesity) into consideration. Another useful end point is observing changes in vital signs such as blood pressure and heart rate in response to the medications you have just administered to counteract the discomfort/pain caused by the ongoing procedure. Another useful end point is the change in respiratory rate in response to drugs given and procedure stimulation.

Summary

The safe and effective administration of moderate and deep sedation by non-anesthesia providers occurs quite frequently in a variety of locations within and outside of the hospital setting. Providing sedation and analgesia for many different types of patients and procedures requires knowledge of the commonly used drugs. An understanding of the pharmacology of the benzodiazepines and opioids as well as their reversal agents is important to assure patient safety. Other drugs used in sedation, such as propofol, ketamine, etomidate, and dexmedetomidine, warrant similar attention prior to their use to maintain safety. Furthermore, techniques to obtain the desired end point with drug administration without undesirable side effects should be kept in mind. Slow titration of a drug while monitoring the patient's response (level of consciousness, respiratory rate, blood pressure, etc.) dictates dosage. Drug choice should be based on the procedure. Painful procedures require analgesia and possibly sedative-hypnotics, whereas nonpainful procedures may only require sedation. Dose requirements vary based on patient characteristics (e.g., height, weight, age) and body habitus. Comorbidities such as hepatic and/or renal failure also frequently affect dose requirements, as does history of alcohol and/or drug use. Generally, decreased doses are required when combining benzodiazepines and/or opioids with other CNS-depressive drugs. Decreased doses should also be used in the elderly and the debilitated.

References

1. Urman R, Vadivelu N. Acute and postoperative pain management. In *Pocket Pain Medicine*. Philadelphia, PA: Lippincott, Williams & Wilkins, 2011.

2. Windle ML. Infiltrative administration of local anesthetic agents. *Medscape Reference* 2011. emedicine.medscape.com/article/149178-overview (accessed June 2011).

3. Arthur GR. Pharmacokinetics. In Strichartz GR, ed., *Handbook of Experimental Pharmacology*, Vol. 81. Berlin: Springer-Verlag, 1987; 165–86.

4. Clarkson CW, Hondeghem LM. Mechanism for bupivacaine depression of cardiac conduction: fast block of sodium channels during the action potential with slow recovery from block during diastole. *Anesthesiology* 1985; **62**: 396–405.

5. Thomas RD, Behbehani MM, Coyle DE, Denson DD. Cardiovascular toxicity of local anesthetics: an alternative hypothesis. *Anesth Analg* 1986; **65**: 444–50.

6. Nath S, Häggmark S, Johansson G, Reiz S. Differential depressant and electrophysiologic cardiotoxicity of local anesthetics: an experimental study with special reference to lidocaine and bupivacaine. *Anesth Analg* 1986; **65**: 1263–70.

7. Weinberg GL. Treatment of local anesthetic systemic toxicity (LAST). *Reg Anesth Pain Med* 2010; **35**: 188–93.

8. American Society of Anesthesiologists Task Force on Sedation and Analgesia by Non-Anesthesiologists. Practice guidelines for sedation and analgesia by non-anesthesiologists. *Anesthesiology* 2002; **96**: 1004–17.

Further reading

Barash PG, Cullen BF, Stoelting RK, Cahalan MK, Stock MC, eds. *Clinical Anesthesia*, 6th edn. Philadelphia, PA: Lippincott Williams & Wilkins, 2009.

Faust RJ, Cucchiara RF, Rose SH, *et al. Anesthesiology Review*, 3rd edn. Philadelphia, PA: Churchill Livingstone, 2002.

Hospira. Dosing guidelines for Precedex®: nonintubated procedural sedation and ICU sedation. Lake Forest, IL: Hospira, 2010. www.precedex.com/wp-content/uploads/2010/02/Dosing_Guide.pdf (accessed June 2011).

Morgan GE, Mikhail MS, Murray MJ. *Clinical Anesthesiology*, 4th edn. New York, NY: McGraw-Hill, 2006.

Riker RR, Shehabi Y, Bokesch PM, *et al.* Dexmedetomidine vs midazolam for sedation of critically ill patients: a randomized trial. *JAMA* 2009; **301**: 489–99.

Stoelting RK, Hillier SC. *Pharmacology and Physiology in Anesthetic Practice*, 4th edn. Philadelphia, PA: Lippincott Williams & Wilkins, 2006.

Stoelting RK, Miller RD. *Basics of Anesthesia*, 5th edn. Philadelphia, PA: Churchill Livingstone, 2007.

Watson DS, Odom-Forren J. *Practical Guide to Moderate Sedation/Analgesia*, 2nd edn. New York, NY: Mosby, 2005.

Chapter 3

Pain assessment and management considerations

Joseph C. Hung, J. Gabriel Tsang, Jamie Wingate,
Martin Kubin, Usman Latif, and Eugenie S. Heitmiller

Introduction

A comprehensive strategy is needed for adequate management of patients through the entire peri-procedure period. Assessments and interventions pre-procedure, peri-procedure, and post-procedure are codependent. For example, failure to recognize an opioid-dependent patient during the initial pre-procedure screening may result in ineffective sedation strategies. Overuse of and/or failure to report long-acting sedative medications used during procedural sedation can result in a delayed and complicated recovery period. This chapter deals with important considerations with regard to pre-procedure, peri-procedure, and post-procedure patient assessment and pain management strategies. For a detailed discussion of patient evaluation and procedure selection, see Chapter 4.

Considerations and patient assessment prior to procedural sedation

Given the magnitude of adverse outcomes that can accompany sedation, it is paramount that before start of any procedure, practitioners evaluate patient characteristics, patient preferences, appropriateness of sedation given the invasiveness of the procedure, special considerations during the procedure (e.g., risk to the patient with movement during the procedure), and patient safety. The primary goal of giving sedation should be to achieve an acceptable level of patient comfort while considering all of these factors.

Practitioner training and experience in administering sedation is also an important consideration. The American Society of Anesthesiologists (ASA) states in its practice recommendations for care of patients receiving sedation that it is often difficult to predict

Moderate and Deep Sedation in Clinical Practice, ed. Richard D. Urman and Alan D. Kaye.
Published by Cambridge University Press. © Cambridge University Press 2012.

how an individual patient will respond to a given dose of sedative medications [1]. All practitioners who administer sedatives should be able to manage complications of patients whose level of sedation is deeper than originally intended. The ASA consensus guidelines for sedation by non-anesthesiologists indicate that a practitioner should be able to control a compromised airway (associated with *deep sedation*) while administering *moderate sedation*, and they similarly specify that a practitioner should be able to manage the cardiovascular instability associated with *general anesthesia* while administering *deep sedation* [1].

Comprehensive perioperative risk stratification is beyond the scope of this chapter. However, with regard to patient characteristics, the expert consensus is strong that careful pre-procedure evaluation of the patient improves patient satisfaction and decreases adverse outcomes [1]. While taking a pre-procedure patient history, the sedation provider should consider the following important patient factors: past experiences with sedation and/or anesthesia, expectations, pain tolerance, anxiety levels/ability to cooperate, drug allergies, time and nature of last oral intake, and overall health (Table 3.1).

In regard to evaluating the patient's overall health, it would be prudent to seek consultation with an expert skilled in perioperative management for patients who have significant organ-system abnormalities and/or those who would be assigned an ASA physical status of 3 or higher (Table 3.2). Sedative drugs and medications are well known to cause critical cardiovascular and hemodynamic perturbations on the deeper end of the sedation scale.

For patients with preexisting painful conditions, it is useful to perform an initial pain assessment prior to the procedure for post-procedure comparison. When evaluating pain characteristics, questions should address a pain rating, location, quality, onset, duration, pattern, alleviating/aggravating factors, and any related symptoms (Table 3.3). A focused physical examination of the pain site should also be performed. Any unusual factors including erythema, swelling, temperature changes, skin changes, pain with non-noxious stimuli, muscle atrophy, and hair growth patterns at the pain site should be noted.

For most patients, pain assessments and establishment of pain treatment goals can be performed by a non-anesthesiologist. However, consultation should be sought for special populations, including the elderly, patients with history of substance abuse, chronic pain patients, pediatric patients, patients with indwelling pain pumps/catheters, and those patients at increased risk from respiratory depression (e.g., sleep apnea, history of airway problems or difficult airway).

The above criteria for pain assessment rely heavily on verbal communication, and adequate pain assessments may not be possible during moderate or deep sedation. In these situations, behavioral pain assessments are useful (see Tables 3.5 and Tables 3.6 below). Many of the behaviors that indicate pain are often obvious, and they may include facial grimacing, writhing or shifting, moaning, agitation, and/or withdrawal from the painful stimulus. In addition, changes in physiologic parameters are also sensitive indicators of pain or discomfort. The patient in pain will often manifest an increase in breathing rate, heart rate, and/or blood pressure. Often, all three physiologic parameters are increased.

Management of the chronic pain and/or opioid-dependent patient can be challenging. Sedation requirements can be extremely variable. In addition to anxiety and depression,

Table 3.1. Important patient history aspects for pre-sedation patient evaluation

Details of past experiences with sedation and/or anesthesia

- Previous effective and ineffective sedation and pain control regimens
- Drug allergies
- Adverse reactions to any medications

Patient expectations

- Anxiety levels/ability to cooperate

Risk and consequences of movement during the procedure

Time and nature of last oral intake

Overall health

- Organ-system abnormalities
  - Airway or respiratory problems or predictors of complications
- History of drug or alcohol abuse
- History of chronic pain and/or chronic opioid use

Table 3.2. American Society of Anesthesiologists (ASA) physical status classification system

ASA physical status	Definition
1	A normal healthy patient
2	A patient with mild systemic disease
3	A patient with severe systemic disease
4	A patient with severe systemic disease that is a constant threat to life
5	A moribund patient who is not expected to survive without the operation
6	A declared brain-dead patient whose organs are being removed for donor purposes

Table 3.3. Criteria for assessing pain

Pain rating (using an appropriate assessment scale)

Location

Quality (sharp, dull, burning, shooting)

Onset (sudden, gradual)

Duration

Pattern (continuous, intermittent)

Alleviating/aggravating factors

Related symptoms

it is not uncommon for this patient population to have other psychiatric disturbances. Furthermore, these patients are often medicated with various anxiolytics, antidepressants, anticonvulsants, and muscle relaxants, all of which can unpredictably impact targeted levels of sedation compared to the typical patient. Unless an adverse drug interaction is foreseen, baseline pain medications should not be withheld in anticipation for any procedure.

Chronic pain patients may also have existing pain control adjuncts such as intrathecal pain pumps and/or spinal cord nerve stimulators. If possible, their use should be continued through the procedure. In the peri-procedure period, it is very important not to reduce baseline methods for controlling pain in any patient population. In all instances, it is imperative for the chronic pain patient to form an acceptable perioperative sedation and pain management strategy with the healthcare delivery team during the evaluation phase. If available, a chronic pain expert should be consulted.

Regional anesthesia techniques (epidural, spinal, and peripheral nerve blocks with or without catheters) can also be employed in conjunction with a regional anesthesia specialist and an acute pain service to avoid titrating large amounts of systemic opioids in opioid-dependent patients. These systems deliver analgesia (usually local anesthetics and/or opioids) directly to target nerves (peripheral nerve catheters) and/or dermatomal regions (neuraxial catheters). Working preexisting neuraxial and nerve catheters can and should be continued through the procedure phase, with recommendations from a regional anesthesia specialist.

Existing patient-controlled analgesia (PCA) intravenous systems may also need readjustment in the procedure phase. Prior to the procedure, the baseline bolus dose can be increased by 20% on PCA systems to cover procedure-related breakthrough pain. Additional increased PCA background infusions may be needed to control long-lasting pain from more invasive techniques. In many centers, PCA adjustments are made only with input from an acute pain specialist.

Overview of pain assessment scales

Appropriate assessment of pain increases caregiver awareness of pain status, allows for the delivery of appropriate interventions, provides for feedback, decreases both patient and caregiver frustration, and improves patient satisfaction. Efficient pain management can result in better wound healing, improved respiratory function, decreased stress, and increased rest. Clinical practice guidelines issued by the Agency for Healthcare Research and Quality (AHRQ) suggest that, like vital signs, pain levels should be checked frequently. These guidelines recommend reassessing pain intensities 30 minutes after parenteral drug administration, 60 minutes after oral drug administration, and with each report of new or changed pain [2].

Since the cognitive functionality, intellectual development, level of alertness, and even educational level can vary dramatically among individual patients, no single all-encompassing method of pain assessment can be used. To address this issue, a wide range of pain assessment tools have been developed and validated over the past 30 years. The following sections will expound upon the most common pain assessment tools in current use in (1) general and (2) special populations. When using any of these tools, it is important to keep in mind that a trend in pain scores is more useful than a single pain score by itself.

General population scales

In the general population, which includes mature children, adults, and the cognitively intact elderly, the use of self-report scales has been validated as the most reliable indicator of pain. The most common self-report scales include the Numeric Rating Scale (NRS), the Verbal Numeric Scale (VNS), the Visual Analog Scale (VAS), and the Faces Pain Scale (FPS).

Numeric Rating Scale (NRS)

The NRS is the most commonly used pain scale. With this scale, patients quantify their pain by pointing to a number on a 0–5 or 0–10 scale, where 0 represents the absence of pain and 5 or 10 represents the worst pain they can imagine. Validated in multiple studies, the NRS is preferred by most adults [3,4]. However, the elderly population may have difficulty with the NRS [2].

Verbal Numeric Scale (VNS)

The VNS is a variation of the NRS that requires the patient to verbally rate pain on a scale of 0 to 10. This scale is most commonly used in clinical practice, and is especially useful with patients who have psychomotor or visual impairment [2]. The VNS is also useful for pain assessment over the telephone or via electronic correspondence.

Visual Analog Scale (VAS)

Similar to the NRS, the VAS is a horizontal or vertical 10 cm line with "no pain" written at one end and "the worst imaginable pain" at the other end [2]. Patients mark a point on the line correlating with pain intensity. The practitioner then measures the distance from "no pain" to the patient's mark to determine a score based on length. The VAS is highly sensitive to change in pain intensity [5]. Like the NRS, this scale is not preferred for use with elderly patients, particularly those with mild to moderate cognitive impairment.

Faces Pain Scale (FPS)

The FPS is a categorical scale that uses visual descriptors, and it has been validated for use in adults and children [5–7]. Patients are shown a scale with seven faces that display different expressions ranging from neutral to grimacing (Figure 3.1). Patients then point to the face that corresponds to their level of pain. Each face correlates with a score between 0 (no pain) and 10 (terrible pain). As the FPS does not require reading ability, this scale is well-suited for and preferred by those with lower education levels or mild cognitive impairment (including the elderly). The FPS has been validated across multiple cultures and has a strong positive correlation with other pain scales [5,8].

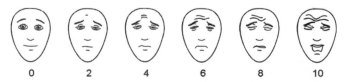

0   2   4   6   8   10

Figure 3.1. Faces Pain Scale (FPS) [9]. This Faces Pain Scale-Revised has been reproduced with the permission of the International Association for the Study of Pain (IASP).

Table 3.4. Pain scale comparison for various patient populations

General population scales	
Normal adult/mature child	NRS preferred by most adults; FPS
Elderly adult	FPS most preferred; VAS least preferred
Mild–moderate cognitive impairment	FPS most preferred; VAS least preferred
Psychomotor impairment	VNS commonly used
Visual impairment	VNS commonly used
Low educational level	FPS most preferred, reading ability not required

NRS, numeric rating scale; VNS, verbal numeric scale; VAS, visual analog scale; FPS, faces pain scale.

In deciding which pain scale to choose, Table 3.4 offers a comparison between various patient demographics.

Special population scales

Although the gold standard for pain assessment is the self-report scale, many instances in clinical practice preclude its use. These scenarios, while quite varied in scope, can most often be generalized into four broad categories:

(1) the young child who has yet to develop verbal communication skills
(2) the individual who is unable to verbalize despite having full cognitive function
(3) the individual who is cognitively impaired due to sedation or delirium
(4) the individual with severe intellectual and developmental delays

Each of these broad categories includes an observational component as part of the assessment. As with the communicative patient, general concepts for assessing procedure-related pain and/or pain during sedation begin in the pre-procedure period with adequate patient preparation. One should always give explanations of the procedure and of any associated sedation plans that are appropriate to the patient's age and cognitive ability. This process can be particularly useful for helping the patient to understand the possibility of pain involvement during the procedure and for enhancing patient cooperation.

Pain assessment in the young child

The Premature Infant Pain Profile (PIPP) and the Neonatal/Infant Pain Scale (NIPS) are commonly used in infants. For children who cannot communicate, (because of either sedation or cognitive impairment) the Faces, Legs, Activity, Cry, Consolability (FLACC) and the Children's Hospital of Eastern Ontario Pain Scale (CHEOPS) are used. In addition, parents can be asked to help assess pain levels [10]. However, this practice may be a logistical challenge in a procedure suite or operating room.

The FLACC scale is one of the most commonly used assessments during sedation (Table 3.5). It is an observer report-based scale that has been validated with low interrater variability [11]. A score of 0–2 is given in each of five categories (face, legs, activity, cry, and consolability). These point values are added together to provide a pain score between 0 and 10. Pediatric sedation is discussed in Chapter 19.

Table 3.5. The FLACC scale

	0	1	2
Face	No particular expression or smile	Occasional grimace or frown, withdrawn, disinterested	Frequent or constant frown, clenched jaw, quivering chin
Legs	Normal position or relaxed	Uneasy, restless, tense	Kicking or legs drawn up
Activity	Lying quietly, moves easily	Squirming, shifting back and forth, tense	Arched, rigid, or jerking
Cry	No cry	Moans or whimpers, occasional complaint	Crying steadily, screams or sobs
Consolability	Content, relaxed	Reassured by occasional touching or talking to, distractible	Difficult to console or comfort

Pain assessment in the nonverbal but cognitive patient

A practitioner may have to manage the pain concerns of an individual who is alert and oriented to his/her surroundings but unable to verbalize that he/she is experiencing pain. Examples include the intubated patient, the patient with neurologic deficits (acute stroke), or any patient with a pathologic condition that influences phonation. Because these patients are alert and aware of their surroundings and condition, most critical care practices recommend the use of self-report scales to assess pain [12,13]. For this subset of patients, a few of the validated self-report scales described above are particularly helpful. These include the NRS, the VAS, and the Verbal Descriptor Scale (VDS).

For the VDS, patients choose the expression that best describes their pain from a written list which contains "no pain," "mild pain," "moderate pain," "severe pain," and "extreme pain." The usefulness of the VDS is limited in the case of patients of lower education levels and those with poor eyesight. Of the NRS, VAS, and VDS, the one found to best correlate with correct assessment of pain is the NRS [14].

Pain assessment in the delirious or sedated patient

The noncommunicative patient population consists largely of elderly patients with severe cognitive impairment. Accordingly, most assessment tools aim to understand pain treatment in this demographic group. However, these same pain scales are also applicable to patients in pain who are in a state of shock, who are suffering from brain injury, or who are deeply sedated. Because direct communication is not possible, assessment tools should aim to address the sensory and behavioral dimensions of pain. These scales rely on behavioral indicators such as restlessness, muscle tension, frowning, grimacing, and vocalizations. Although several different pain scales have been validated, the most effective assessment tool in the population subset is the Behavioral Pain Scale (BPS) [15–17]. To use the BPS, a patient is observed for 1 minute. Evaluation of pain status is based on the sum of three subscales: facial expression, upper limb movement, and compliance with mechanical ventilation (Table 3.6). Each subscale is scored from 1 to 4

Table 3.6. The Behavioral Pain Scale (BPS)

Item	Description	Score
Facial expression	Relaxed	1
	Partially tightened	2
	Fully tightened	3
	Grimacing	4
Upper limbs	No movement	1
	Partially bent	2
	Fully bent with finger flexion	3
	Permanently retracted	4
Compliance with ventilation	Tolerating movement	1
	Coughing but tolerating ventilation for most of the time	2
	Fighting ventilator	3
	Unable to control ventilation	4

based on response. Thus the cumulative BPS score is between 3 (no pain) and 12 (maximal pain).

Pain assessment in the intellectually and developmentally delayed

Assessing pain in individuals with intellectual and/or developmental delay can be particularly challenging. Although the pain scales currently in use have been validated, their interpretation can be complicated. Two commonly used scales in this population include the Non-Communicating Children's Pain Checklist (NCCPC) in the pediatric population and the Non-Communicating Adult Pain Checklist (NCAPC) in the adult population.

In brief, the NCCPC is based on a 27-item scale representing six subcategories of pain behavior that include vocal reaction, emotional reaction, facial expression, body language, protective reaction, and physiological reaction. The total score ranges from 0 to 81. The NCAPC is a modified version of the NCCPC that is based on an 18-item scale with a total score that ranges from 0 to 54. In general, the use and interpretation of these assessment tools requires special training, and they are beyond the scope of this chapter.

Recovery and discharge

Common postoperative factors that result in discharge delay include pain, postoperative nausea and vomiting (PONV), drowsiness, and lack of a patient escort. Concern over inadequate pain control is a major source of anxiety for patients undergoing procedures. Moreover, uncontrolled pain itself is associated with increased complaints of nausea, vomiting, delirium, readmission to the hospital, and delayed resumption of normal activities at home [18].

The American Society of PeriAnesthesia Nurses (ASPAN) has published clinical guidelines for dealing with post-sedation pain [19]. Care is broken down into three phases: *assessment*, *intervention*, and *expected outcomes*. The assessment portion should include a history of any pre-procedure pain and any previous interventions with clinical outcome.

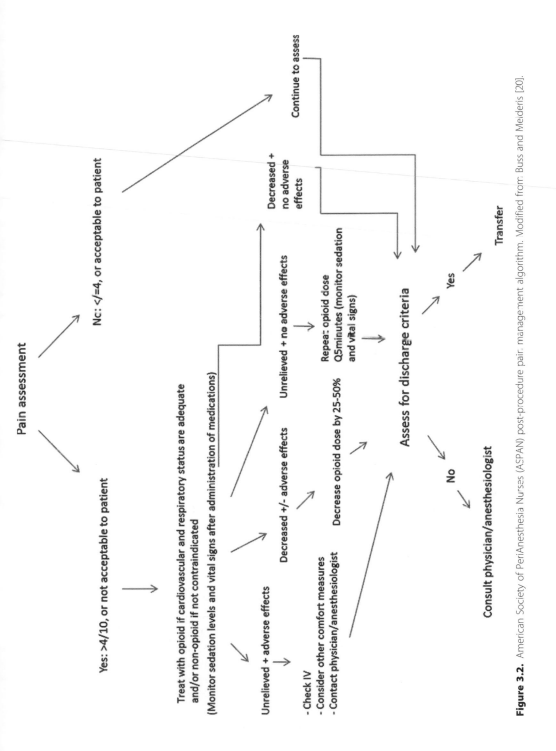

Figure 3.2. American Society of PeriAnesthesia Nurses (ASPAN) post-procedure pain management algorithm. Modified from: Buss and Melderis [20].

With any patient intervention, vigilance with proper monitoring for adverse effects is critical. Familiarity with the procedure requiring sedation can also help guide therapy and outcomes. For example, a patient complaining of arm pain after an abdominal procedure might have had a positioning injury or existing arthritis prior to the procedure.

When treating post-sedation patients, ASPAN suggests the use of nonopioid medications for patients experiencing mild to moderate pain. For moderate to severe pain, multimodal therapy is often necessary. Different classes of effective analgesics used may include opioids, NSAIDs, tricyclic antidepressants, and anticonvulsants. When using nontraditional therapies or dealing with refractory pain, a pain expert should be consulted. Buss and Melderis [20] offer a practical pain treatment algorithm for pain in the post-anesthesia care unit (PACU) (Figure 3.2). If no contraindications exist and vital signs are stable, pre-procedure baseline pain regimens should always be continued in the recovery period. Taking care of psychosocial needs (allowing visitation from family members) may also be beneficial for recovery.

In general, the use of opioid medications (both during sedation and in the recovery phase) must be balanced against their side effects (sedation, constipation, nausea and vomiting, and respiratory depression). Overuse of opioids may in fact significantly prolong recovery times because of their side effects.

Comprehensive post-procedure discharge criteria are beyond the scope of this chapter and patient discharge considerations are discussed in Chapters 4 and 8. However, specific considerations for discharge readiness from a pain management perspective include: allowance of sufficient time to elapse (2 hours) after the last administration of sedation reversal agents (naloxone, flumazenil) to ensure patients do not become re-sedated; providing ambulatory patients and their designated escorts with instructions regarding diet, medications, activities post-sedation, and telephone contact number in case of emergency; and counseling parents/guardians on the possibility of airway obstruction in children if the head falls forward when the child is secured in a car seat.

Summary

A key factor related to successful pain management in the peri-procedure period is recognizing the need for a collaborative team effort between the patient and all involved healthcare team members. In addition, it is important to realize that the peri-procedure pain experience is a dynamic process that requires constant assessment and adjustment. With appropriate vigilance, planning, and continuous communication between team members, many of the barriers involved in planning and executing an effective pain management strategy can be overcome.

References

1. American Society of Anesthesiologists Task Force on Sedation and Analgesia by Non-Anesthesiologists. Practice guidelines for sedation and analgesia by non-anesthesiologists. *Anesthesiology* 2002; **96**: 1004–17.

2. Berry PH, Covington E, Dahl J, Katz J, Miaskowski C. *Pain: Current Understanding of Assessment, Management and Treatments*. Reston, VA: National Pharmaceutical Council and the Joint Commission on Accreditation of Healthcare Organizations, 2006.

3. Gagliese L, Weizblit N, Ellis W, Chan VW. The measurement of postoperative pain: a comparison of intensity scales in younger and older surgical patients. *Pain* 2005; **117**: 412–20.

4. Herr KA, Spratt K, Mobily PR, Richardson G. Pain intensity assessment in older adults: use of experimental pain to compare

psychometric properties and usability of selected pain scales with younger adults. *Clin J Pain* 2004; **20**: 207–19.

5. Bieri D, Reeve RA, Champion GD, Addicoat L, Ziegler JB. The Faces Pain Scale for the self-assessment of the severity of pain experienced by children: development, initial validation, and preliminary investigation for ratio scale properties. *Pain* 1990; **41**: 139–50.

6. Taylor LJ, Harris J, Epps CD, Herr K. Psychometric evaluation of selected pain intensity scales for use with cognitively impaired and cognitively intact older adults. *Rehabil Nurs* 2005; **30**: 55–61.

7. Stuppy DJ. The Faces Pain Scale: reliability and validity with mature adults. *Appl Nurs Res* 1998; **11**: 84–9.

8. Matsumoto D. Ethnic differences in affect intensity, emotion judgments, display rule attitudes, and self-reported emotional expression in an American sample. *Motiv Emotion* 1993; **17**: 107–23.

9. Hicks CL, von Baeyer CL, Spafford PA, van Korlaar I, Goodenough B. The Faces Pain Scale-Revised: toward a common metric in pediatric pain measurement. *Pain* 2001; **93**: 173–83.

10. Stallard P, Williams L, Lenton S, Velleman R. Pain in cognitively impaired, non-communicating children. *Arch Dis Child* 2001; **85**: 460–2.

11. Merkel SI, Voepel-Lewis T, Shayevitz JR, Malviya S. The FLACC: a behavioral scale for scoring postoperative pain in young children. *Pediatr Nurs* 1997; **23**: 293–7.

12. Jacobi J, Fraser GL, Coursin DB, *et al.* Clinical practice guidelines for the

sustained use of sedatives and analgesics in the critically ill adult. *Crit Care Med* 2002; **30**: 119–41.

13. Sauder P, Andreoletti M, Cambonie G, *et al.* [Sedation and analgesia in intensive care (with the exception of new-born babies). French Society of Anesthesia and Resuscitation. French-speaking Resuscitation Society.]. *Ann Fr Anesth Reanim* 2008; **27**: 541–51.

14. Chanques G, Viel E, Constantin JM, *et al.* The measurement of pain in intensive care unit: comparison of 5 self-report intensity scales. *Pain* 2010; **151**: 711–21.

15. Payen JF, Bru O, Bosson JL, *et al.* Assessing pain in critically ill sedated patients by using a behavioral pain scale. *Crit Care Med* 2001; **29**: 2258–63.

16. Aissaoui Y, Zeggwagh AA, Zekraoui A, Abidi K, Abouqal R. Validation of a behavioral pain scale in critically ill, sedated, and mechanically ventilated patients *Anesth Analg* 2005; **101**: 1470–6.

17. Ahlers SJ, van Gulik L, van der Veen AM, *et al.* Comparison of different pain scoring systems in critically ill patients in a general ICU. *Crit Care* 2008; **12**: R15.

18. Joshi GP. Pain management after ambulatory surgery. *Ambulatory Surgery* 1999; **7**: 3–12.

19. ASPAN pain and comfort clinical guideline. www.aspan.org/Portals/6/docs/ClinicalPractice/Guidelines/ASPAN_ClinicalGuideline_PainComfort.pdf (accessed June 2011).

20. Buss HE, Melderis K. PACU pain management algorithm. *J Perianesth Nurs* 2002; **17**: 11–20.

Patient evaluation and procedure selection

Debra E. Morrison and Kristi Dorn Hare

Patient evaluation

Pre-screening

Patient evaluation for a sedation procedure can begin with the first telephone contact. When the patient first calls to schedule an appointment, an administrative assistant or scheduler may ask simple screening questions about snoring/sleep apnea, age, height and weight, the presence of common comorbid diseases such as diabetes, heart and lung disease, and routine use of narcotics or sedatives. Although a clerical person may not have the clinical education to question patients in detail or follow up positive findings with further questions, initial screening will allow separation of patients into those who are good candidates for sedation and those who are not. This determination will help to schedule and consent patients appropriately, for sedation versus sedation with anesthesia backup versus anesthesia.

This is especially helpful when patients, in particular inpatients and others who are scheduled "only" for diagnostic procedures, are not routinely seen and evaluated until the day of the procedure. Patients who are referred for procedures in radiology and transferred from private gastroenterologists for interventional gastroenterology procedures are often not seen by the physician performing a procedure until the day of the procedure, when it may be too late to provide an alternative to sedation. Inpatients who are scheduled for "minor" procedures in radiology may not be seen until they arrive in the radiology suite. The pre-sedation evaluation may be at extremely short notice in the emergency department or the cardiac cath lab when the procedure is urgent or emergent.

Patients for elective procedures may be referred by their primary care physician or may be self-referred. In either circumstance, the referral may not be associated with an informative history and physical by the physician who knows the patient best. The surgeon/practitioner/physician who receives the referral may not be able to determine whether the referral is a query alone ("Does this patient need a procedure? Just wondering, but there are

Moderate and Deep Sedation in Clinical Practice, ed. Richard D. Urman and Alan D. Kaye.
Published by Cambridge University Press. © Cambridge University Press 2012.

other unresolved medical issues, so send the patient back before scheduling anything") or a query accompanied by a clinical green light to proceed ("If this patient needs a procedure, the patient is optimized to proceed with whatever you think is necessary, and the evidence is attached"). It is helpful to request clarification of this issue from referring physicians, but the problem remains when the patient is self-referred.

If there is time, particularly if the procedure is elective, a formal screening questionnaire can be employed. A screening questionnaire filled out prior to the first encounter (completed at home and mailed in, or over the internet, or while the patient is waiting to be seen) will facilitate evaluation. The screening questionnaire can be followed up by a nurse practitioner or an experienced sedation RN, depending on the urgency of the case.

The interviewer asks important historical questions about medication use, exercise tolerance, medical history, surgical history, allergies, drug intolerance, social habits, and expectations regarding the procedure and sedation. The interviewer can discover the patient's previous experiences with anesthesia, sedation, and other procedures. It is important to uncover intolerances to medications, positioning issues (ability to lie flat, neck range of motion), sleep apnea/snoring, difficult intubation or any history of unexpected events during procedures. The patient will not always know what historical information is important. It is important for an experienced nurse to ask the right questions in a kind, nonthreatening and nonjudgmental way and to know, from clinical experience, which answers necessitate further investigation. The patient may be more likely to confide in the nurse, while telling the physician what he/she thinks the physician wants to hear. The physician can be notified of patients who present more of a clinical challenge and must be evaluated further or scheduled differently.

History and physical

If necessary, the patient can be referred to his/her primary care physician for a pre-procedure history and physical (H&P) or medical clearance between the date of initial encounter and the day of the procedure. If appropriate, the surgeon/practitioner/physician who is to perform the procedure should perform the H&P. In any case, the H&P should be less than 30 days old prior to moderate sedation and less than 48 hours old prior to deep sedation.

Patient instructions

It is important that the patient be at his/her baseline "steady state" for the procedure. Even if the patient is NPO the night before, required medications may be taken with sips of water in the early morning to ensure that blood pressure, heart rate, and other medical conditions are controlled prior to the procedure. The phrase "NPO after midnight" should always be accompanied by the statement "except the following necessary medications with sips of water or other clear liquid."

Patients should/may be informed that they may continue to drink clear liquids up until 2 hours before they arrive at the facility. This allows for bowel preps to be completed, adequate hydration, patient satisfaction, and, for the diabetic patient, maintenance of adequate blood glucose. Clear liquids may include tea or coffee without milk or cream, clear juices and sodas without particulate matter, fat-free broth, water, or perhaps only bowel prep.

Any procedure is an anxiety-producing event. If the patient takes medication for baseline anxiety or pain, these medications should be continued to avoid a distressing spike in anxiety or pain level on the morning of the procedure. If the patient is NPO, he/she should not take oral diabetic medications or the usual dose of short- or intermediate-acting insulin, in order to avoid hypoglycemia. Insulin pumps or the dose of long-acting non-peaking insulin (glargine or levemir) should be adjusted to cover only basal requirements. The patient may require the assistance of his/her primary care physician to adjust insulin appropriately. He/she may bring short- or intermediate-acting insulin to the facility to be administered as needed during the peri-procedure period.

Screening, evaluation, and instruction of patients requires clinical experience, and clerical staff members should not be performing any more than simple initial screening or instructing patients as to time, location, and routine standard instructions. Lack of critical information or incorrect instruction can cause a procedure to be canceled or rescheduled, or allow an adverse event to occur during or after the procedure. Patients should be optimized and adequately informed for the procedure, so that everything proceeds as planned.

Evaluation on day of procedure

Not all procedure areas allow or require pre-procedure screening or interviews. The patients are evaluated when they arrive on the day of the procedure or are brought to the procedure area as inpatients. To avoid surprises, it is useful to require the referring physician to provide critical information. It seems to be a common belief that radiology in particular is a "black box" into which even a very sick patient can be deposited, later to emerge unscathed with a diagnosis or an inferior vena cava filter. The referring service cannot begin to imagine what takes place while the patient is in the procedure area. It is difficult to accustom referring physicians to providing needed information, but the effort is well worth it in the end.

Initial evaluation

It is the procedural RN who will perform the initial evaluation on the day of the procedure. There should be a standard history form that he/she fills out, based also on any initial screening, while talking with the patient. It should include all of the elements: medication use, exercise tolerance, medical history, surgical history, allergies, drug intolerance, and social habits.

The interviewer can discover the patient's previous experiences with anesthesia, sedation, and other procedures and his/her expectations regarding the procedure and sedation. It is important to uncover intolerances to medications, positioning issues (ability to lie flat, neck range of motion), sleep apnea/snoring, difficult intubation or any history of unexpected events during procedures.

The pre-procedural assessment usually also addresses religion, whether or not the patient has a ride home (if applicable), who to call in an emergency, and some discharge planning.

Data should include height, pain score (1–10/10) weight, blood pressure, heart rate, respiratory rate, temperature, oxygen saturation, whether room air or oxygen (and how much oxygen), pertinent labs (including very recent glucose or potassium if the patient is a diabetic or in renal failure), studies, ECG or chest x-ray if appropriate.

Table 4.1. Richmond Agitation–Sedation Scale (RASS)

Score	Description
+4	Combative, violent, danger to staff
+3	Pulls or removes tube(s) or catheter(s); aggressive
+2	Frequent nonpurposeful movement, fights ventilator
+1	Anxious, apprehensive, but not aggressive
0	Alert and calm
−1	Awakens to voice (eye opening/contact) > 10 seconds
−2	Light sedation, briefly awakens to voice (eye opening/contact) < 10 seconds
−3	Moderate sedation, movement or eye opening; no eye contact
−4	Deep sedation, no response to voice, but movement or eye opening to physical stimulation
−5	Unarousable, no response to voice or physical stimulation

The assessment should include baseline level of consciousness/sedation score, which should also be monitored and documented during sedation (Table 4.1). In addition, it should include a baseline modified Aldrete score or the equivalent, so that the patient can be compared against baseline in the recovery area in order to determine criteria for discharge from post-sedation monitoring (Table 4.2).

The RN also makes important visual observations about the patient and any accompanying family members: eye contact, anxiety, strength, agility, fragility, steadiness, pain, distress, color, family relationships, and general health status. An astute RN begins planning appropriate sedation for the specific procedure from the moment she/he meets the patient. She/he will know if the patient will need lifting or positioning help, constant reassurance, or an attendant of a certain age or gender. It is important to put the patient at ease and to reassure him/her that he/she is important and will be well cared for. Questions and concerns should be solicited, welcomed, and addressed.

If the procedure is to be done in an inpatient ICU room, the unit RN may be called upon to be the sedation/procedure RN. The ICU RN needs to understand this role and be prepared to perform it, including completion of a thorough pre-procedure assessment.

Physician exam, informed consent, and attestation

The United States Centers for Medicare and Medicaid Services (CMS) requires that the procedure physician participate in the pre-procedure evaluation as well. A licensed physician or allied health professional (fellow, resident, physician assistant, or nurse practitioner) may complete the initial assessment and sedation plan, including the physical exam, which should include heart and lung exam and an appropriate neurological exam as well as any other pertinent physical abnormalities. An airway exam should be completed (Table 4.3), and Mallampati scoring should be performed (Figure 4.1).

High Mallampati score, short distance between chin and thyroid cartilage (small chin), poor mouth opening, short thick neck and other abnormalities predict difficult

Table 4.2. Adult Aldrete score (modified): a minimum score of 10 (or baseline), with no score less than 1 in any category, is required for discharge from sedation monitoring

Variable		Pre	Post
Activity: can move voluntarily or on command	4 extremities	2	2
	2 extremities	1	1
	0 extremities	0	0
Respiration	Can deep breathe/cough freely	2	2
	Dyspnea/shallow or limited breathing/tachypnea	1	1
	Apneic/mechanical ventilator	0	0
Circulation (preoperative BP _____ mmHg)	BP ± 20% of pre-sedation level	2	2
	BP ± 20–49% of pre-sedation level	1	1
	BP ± 50% of pre-sedation level	0	0
Consciousness	Fully awake	2	2
	Arousable on calling	1	1
	Not responding	0	0
Oxygen saturation %	> 92% on room air	2	2
	Needs O_2 to remain > 90%	1	1
	< 90% with O_2	0	0
	Total score		

Based on Aldrete JA, Kroulik D. A postanesthetic recovery score. *Anesth Analg* 1970; **49**: 924–34.

Table 4.3. A guide to airway examination

Nonintubated patient	Intubated patient
	☐ **Endotracheal tube** ☐ **Tracheostomy**
☐ Cooperative patient ☐ Uncooperative patient	☐ Cooperative patient ☐ Uncooperative patient
Mouth opening/TMJ excursion ☐ 0 ☐ 1 ☐ 2 ☐ 3 pts FB	*Anatomy externally* ☐ normal ☐ abnormal
Mallampati class ☐ 1 ☐ 2 ☐ 3 ☐ 4	*History of airway problems* ☐ no ☐ yes
Thyromental distance/chin ☐ 0 ☐ 1 ☐ 2 ☐ 3 pts FB ☐ beard	
Teeth ☐ intact/normal for age ☐ poor repair ☐ loose ☐ missing	
Denture ☐ in ☐ out	
Neck extension/ROM ☐ full ☐ limited ☐ Thick obese short neck	
Remarks:	

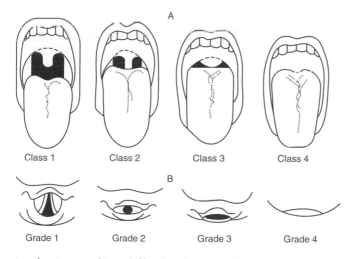

Figure 4.1. (A) Mallampati scoring classes during an airway examination (1–4); (B) Visualization grades during direct laryngoscopy (1–4).

A

Class 1   Class 2   Class 3   Class 4

B

Grade 1   Grade 2   Grade 3   Grade 4

intubation and/or difficulty/impossibility of mask ventilation and should alert the surgeon/practitioner/physician that the patient is a poor candidate for moderate or deep sedation, or may be difficult to intubate in an emergency. Other indicators include but are not limited to the presence of a beard (which may cover a small chin or make mask ventilation difficult), protruding upper teeth (maxilla relatively large, making mandible relatively small, predictive of a difficult airway), narrow jaw, history of radiation to the neck or larynx, and loose teeth. If the patient is uncooperative, the airway exam must be based on external appearance alone. If the patient has an established airway (tracheostomy or endotracheal tube), airway patency is more or less assured under most circumstances.

The attending physician is required to review the assessment and exam, talk to the patient and/or family about the procedure and the sedation plan (including a contingency plan in the event of failed sedation, which may include consent for anesthesia), and sign declaring that the patient is a good/appropriate candidate for the procedure and sedation planned.

An ASA score should be assigned, and the implications of the assigned score should be considered before proceeding with sedation. Even if the procedure is simple and short, a moribund patient with a difficult airway who has a massive deep venous thrombosis may not be a candidate for an inferior vena cava (IVC) filter under minimal or moderate sedation in radiology. The ASA score (American Society of Anesthesiologists physical status class) predicts the possibility of adverse events:

- **Class 1** patients are healthy with no systemic disease, and the pathologic process for which the operation is to be performed is localized, without systemic effect. *Example:* a healthy athlete scheduled for knee surgery.
- **Class 2** patients have mild to moderate systemic dysfunction caused by a coexisting systemic disease or by the pathologic process for which the operation is to be performed. *Examples:* controlled hypertension, controlled diabetes, upper respiratory infection, smoking, thyroid tumor that does not threaten the airway. Pregnancy and extremes of age are sometimes included in this category.
- **Class 3** patients have multiple-system disease or controlled major system disease that affects activity. *Examples:* chronic obstructive pulmonary disease, chronic stable angina,

obesity (which is a multisystem disease), lung tumor that decreases pulmonary function, pheochromocytoma after medical optimization.

- **Class 4** patients have severe systems disorders that are life-threatening and may not be correctable by medical management or operation. *Examples:* congestive heart failure, unstable angina, severe pulmonary or hepatic dysfunction, major trauma, prematurity with respiratory distress and necrotizing enterocolitis, pheochromocytoma prior to medical optimization.
- **Class 5** patients are moribund, with little chance of survival with surgery, and no chance of survival without surgery. *Examples:* ruptured aortic aneurysm, major trauma, massive intracerebral injury.
- (**Class 6** is used to denote a brain-dead organ donor.)
- **E** is used as a modifier to denote emergency operation, with no time to optimize medical condition. A healthy patient with an acute appendicitis would be classified 1E. E implies increased risk.

Class 4 and 5 patients are at increased risk for morbidity and mortality, with mortality rates of 7–50%.

RN affirmation

At the authors' institution, the registered nurse (RN) as the gatekeeper also signs the bottom of the pre-procedure evaluation form along with the nursing history form only after she/he has ascertained that the physician portion is complete. Sedation and procedure may not commence until the nurse declares the pre-procedure evaluation to be completed.

Final review

The physician and the RN do a miniature "time-out" at the bedside here to concur that the evaluation is complete and it is safe to proceed. This could be a time for the entire team to come together for a pre-procedure "huddle" to review patient status and any concerns before moving the patient into the procedure room. There are successes reported in the literature related to team building and culture of safety resulting from these huddles.

Procedure selection

Patient selection

Before proceeding to procedure selection, it must be restated that patient selection and procedure selection go hand in hand. After patients are screened, and even after evaluation on the day of the procedure, only those patients who are appropriate candidates for sedation should be scheduled for or proceed with procedures under sedation. It is never too late to change plans when new information or findings become evident.

Avoid complications and sedation failure by selecting only patients who are amenable to easy and safe sedation. Consider scheduling patients with the characteristics listed below under anesthesia rather than under sedation, unless the procedure is amenable to local anesthesia with minimal sedation, or schedule for sedation with anesthesia backup consented for and immediately available.

A good candidate for sedation is a person with good overall health status, and no significant comorbid conditions, serious multiple allergies, or known contraindications.

Adverse events that occur during sedation most often involve the respiratory or cardiovascular systems. The following should always trigger concerns, even if they are discovered at the last moment:

- obesity
- difficult airway/significant craniofacial abnormalities
- beards (small chins both predict difficult airways and lead patients to grow beards)
- sleep apnea
- malignant hyperthermia
- coagulopathy/hypercoagulability
- heart or lung disease that is a threat to life
- significant neurological disease
- other organ-system disease that presents a significant hazard, such as diabetes
- history of anesthesia/sedation complications or sedation failure
- intolerance of medications routinely used for sedation
- routine medications or drugs that may react with sedation agents
- chronic pain or anxiety with a baseline need for analgesics or anxiolytics
- pediatric patients, who are not consenting individuals and are thus not obligated to cooperate
- extremes of age

Procedure and location selection

The scope of practice of the surgeon/practitioner/physician(s) involved and the individual facility determine the range of procedures possible. The setting may be quite flexible and general (an operating room) or very specifically designed and equipped (e.g., diagnostic or interventional radiology, diagnostic or interventional gastroenterology, or cardiac catheterization lab).

Facilities may also be distinguished by their proximity to the highest level of medical care. Locations may include those within the hospital that are routinely amenable to anesthesia or deep sedation (operating rooms, emergency department, intensive care units), those within the hospital designed specifically for diagnostic and interventional specialty practices including gastroenterology, radiology, and cardiology (where procedures usually take place in the dark!), the detached outpatient surgery center on the medical center campus, one of many other diagnostic and/or procedural areas on or near the medical center campus, a detached outpatient surgery center with or without facilities for overnight observation, or a procedure room in a physician's private office that serves as its own recovery area.

Procedures should be scheduled in the setting equipped for the specific requirements and complexity of the procedure, specifics of the recovery, and the anticipated length of recovery/time to discharge.

Within the hospital itself, there is a range of immediate access to the highest level of care. Outpatient surgery centers on a medical center campus have access to in-hospital recovery facilities and 23-hour observation/limited-stay units as well as inpatient floors and intensive care units. Some detached outpatient surgical centers are equipped for overnight recovery and observation, although most are equipped only for day surgery. Office practice locations may be equipped only for recovery in the procedure room itself, allowing procedures to be scheduled no earlier than the end of the recovery period of the previous patient.

There should be a finite and known set of designated locations where procedures and/or sedation can take place within a facility or building, with designated recovery areas for each location, even if the setting is the physician's private office. Benefits of designating locations include the ability to monitor quality of care and the ability to direct rescue personnel quickly. Potential locations include the following:

- Main hospital operating rooms are usually not a site for procedures under sedation, but there may be occasions where a surgeon has a series of cases, one of which may be amenable to local anesthesia, with minimal or moderate sedation. An example is a surgical oncologist who is removing a small lesion or a portacath, with one of the post-anesthesia care unit (PACU) RNs administering sedation and monitoring the patient.
- Vascular multi-use hybrid angiography/operating suites adjacent to or part of the main operating room can be a site for diagnostic angiography under local with minimal or moderate sedation. An IVC filter might be placed in a very sick patient with local alone, with a sedation nurse to monitor, comfort, and reassure the patient.
- Main hospital PACUs or preoperative holding areas may have small monitored procedure rooms where an emergency thoracostomy might be placed on a patient who has a pneumothorax discovered on the postoperative chest film under local anesthesia and minimal or moderate sedation, or a lumbar puncture might be performed with local anesthesia and minimal sedation. Bone marrow biopsies may be "orphan" procedures, only occasionally performed under more than local and minimal sedation (moderate sedation or even general anesthesia), and they might easily be performed in the PACU or preoperative holding area.
- The emergency department is a site for a number of procedures, including lumbar punctures, suturing of wounds, and reducing fractures and dislocations. Most emergency physicians perform at least moderate sedation, and those with advanced airway skills can perform deep sedation, with end-tidal CO_2 monitoring. Trauma patients who are already intubated can undergo even deep sedation, although hemodynamic instability poses a significant concern. In a trauma center, all manner of emergency procedures may take place in the emergency department. Relief of pain and/or anxiety may uncover the symptoms of hypovolemia and shock.
- Intensive care units, including but not limited to the surgical ICU, medical ICU, cardiac care unit, neuroscience ICU, neonatal ICU, pediatric ICU, and burn ICU, are common sites of procedures under sedation, including but not limited to thoracostomy placement, wound debridement, tracheostomy, PEG tubes, placement of invasive monitoring catheters, and ventriculostomies. If patients are not intubated and procedures such as ventriculostomies are too painful for moderate sedation, intubation should be considered or a physician (intensivist) who is credentialed for deep sedation should be present to administer sedation while the neurosurgeon performs the ventriculostomy. If the patient is hemodynamically unstable or at risk of aspiration, as is often the case with an acute upper gastrointestinal bleed, the airway should be secured before attempting sedation, and the procedure may need to be performed in the operating room rather than the intensive care unit if massive transfusion is anticipated. Gastroenterologists find it challenging to cauterize and clip while directing sedation as well as transfusion, and benefit from a second senior physician (the anesthesiologist, since an intensivist may not be readily available in

the middle of the night) stabilizing the patient and transfusing blood products. A patient may be transferred to the operating room, or an anesthesiologist may be available to bring the benefits of the operating room to the patient. This circumstance underscores the importance of consenting for multiple contingencies. A patient who needs a foreign body removed from the stomach might also best be scheduled under anesthesia in the operating room rather than in the ICU, since movement will make the task more challenging.

- The ENT clinic procedure room may be a site of long procedures, including rhinoplasty, that are amenable to local anesthesia and moderate sedation. Despite the length of some of the procedures, patients are kept fairly comfortable in the minimal to moderate sedation range.

- In the urology clinic, routine brief diagnostic cystoscopy is possible with local anesthesia and minimal to moderate sedation. Patients may be recovered by the RN in the procedure room itself.

- Inpatient and outpatient echocardiography labs may commonly be sites for transesophageal echocardiography with local anesthesia and moderate sedation. Viscous lidocaine is gargled and swallowed while the patient is still awake to minimize the stimulating effect of the echo probe. Benzocaine spray is associated with methemoglobinemia and its use is not advised since it is impossible to regulate the dose. If a cardioversion may be required after transesophageal echocardiography, the patient is pre-consented and evaluated for anesthesia prior to sedation. The two procedures can take place at the same time in the ICU, or the cardioversion can follow in the ICU after the echocardiogram in the echo lab.

- The cardiac catherization lab is the site of a range of diagnostic and interventional procedures. Angiography and percutaneous transluminal coronary angioplasty (PTCA) are usually performed under sedation, as is pacemaker placement. The patient can be pre-assessed and consented for a brief general anesthesia (with propofol) for the actual testing of the pacemaker, which takes only a few minutes, after which the patient is returned to the care of the RN administering sedation. Other diagnostic and interventional studies are scheduled for sedation or anesthesia after pre-screening and assessment by the cardiologist. In some circumstances, the patient is evaluated and consented for anesthesia, which is canceled in favor of sedation if the patient seems to tolerate sedation without problems. This works well if the cardiologists and the anesthesiologists communicate effectively. Because the cardiologists work in the dark and have excellent technology at the authors' institution, they voluntarily utilize end-tidal CO_2 monitors in the cath lab to detect apnea.

- Interventional radiology is the site of a range of procedures including CT- and fluoroscopy-guided biopsies, cryotherapy, placements of drains and stents, embolization of damaged blood vessels, and neurointerventional procedures. Both patient and procedure considerations must be taken into account. If the patient is unstable or potentially unstable, the airway should be secured in advance and an anesthesiologist should be present to manage the patient, unless the patient is already intubated and the trauma team is present. A trauma patient who is not yet unstable but is potentially unstable should not be sent optimistically to radiology with an unsecured airway and inadequate IV access for diagnostic/possible interventional procedure in the middle of the night without a contingency plan. If the patient must not move during the procedure, if it necessitates a prone position, or if it is likely to be very painful, the procedure should probably be performed under anesthesia. Even if the procedure is "minor" but the patient is ASA 3–5, any sedation other than reassurance may be unwise, and a contingency plan should be created in advance. Local anesthetic with assurance and vigilant monitoring is in the end kinder than precipitating a crisis. Because so many procedures take place in the dark, making it difficult to observe patients, end-tidal CO_2 monitoring can be beneficial in this setting.

- Diagnostic radiology is the site of many routine procedures (CT, MRI, nuclear medicine/PET scans, ultrasound) and is easily tolerated by most consenting adults, but some patients require at least oral sedation and distraction with music or talking. Patients who have trouble cooperating may or may not be more cooperative with sedation. Challenging patients might be scheduled under anesthesia or an anesthesiologist-led nurse sedation team on specific days. A protocol should be developed to manage recurring sedation challenges so that care is consistent.

- Interventional gastroenterology can be the site of both simple diagnostic procedures (e.g., upper and lower diagnostic endoscopies, enteroscopies) and complex diagnostic and interventional procedures (including but not limited to endoscopic ultrasound, ERCP, stent placement, foreign body removal). Even a simple diagnostic procedure is hazardous if the patient is fragile or obese or has sleep apnea, and again, since procedures take place in the dark, end-tidal CO_2 monitoring should be considered even for moderate sedation. Again, both the patient and the procedure must be considered when determining whether sedation or anesthesia is appropriate. At many institutions, as patient acuity and comorbidities as well as procedure complexity have increased, the percentage of cases done under anesthesia has risen from 40% to 60%, after patient and case pre-selection by the team at the facility. With high demand for time, most, or all, of the cases must proceed as planned, without failed sedation or unanticipated adverse events. Patients who are extremely ill should be scheduled for the main operating room rather than a detached location.

- Aesthetics and plastic surgery practices may distribute their time between the main hospital operating rooms, a detached outpatient suite on the campus of the medical center, a detached outpatient suite off but associated with the medical center campus, a private detached outpatient suite, and a private office. Again, pre-screening allows procedures and patients to be scheduled in the appropriate location.

- An outpatient chronic pain clinic may be the site of procedures, but the patients are known to the practitioners, and pre-screening is guaranteed. These patients are already on chronic pain medications, which should not be discontinued, and do not "count" as part of the sedation given during the procedure. Patients who are not likely to tolerate sedation should be scheduled in an operating room.

- An outpatient laser facility for procedures on eyes or skin may be a site for local anesthesia with minimal or moderate sedation, or even general anesthesia. Patients can be pre-screened for type of sedation or anesthesia required, with inability to cooperate (e.g., pediatric patients) a first consideration.

- The pulmonary lab is mostly a site for flexible bronchoscopy, although pulmonologists also perform bronchoscopies in the intensive care units. Diagnostic flexible bronchoscopies can be performed with moderate sedation, while rigid bronchoscopies and flexible bronchoscopies with bronchial ultrasound and biopsies are best performed under general anesthesia. Many of these patients are extremely fragile with threatened loss of airway, and the procedures are often urgent.

- An outpatient surgery center on the campus of a medical center has access to the hospital itself, but patients should be pre-screened to avoid cancelations, delays, and problems. Patients can be scheduled under any type of anesthesia or sedation, and it is possible to schedule and consent a patient for sedation with anesthesia backup since most patients are scheduled under anesthesia. Patients can easily be transferred to the main hospital for planned or unplanned admission, although the majority of patients should recover and be discharged home.
- A freestanding surgery center detached from the medical center campus must be more self-sufficient, although there may often be access to anesthesia care as well as sedation. Patients should be pre-screened and cases should be scheduled appropriately. Some centers may be staffed and equipped for 23-hour overnight observation, but most patients are expected to recover and be discharged home. This is not the ideal setting for the patient who is fragile or ill, or for procedures involving significant fluid shifts and blood loss. Any member of the team should feel empowered to call emergency ambulance services if she/he feels a patient is in danger.
- The physician's private office is extremely isolated, and, in general, only very simple procedures with local or minimal sedation are appropriate in this setting. Mohs procedures, biopsies, vasectomies, and lumbar punctures are procedures which are amenable to local anesthesia with minimal sedation. When such a procedure is routinely performed in a facility equipped and staffed for the procedure, most patients do well.

Criteria for selection

Consider the length of each procedure. Schedule procedures in locations detached from the medical center campus only if the procedure and recovery period can be completed within the working day (which may include overnight observation in some facilities). Consider how long a patient can comfortably lie still in a given position, and the cumulative dose of local anesthetic, sedative, and/or opioid that will be required before the procedure is completed.

Schedule procedures in locations equipped both for the procedure and for sedation and any contingencies that can be routinely expected as a result of either the procedure or the patient. Always consider the patient when choosing the location.

If a procedure involves or may involve blood loss, schedule it in a facility where transfusion is an option.

Procedures taking place out of the operating room setting should be amenable to local anesthesia with minimal or moderate sedation unless they are to take place in the emergency department or intensive care unit with physicians credentialed and skilled in deep sedation or anesthesia. Schedule procedures that require deeper sedation or anesthesia, even if appropriate for the location, for a day and in a setting when deep sedation or anesthesia care can be provided.

Procedures where it is critical that the patient does not move (with or without requiring cooperation from the patient) should not be scheduled under significant sedation. A significantly sedated patient may not be relied upon to remember to cooperate, and a patient cannot be guaranteed to stay still unless he/she is unable to be uncooperative, and the latter circumstance is beyond the scope of sedation practice. More sedation is rarely the solution to restlessness, agitation, or lack of cooperation.

If a procedure may be amenable to sedation in some patients, but not certainly amenable to sedation in all patients, it is reasonable to schedule patients on a day when both sedation and anesthesia are available. Evaluate patients and consent them for both contingencies. This allows a greater range of options without aborting the procedure and rescheduling.

Summary

The chapter covers pre-screening, history and physical for evaluation of patients who are potential candidates for procedures under sedation, as well as instructions for patients. Reevaluation of patients on the day of the procedure is a requirement and should be documented, along with exam by the proceduralist physician, informed consent, and affirmation by the RN that all is in order prior to initiation of sedation. Patient and procedure should be determined to be appropriate for sedation, and selection criteria are discussed.

Further reading

American Society of Anesthesiologists Task Force on Preanesthesia Evaluation. Practice advisory for preanesthesia evaluation. *Anesthesiology* 2002; **96**: 485–96.

AORN position statement on allied health care providers and support personnel in the perioperative practice setting. AORN, 2011. www.aorn.org/PracticeResources/AORN PositionStatements (accessed June 2011).

AORN position statement on creating a practice environment of safety. AORN, 2011. www.aorn.org/PracticeResources/ AORNPositionStatements (accessed June 2011).

AORN position statement on one perioperative registered nurse circulator dedicated to every patient undergoing a surgical or other invasive procedure. AORN, 2007. www.aorn.org/PracticeResources/AORN PositionStatements (accessed June 2011).

Frank RL. Procedural sedation in adults. *UpToDate* 2011. www.uptodate.com/ contents/procedural-sedation-in-adults (accessed June 2011).

Morrison DE, Harris AL. Preoperative and anesthetic management of the surgical patient. In Wilson SE, ed., *Educational Review Manual in General Surgery*, 8th edn. New York, NY: Castle Connolly, 2009.

Ogg M, Burlingame B. Clinical issues: recommended practices for moderate sedation/analgesia. *AORN J* 2008; **88**: 275–7.

University HealthSystem Consortium Consensus Group on Deep Sedation. *Deep Sedation Best Practice Recommendations.* Oak Brook, IL: UHC, 2006.

University HealthSystem Consortium Consensus Group on Moderate Sedation. *Moderate Sedation Best Practice Recommendations.* Oak Brook, IL: UHC, 2005.

Patient monitoring, equipment, and intravenous fluids

Erika G. Puente, Maria A. Antor, and Sergio D. Bergese

Patient monitoring and equipment
Standard monitoring
Monitoring is one of the most important aspects of the practice of sedation. An appropriately trained and experienced healthcare provider is considered the only indispensable monitor for the immediate supervision of the staff as well as the observation of the patient. Indeed, a qualified healthcare provider is the main determinant of patient safety during sedation and anesthesia [1–4]. Therefore, any physician or other healthcare provider who will be involved in patient care during any procedure requiring sedation should be clinically competent in the practice of resuscitation and monitoring. The reader is referred to the Guidelines and Standards section of the book, and needs to be familiar with specialty-specific monitoring practice advisories.

Furthermore, healthcare providers should be familiar with monitoring equipment and be able to interpret the data obtained from it. Mechanical and electronic monitors are a good resource and can provide useful information to assist the healthcare provider in ensuring the integrity of vital organs and proper perfusion and oxygenation of tissue [1]. Although monitoring will not prevent all adverse events or accidents in the perioperative period, there is vast evidence that it will improve patient safety by detecting the consequences of errors and by giving early warning that the condition of a patient is deteriorating.

The monitoring process, basically "data collection," involves vigilant observation of the patient's signs and symptoms and interpretation of data provided by the monitors. Initiation of corrective action and timely therapeutic intervention are required if any parameters are found to be out of range and clinically significant.

Moderate and Deep Sedation in Clinical Practice, ed. Richard D. Urman and Alan D. Kaye.
Published by Cambridge University Press. © Cambridge University Press 2012.

Table 5.1. Patient monitoring and supplementary devices

Basic monitoring
Pulse oximeter
Electrocardiography (ECG)
Automatic noninvasive blood pressure measuring device
Capnography (increasingly utilized for moderate/deep sedation)
Respiratory monitorig devices
Additional monitoring (as required)
Brain function monitor (e.g bispectral index monitor)
Transesophageal echocardiography
Invasive blood pressure monitoring (peripheral arterial, central venous, pulmonary arterial)
Temperature measurement
Supplementary Equipment (immediately available)
Stethoscope
Appropriate lighting
Defibrillation and other resuscitation equipment
Drug and fluid infusion devices

In the past, the availability of technology and monitoring devices was limited to the most primitive monitoring equipment in medicine such as the stethoscope and the manual blood pressure cuff. The data obtained from these devices were interpreted by an experienced physician and utilized for the application of therapeutic interventions. In the present, data collection can be accomplished either manually or automatically. With the development of new and advanced technologies, basic automatic data collection monitoring devices are available to most sedation and anesthesia providers, and to healthcare institutions at almost every level.

While automatic data collection systems provide continuous data on several patient parameters allowing more time for the provider to make a clinical decision, these systems also have built-in alarms. These may give false or no alarm, contribute to "alarm fatigue", display distorted data, or even malfunction in the middle of a case [3,5]. Therefore, the use of these monitoring devices has to be under the premise that they will never be a substitute for a trained healthcare provider and the initial manual monitoring techniques. Monitoring equipment can range from very basic to more sophisticated (Table 5.1), dictated by patient's condition and the procedure being performed.

It is important to emphasize that when administering a sedative/analgesic to a patient, this must occur in an adequately equipped facility. The minimally required equipment for patient monitoring, drugs, and other supplies must be readily available, including life support and emergency resuscitation equipment [1] (Table 5.1).

Monitoring should be tailored to the specific operative procedure, the patient's risk factors, underlying medical conditions, and the type of sedation/anesthesia to be administered [5] (Table 5.2).

Table 5.2. Monitoring requirements for different anesthetic and sedation techniques

Monitoring during deep sedation and general anesthesia
Blood pressure (noninvasive or invasive; CVP, PAP, if applicable)
Pulse oximeter
Electrocardiography
Temperature probe
Capnography
Exhaled/inhaled anesthetic gas concentration (intubated patients)
Circuit low pressure alarm (intubated patients)
Additional ventilator parameters (intubated patients)
Monitoring during moderate sedation
Blood pressure (noninvasive or invasive)
Pulse oximeter
Electrocardiography
Capnography (see ASA and other professional society guidelines)
Additional monitoring for intubated patients (see above)

CVP, central venous pressure; MAC, monitored anesthesia care; PAP, pulmonary artery pressure; ASA, American Society of Anesthesiologists.

Monitoring outside the operating room is becoming more frequent and necessary. Advances in technology for surgical, therapeutic, and diagnostic procedures are increasingly opening new possibilities and new procedural sites away from the operating room that nevertheless require adequate and reliable patient monitoring. Although these procedures are generally shorter in duration and may be done on an outpatient basis, they may be complex and involve medically challenging patients. Thus, patient monitoring requirements should be the same in these remote locations, since the monitoring is no less important than when patients undergo procedures in the operating room or when they require postoperative hospitalization [6].

It is the responsibility of the healthcare provider who will be administering sedation and monitoring the patient to check all equipment before starting each case and, if possible, to complete an equipment checklist. Healthcare providers must be familiar with the equipment that they will be using, and they must verify adequate functioning of the following, as applicable: oxygen supply, suction, monitoring devices, breathing systems, vapor analyzer (if applicable), infusion devices, and alarms.

Monitoring must be performed during all phases of sedation. It involves the observation of the data provided by the monitoring devices as well as clinical observation of the patient's mucosal color, pupil size, response to procedure stimuli, and movements of the chest wall. During the start and maintenance of sedation the following must be utilized and monitor readings periodically recorded: pulse oximeter reading, blood pressure reading, electrocardiography, measurement of airway gases such as inspired oxygen flows/concentration and exhaled carbon dioxide (if used), and airway pressures and tidal volumes (if the patient is intubated) [2].

Cardiovascular and hemodynamic monitoring
Arterial blood pressure monitoring

Blood pressure is an indirect way to measure and monitor adequate organ perfusion. During the procedure blood pressure may vary and organ perfusion may be compromised. The accurate measurement of blood pressure is of extreme importance to guide the therapeutic approach of the care provider. Normal blood pressure ranges are considered those under 120 mmHg systolic and 80 mmHg diastolic. Values over these parameters are considered hypertension, and the JNC-7 (Joint National Commission, 7th report) has classified elevated blood pressure into the categories shown in Table 5.3 [7]. Hypertension increases the risk of patients developing cardiac arrhythmias, increased myocardial oxygen consumption, bleeding, increased systemic vascular resistance and heart rate [3]. Therefore, hypertension should be addressed prior to procedure to prevent these complications. The ultimate goal should be to manage and control blood pressure at the same time by balancing the effects of the body's autoregulatory mechanisms and the use of antihypertensive and sedative medications, in order to maintain blood pressure within the desired range. Adequate hemodynamic control may not only limit postoperative complications but also provide improved long-term outcomes. Monitoring plays an important role in enabling the clinician to predict the blood pressure response, rapidly and flexibly control it, and ultimately adjust the treatment to each individual's needs [8].

Nevertheless, attention should also be directed towards detecting lower than normal blood pressure, or hypotension. Although hypotension has not been classified as precisely as hypertension, in general, hypotension is considered a drop in blood pressure to levels that affect blood flow to organs enough to generate symptoms and/or signs of low blood pressure. The amount of pressure required for a patient to maintain adequate blood flow to a vital organ varies among individuals. Therefore, clinically significant hypotension has been defined as a drop in systemic arterial blood pressure of more than 20–30% below the preoperative blood pressure, or a mean arterial pressure of less than 60 mmHg. The aim should be to keep the mean arterial pressure above 75% of the patient's baseline value. Hypotension may occur in response to hypovolemic states, reduced cardiac output, myocardial ischemia, sepsis, effect of drugs and anesthetic agents, vagal responses, or acidosis [3,9]. Management of hypotension will be tailored to the underlying cause while providing adequate oxygenation, volume replenishment, and correction of the metabolic changes.

Table 5.3. JNC-7 blood pressure classification in adults (≥ 18 years old) [7]

Blood pressure categories	Systolic	Diastolic
Normal	< 120 mmHg	< 80 mmHg
Prehypertension	120–139 mmHg	80–89 mmHg
Stage 1 hypertension	140–159 mmHg	90–99 mmHg
Stage 2 hypertension	≥ 160 mmHg	≥ 100 mmHg

Table 5.4. Noninvasive and invasive blood pressure monitoring techniques

Noninvasive blood pressure monitoring
Auscultation of Korotkoff sounds
Palpation of arterial pulse
Doppler ultrasonic flow probes
Oscillotonometry
Automated devices
Invasive blood pressure monitoring
Arterial cannulation
Central venous catheter
Pulmonary artery catheters

Blood pressure can be monitored and measured by many different methods, mainly classified into noninvasive and invasive (Table 5.4).

Noninvasive arterial blood pressure monitoring

Noninvasive monitoring involves applying external pressure with a manual blood pressure cuff over the proximal upper or lower limb. The standard location for blood pressure measurement is usually considered the brachial artery. The cuff is applied to the proximal part of the arm just above the elbow and inflated, transiently interrupting arterial blood flow until the distal pulse of the limb disappears. Then it is slowly deflated until the pulse reappears. In the clinical setting, the gold standard and the most frequent interpretation method used by physicians is the Korotkoff sounds method. This requires the use of a mercury sphygmomanometer and a stethoscope to listen to the sounds that are generated from the turbulence of the blood as it begins to flow again through the artery, and as the pressure from the inflated cuff decreases. The first sound generally corresponds to the systolic blood pressure, while the moment the sound disappears corresponds with the diastolic blood pressure. When performed properly, this method is considered one of the most accurate, although there is still some degree of error common to all manual techniques. It is important to keep in mind that the size of the pressure cuff in relation to the patient's limb diameter may influence the accuracy of the pressure measurement. A cuff that is too narrow may give higher than normal measurements, and a cuff that is too wide may give lower values. Normally, the cuff should cover around two-thirds of the proximal limb or measure 20% more than the diameter of the limb (Table 5.5). Also, if the cuff is deflated too fast, this can result in higher blood pressure measurements. The recommended cuff deflation rate is 3–5 mmHg per second [4,11,12]. Other variations in blood pressure may also result from changes in the location of the blood pressure measurement and changes in posture. The more distal the artery, the more the systolic pressure increases and the diastolic pressure decreases [12]. Diastolic blood pressure measurements tend to be slightly higher in patients who are sitting versus supine [4].

The oscillotonometric method is a technique consisting of observing the oscillations of pressure on the sphygmomanometer cuff during gradual deflation. The point where maximal oscillations are observed has been shown to correspond with the mean arterial

Table 5.5. Mercury sphygmomanometer cuff sizes

Indication	Bladder	Arm
	Width × length	Circumference
Small adult/child	12 × 18 cm	< 23 cm
Standard adult	12 × 16 cm	< 33 cm
Large adult	12 × 40 cm	< 50 cm
Adult thigh cuff	20 × 42 cm	< 53 cm

Reproduced with permission from Williams *et al.* [10].

Table 5.6. British Hypertension Society recommendations for blood pressure measurement by standard mercury sphygmomanometer or semiautomated device

Verify that the device is validated and properly calibrated
Preferably measure blood pressure in the sitting position
In elderly and diabetic patients obtain an initial measurement for comparison
Ensure patient is comfortable by removing tight clothing
Raise arm to heart level and ask the patient to relax the limb
Ask the patient to remain silent during the measurement procedure
Verify that the cuff size is appropriate for the patient
Deflate the cuff slowly by lowering the mercury column at a rate of 2 mm/s
Measure and record blood pressure to the nearest 2 mmHg
Consider diastolic blood pressure at the point of sound disappearance (phase V)
Take two readings and use the mean
An isolated reading should not be considered enough basis to initiate treatment

Reproduced with permission from Williams *et al.* [10].

pressure. This technique has been used for the development of ambulatory blood pressure monitors and home monitors.

Ultrasound techniques are used when patients have very weak or inaudible Korotkoff sounds. An ultrasound transmitter is placed over the artery under a sphygmomanometer cuff. The transmitter will detect the motion of the blood vessel as the flow increases, and also the decrease in motion of the artery as it reaches diastolic blood pressure levels [11,12]. The guidelines for management of hypertension from the British Hypertension Society describe the appropriate method to be followed for the accurate measurement and interpretation of blood pressure values [10] (Table 5.6).

Blood pressure measurement equipment

- **Mercury sphygmomanometers**, based on mercury displacement, are considered the gold standard for clinical measurement of blood pressure. This device has hardly changed for the past 50 years and has not been surpassed by any other device in terms of

Table 5.7. Arterial line insertion technique

(1) Immobilize the forearm and hand

(2) Hyperextend the wrist

(3) Palpate the radial artery and prep the skin

(4) Administer 1% lidocaine locally

(5) Select catheter size: 18–20 adults, 22–24 infants

(6) Place the catheter: direct threading or transfixing methods

(7) Securely attach the catheter and T-connector to the skin

(8) Join the T-connector to the transducer system

(9) Flush the line with approximately 3 mL saline

accuracy and satisfaction. The current tendency is to withdraw mercury from its use in sphygmomanometers, as has happened with thermometers. The major concern is the metal's toxicity and safety. The downside is that there has not been a more accurate device developed to replace it.

- **Aneroid devices** (aneroid means "without fluid") are devices capable of measuring the pressure of liquid, as well as of gas. These have been less popular because of significant concerns about their accuracy [13].
- **Automated devices or electronic monitors** are used frequently in the clinical setting because of their ability to provide periodic blood pressure measurements. These readings can be scheduled or timed according to the frequency required. The American Society of Anesthesiologists Task Force on Sedation and Analgesia by Non-Anesthesiologists recommends that blood pressure should be measured at a minimum of 5-minute intervals during the procedure, unless such monitoring interferes with the procedure [14]. Some devices allow readings as frequently as every minute, although such short cycles should be avoided for routine monitoring [11].

Invasive arterial blood pressure monitoring

Invasive arterial BP monitoring is a method of direct arterial pressure monitoring by means of a peripheral arterial catheter that connects to an external transducer [4,11]. Direct blood pressure measurement is indicated in cardiopulmonary bypass surgeries and hemodynamically unstable patients when ample variability in blood pressure is expected. Also, a tight control of blood pressure may be required in patients with intracranial aneurysms, severe carotid or coronary artery disease, induced hypotension cases, and when there is a need for numerous arterial blood gas samples. The most common site chosen for cannulation is the radial artery. Some complications associated with the placement of the line are thrombosis, distal ischemia (< 0.1%), infection, hemorrhage, and fistula or aneurysm formation [4,11]. The insertion technique is summarized in Table 5.7.

Electrocardiography (ECG)

The ECG is an indirect method of measuring cardiac electric activity by means of a visual display. Monitoring the ECG signals in the sedated patient offers the ability to detect cardiac arrhythmias, myocardial ischemia, electrolyte imbalances, and the presence of pacemaker

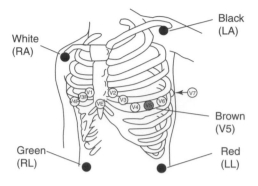

White
(RA)

Black
(LA)

Brown
(V5)

Green
(RL)

Red
(LL)

Figure 5.1. Proper placement of the ECG leads.

function [3]. The most important aspect of ECG monitoring is correct electrode placement (Figure 5.1). Two sensing electrodes and one ground electrode are required as a minimum, although four- or five-lead monitoring is also frequently used. Special attention should be paid to both electrode positioning and placement, since the improper application of the electrodes could predispose to electrical noise and inadequate graphing of the signals [11]. Lead I, II, or III are generally used for procedural monitoring and recovery. Lead II is most commonly used because it allows good visualization of the P waves and facilitates the detection of arrhythmias. Lead V_5 is preferred for the detection of myocardial ischemia [3,15] (Table 5.8).

Respiratory monitoring

Monitoring respiratory activity can be achieved by capnography or auscultation of breath sounds. A method of indirectly monitoring respiratory activity by chest observation alone does not guarantee adequate air exchange. Automated apnea monitoring and appropriate alarms are especially useful when the patient is physically separated from the healthcare provider. Since ventilation and oxygenation are distinct physiologic processes, the monitoring of both respiration and oxygenation should be considered.

Monitoring of oxygenation

Pulse oximetry was developed in the early 1980s and is now the primary source of oxygen saturation monitoring in any clinical setting. Pulse oximetry indirectly measures arterial oxygen saturation of the blood, noninvasively and continuously. It has been shown to be effective to detect desaturation and hypoxemia earlier than clinical observation of the patient alone. The hemoglobin saturation is determined by light-absorbance techniques that measure the transmitted light by oxyhemoglobin and deoxyhemoglobin combined. A normal SpO_2 (95–100%) indicates adequate oxygenation of the lungs and peripheral tissues. It must not be assumed, however, that this is an indication of the amount of oxygen that is actually being delivered. A low SpO_2 may indicate a problem with the patient or with the monitor. It is important to consider the possibility of artifacts in the measurements. Some of the artifacts can be related to the use of contrast dyes (methylene blue, indocyanine green, indigo carmine), increased carboxyhemoglobin, presence of large amounts of methemoglobin, and noise generated by the surgical electrocautery or other electrical devices in the operating room [3,11].

Table 5.8. ECG monitoring

ECG analysis	Possible abnormalities
Rate	Regular or irregular
P–P interval	Tachycardia or bradycardia
Rhythm	Sinus rhythm determined by the presence of P waves Atrioventricular conduction blocks: absence of P waves
Premature depolarizations	Extrasystoles Atrial Ventricular
Fibrillation	Atrial Ventricular
Ectopic tachycardias	
Myocardial ischemia	
ST segment elevation or depression	
Detect changes in the QRS complex – Q wave	
Electrolyte imbalance	
Hyperkalemia	Tall peaked T waves ($\geq$ 6 mEq/L) Prolongation of PR interval ($\geq$ 7 mEq/L) Absent P wave with wide QRS complex ($\geq$ 8 mEq/L) Ventricular fibrillation, "sine wave pattern," asystole
Hypokalemia	T wave depression Prominent U waves
Pacemaker function	
Sharp electrical spikes where one would expect P waves	
Other ECG patterns possible, depending on the type of pacemaker	

Based on information from Webster *et al.* [15].

Temperature monitoring

Although patients undergoing sedation are not exposed to potent inhalation agents used for general anesthesia, the importance of temperature monitoring should not be underestimated. Patients undergoing minor surgical procedures are generally exposed to the ambient environment. Therefore, they are prone to core heat loss by redistribution effects and peripheral heat loss through all the physical mechanisms of heat transfer (radiation, conduction, convection, and evaporation). Hypothermia can impact patient recovery and outcomes. Shivering can increase oxygen demand, and can cause hypertension and tachycardia. Wound healing and coagulation may also be affected by low body temperatures [4].

If necessary, temperature can be monitored at several anatomical sites. The most common ones are the most readily available and practical, such as the skin, axilla, rectum, esophagus, nasopharynx, tympanic membranes, and bladder. Each of these sites presents advantages and disadvantages (Table 5.9).

Table 5.9. Temperature monitoring sites

Site	Considerations
Skin (3–4 °C < core temperature)	Changes in skin temperature may not directly reflect changes in core temperature
Axilla (1 °C < core temperature)	Prone to dislocation of the temperature probe and increased error
Rectum	Less accurate in detecting early changes in normal body temperature
Esophagus	Accurate in reflecting core and blood temperature but less practical
Nasopharynx	Accurate measure of brain temperature. Contraindicated in patients with coagulopathies, head trauma, or CSF rhinorrhea, and in pregnant women
Tympanic membrane	Measure of core temperature. Practical and accurate. Perforation of the tympanic membrane may occur
Bladder probe	Accurately measures core temperature, but is less practical and requires a special probe.

Carbon dioxide measurement

The measurement of exhaled carbon dioxide produced in tissues, which is eliminated via the pulmonary circulation in exchange for oxygen, is an indirect indicator of pulmonary perfusion, alveolar ventilation, and respiratory patterns. While pulse oximetry serves as a good measure of oxygenation, capnography can provide a more sensitive measure of ventilation. In fact, apnea may not be detected by the pulse oximeter alone until 30–60 seconds after it occurs. On the other hand, capnography can detect hypoventilation and apnea almost immediately. Capnography can be used to monitor the adequacy of ventilation in both intubated patients on a ventilator and nonintubated patients breathing spontaneously.

The maximum concentration of carbon dioxide is reached at the end of exhalation, and then identified as end-tidal CO_2 ($ETCO_2$). Normal values for $ETCO_2$ are approximately 5% of alveolar concentration, or 35–37 mmHg. The gradient between arterial CO_2 and $ETCO_2$ is around 5–6 mmHg. In intubated patients, the measurement of $ETCO_2$ is useful in the clinical setting to verify proper placement of the endotracheal tube, to assess ventilation, and to monitor for complications such as pulmonary embolism and airway obstruction. It can also assist in the detection of any problems with the ventilator or the endotracheal tube, whether this is caused by obstruction due to secretions or by the presence of leaks in the circuit [11].

The $ETCO_2$ can be measured by several methods or devices, named according to the mechanism used to measure the $ETCO_2$. Capnography and capnometry are usually digital monitors that measure either partial pressure of CO_2 or percentage of CO_2 in exhaled gas through methods such as infrared, Raman, molecular correlation, mass, and photoacoustic spectroscopy. Capnography involves the measurement of the $ETCO_2$ value and the representation of the CO_2 waveform, graph, or capnogram, and it uses a capnograph device (Figure 5.2). Capnometry, measured by a capnometer, is the measurement of the $ETCO_2$ value only and does not display the waveform graph. The measurement of exhaled CO_2 can be accomplished by using either a mainstream or a sidestream method. The difference between these methods lies in the location at which the sample of the exhaled CO_2 is obtained. With the mainstream monitor, the sensor is located at the patient–ventilator

(a)

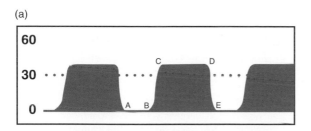

(b)

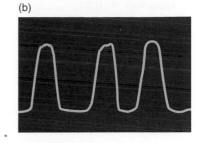

The "normal" capnogram shape cosists of the following:

A-B   **Zero baseline** – the beginning of exhalation
B-C   **Rapid, sharp rise** – anatomical dead space gas replaced by more
      distal airway gases that contain more CO_2
C-D   **Alveolar "plateau"** – contains mixed alveolar gases
D   **End-tidal CO_2** – highest concentration of exhaled CO_2
D-E   **Rapid, sharp downstroke** – inhalation phase; fresh gas rapidly
      replaces CO_2

Figure 5.2. Typical exhaled CO_2 tracing in intubated and nonintubated patients: (A) normal CO_2 waveform in an intubated patient; (B) typical CO_2 waveform in a spontaneously breathing patient.

Mainstream

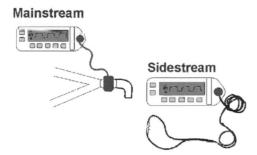

Sidestream

Figure 5.3. Mainstream (attached to the ventilator circuit) and sidestream (attached to nasal cannula) exhaled CO_2 monitoring devices.

circuit interface, close to the patient (Figure 5.3). Potential advantages of the mainstream monitor are more precise graphical representation of the capnogram, less rebreathing, and less chance of sample line occlusion. With the sidestream monitor, the sample is obtained from the patient–ventilator circuit interface but is then transported through connecting tubing to the monitor for analysis (distal-diverting from the patient) [11,16,17]. One advantage of sidestream capnography is the ability to monitor nonintubated patients, since the sampling of expiratory gases can be obtained from the nasal cavity using nasal adaptors or cannulae. One disadvantage is that there is a delay in recording CO_2 measurement, because the exhaled gas needs to travel through long sampling tubing, and the tubing is subject to disconnection or occlusion. Note that in nonintubated patients breathing spontaneously, the CO_2 wave forms may not be as "perfect" in shape as those seen in intubated patients (Figure 5.2). However, in non-intubated patients, it is recommended to follow changes in the shape or frequency of the CO_2 waveform to help guide sedation and prevent drug overdosing and hypoventilation. The quality of the expired CO_2 tracing, costs associated with the use of the specific device, and patient comfort while wearing the device are all important considerations. Table 5.10 below summarizes the pros and cons of routine exhaled CO_2 monitoring in nonintubated patients.

Table 5.10. Routine exhaled CO_2 monitoring in nonintubated patients: Pros and Cons

Pros	Cons
Non – invasive	Results in higher costs
Relatively simple to interpret	Requires the use of a special nasal-oral cannula
Provides accurate information on the quality of ventilation breath-by-breath	May display sporadic artifacts and false positives caused by patient movement, verbalization or crying and/or nasal cannula displacement
Provides early warning of respiratory depression before evident clinical manifestations	A few of early alerts may be false positives and not clinically relevant
Useful during sedation procedures where direct patient observation is not feasible	Patient is unable to tolerate the nasal cannula (specially in pediatric population)
Reduces moderate and severe hypoxemic events during sedation	Requires training of the staff for proper use and interpretation
Helps prevent oversedation	

Table adapted from Green SM and Pershad J. Should Capnographic Monitoring be Standard Practice During Emergency Department Procedural Sedation and Analgesia? Pro and Con. *Annals of Emergency Medicine* 2010; 55: 265–67.

Brain function monitoring

Measurement of the electrophysiologic activity of the cerebral cortex has been correlated to depth of anesthesia. Bispectral Index (BIS) monitors measure the level of cerebral cortex activity in patients undergoing anesthesia. These devices provide a measurement of the depth of sedation/anesthesia that patients reach while undergoing a surgical or interventional procedure. These monitors have been used in the setting of moderate or deep sedation, although they are more frequently used in the operating rooms during general anesthesia to prevent incidence of drug overdose and intraoperative awareness. Some studies have shown a good correlation between BIS values and the Observer's Assessment of Alertness/Sedation (OAA/S) scale [18]. Although the use of these monitors has not yet been standardized, and they are not yet specifically recommended in the monitoring guidelines for anesthesiologists or non-anesthesia sedation providers, their incorporation into patient monitoring practices may have benefits. The downside of this technology is that there are several different monitors available, and the interpretation of the measurements obtained, although they may correlate, has not been standardized. A study comparing the BIS VISTA technology and the SNAP II monitor determined that even though the indices from both monitors are correlated, they are not interchangeable, with the SNAP II index (SI) consistently higher in value than the corresponding BIS [19]. These values should be interpreted according to the range indices provided for each individual monitor. For the BIS monitor, sedation for a patient under general anesthesia should be targeted to a BIS between 40 and 60 [17,19]. The role of brain function monitoring in moderate and deep sedation has not been established, because of low accuracy in distinguishing between the different levels of sedation (see Chapter 12).

Intravenous fluids

Fluid compartment physiology and intravenous fluids

Sixty percent of total body weight is accounted for by water. That is, for an adult of 75 kg the estimated total body water is approximately 45 L. The total body fluid is distributed into the intracellular and extracellular fluid compartments:

- intracellular fluid (ICF): approximately two-thirds of total body water
- extracellular fluid (ECF): approximately one-third of total body water

The extracellular and intracellular compartments are divided by the cell membranes. The extracellular fluid is further divided into the interstitial compartment (ISF: fluid that lies in the interstices of all body tissues), the intravascular compartment (composed by blood cells such as: red cells, white cells and platelets), and the plasma compartment (the major fluid compartment in which blood cells are suspended) (Figure 5.4). Transcellular fluid is secreted by epithelial cells and constitutes the cerebrospinal fluid, intraocular fluid, and digestive fluids.

Since the plasma membranes of the cells are highly permeable to water, fluids move easily and quickly through cell and vessel walls and disperse throughout all the compartments. Cations and anions are also distributed between ECF and ICF. Sodium (Na^+) and chlorine (Cl^-) are extracellular ions, whereas potassium (K^+) is a major ion of the ICF. The energy-dependent Na/K adenosine triphosphatase pump in cell walls extrudes Na and Cl and maintains a sodium gradient across the cell membrane. Also, the ionic composition is similar in the major components of the ECF. There is an ionic equilibrium in all compartments.

A change in anionic concentration, which can cause problems with normal cell functioning and volume, results in a rapid water movement in order to maintain an osmotic equilibrium. Fluid shifts occur only if the perturbation of the ECF alters its osmolarity. A measurement of plasma osmolarity provides a measure of ECF and ICF osmolarity. Plasma osmolarity is a measure of the concentration of substances such as sodium, chloride, potassium, urea, glucose, and other ions in blood. It is calculated as the number of osmoles (Osm) of solute per liter. Osmolarity of blood increases with dehydration and decreases with overhydration.

Capillary membranes are freely permeable to all natural substances dissolved in the plasma, except for proteins such as albumin and colloids.

Patients undergoing surgery can have a series of underlying conditions that will ultimately predispose them to altered fluid distributions. Several factors such as hypertension, dehydration, intraoperative fluid losses, and the patient's overall hemodynamic status will determine the approach to fluid replacement. In some situations it is necessary to

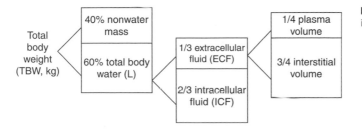

Figure 5.4. Fluid compartments in the human body.

consider restoration of intravascular volume to optimize cardiac output, in order to ensure adequate tissue oxygenation and hemodynamic stability [20–22].

The use of intravenous access and solutions allows for the maintenance of fluid and electrolyte balance in surgical cases. Intravenous solutions can be generally classified into two categories, crystalloids and colloids. During sedation, the use of crystalloid solutions is generally recommended for the intravenous replacement of fluids.

Crystalloid solutions

Crystalloids are solutions composed of inorganic ions and small organic molecules dissolved in water. The predominant solute is either glucose or sodium chloride (saline), and it is generally selected based on osmolarity. The value of the osmolarity of the extracellular fluid, which is determined by measuring solute concentration of the blood, is 280–300 mOsm/L in normal serum. One of the main properties of electrolyte solutions (crystalloids) is that they are capable of conducting an electrical current. Thus, cations (K^+ and Na^+) will maintain a positive charge, and anions (Cl^-) a negative charge.

The tonicity of crystalloids is also an important factor in the selection of intravenous fluids. These solutions may be isotonic (same osmotic pressure as plasma), hypotonic (lower osmotic pressure than plasma), or hypertonic (greater osmotic pressure than plasma). The benefits of crystalloid solutions are that they are safe, effective, nontoxic, reaction-free, easy to store, free of religious disagreement concerning their use, and inexpensive. The major disadvantages of hypotonic and isotonic crystalloids are that they have limited ability to remain within the intravascular space. This predisposes patients to swelling and extravasation of fluids into the interstitial compartment. Therefore, edema formation is not uncommon when large volumes of crystalloid solutions are provided to maintain intravascular fluid and to increase blood pressure.

Infusions of isotonic fluids, such as saline, with a concentration of 0.9% wt/vol (0.9% normal saline or Lactated Ringer's) result in an even and equal distribution of this fluid throughout the extracellular compartment due to the very similar ionic composition to that of plasma (300 Osm/L). Furthermore, with the administration of hypotonic solutions (0.45% saline), cells have a tendency to swell. When hypotonic solutions are incorporated into the extracellular fluid, the osmolarity begins to decrease, driving water to enter the cells in an area of higher osmolarity. On the other hand, hypertonic solutions (3% saline) tend to increase osmolarity of the surrounding extracellular fluid and drive water out of the intracellular compartments into extracellular fluid, causing cellular dehydration and shrinkage.

Other solutions, such as glucose solutions, are also available as isotonic or hypertonic solutions. In isotonic solutions, there is only a small amount of glucose, which is rapidly metabolized, thus allowing the solvent water to be distributed freely throughout the total body water. This type of solution should be utilized to treat simple dehydration and for water replacement. In the case of the hypertonic glucose solutions, these are mostly given when patients require glucose administration as a metabolic substrate in hypoglycemia or as an adjuvant to insulin therapy. The composition of various crystalloid solutions is given in Table 5.11 [20,21].

Colloid solutions

Colloids are homogeneous noncrystalline substances consisting of large molecules dissolved in another substance. Colloid solutions increase the intravascular compartment and are therefore useful as volume expanders. Some disadvantages of colloids are that they are

Table 5.11. Comparison of the composition and osmolarity of crystalloid solutions for intravenous administration

Solution	Osmolarity (mOsm/L)	Na$^+$ (mmol/L)	Cl$^-$ (mmol/L)	K$^+$ (mmol/L)	Ca^{2+} (mmol/L)	Glucose (mg/L)	HCO$_3^-$ (mmol/L)	Lactate (mmol/L)	Energy (kCal/L)
Glucose 5%	252	—	—	—	—	50	—	—	400
Glucose 25%	1260	—	—	—	—	250	—	—	2000
Glucose 50%	2520	—	—	—	—	500	—	—	4000
Sodium chloride 0.9%	308	154.0	154.0	—	—	—	—	—	—
Sodium chloride and glucose	264	31.0	31.0	—	—	40	—	—	320
Ringer's solution	309	147.0	156.0	4.0	2.2	—	—	—	—
Compound sodium lactate^a	278	131.0	111.0	5.0	2.0	—	—	29.0	—
Plasmalyte B	298.5	140	95	5	—	—	50	—	—
Normasol^b	280	140	98	5	—	—	—	—	—

^{a} Hartmann's solution or Lactated Ringer's solution.
^{b} Normasol contains acetate 27 mmol/L and gluconate 23 mmol/L.
Reproduced with permission from Grocott et al. [21].

expensive, may result in a hypersensitivity reaction, and some have specific storage requirements and a short shelf-life.

There are several colloid solutions used in clinical practice for fluid therapy, such as albumin, fresh frozen plasma, hydroxyethyl starches, and dextran. These can be classified into semisynthetic and naturally occurring human plasma derivatives. Semisynthetic colloids differ in the magnitude and duration of their plasma volume expansion properties, their effect on blood flow properties and its elements, coagulation, inflammation, adverse reactions to drugs, and cost. Even though the human-derived colloids exhibit similar effectiveness in maintaining colloid oncotic pressure, differences in safety profiles are well-recognized disadvantages [21,23]. A comparison of the composition of different intravenous colloid solutions is shown in Table 5.12.

Intravenous therapy

The main objective of obtaining intravenous access is to allow for the safe, effective, direct, and immediate delivery of medications and supplemental fluids to patients. Intravenous access is the main route of administration of sedation medications and intravenous fluid management and therapy. This access not only allows for the adequate administration of proper sedative agents, but also provides access for the replacement of fluid and pharmacological management of patients who might decompensate or present with an acute complication.

Intravenous insertion technique

For the initiation of intravenous access, an appropriately-sized angiocatheter (16-22G) should be obtained. Gather the required equipment and supplies and have them near the patient's bedside, close enough to reach without having to change positions. Place the tourniquet on the selected limb (most frequently an upper extremity) and proceed with the selection of a vein.

Supplies and equipment required for the intravenous insertion are as follows:

(1) disposable gloves
(2) alcohol and povidone–iodine (PVPI) topical antiseptic (ie. Betadine)
(3) tourniquet
(4) intravenous catheter: over the needle catheter, through the needle catheter, and hollow needle/butterfly needle
(5) lidocaine
(6) local anesthetic cream for pediatric patients
(7) paper tape
(8) tuberculin syringe
(9) assortment of syringes
(10) infusion sets: 10 or 15 gtt/mL (large/macro drip), 60 gtt/mL (small/micro drip)
(11) intravenous solutions
(12) restricting band
(13) tape or transparent dressing (ie. Tegaderm)
(14) catheter-securing device (ie. Veni-Gard)
(15) armboard (optional)
(16) labels
(17) sterile dressings

Table 5.12. Comparison of the composition of colloid solutions for intravenous administration.

Solution	Colloid	MWw (Da)	MWn (Da)	Degree of substitution	Na⁺ (mmol/L)	Cl⁻ (mmol/L)	K⁺ (mmol/L)	Ca²⁺ (mmol/L)	Mg²⁺ (mmol/L)	Glucose (mg/L)
Gelofusine (4%)	Succinylated gelatin	30,000	22,600	—	154	125	—	—	—	—
Haemaccel (3.5%)	Polygeline	35,000	24,300	—	145	145	5.1	6.25	—	—
Voluven	Tetrastarch	130,000	60,000	0.4	154	154	—	—	—	—
Pentaspan	Pentastarch	264,000	63,000	0.45	154	154	—	—	—	—
HAES-steril 6% or 10%	Pentastarch	200,000	60,000	0.5	154	154	—	—	—	—
EloHase 6%	Hexastarch	200,000	60,000	0.6	154	154	—	—	—	—
Hespan 6%	Hetastarch	450,000	70,000	0.7	150	150	—	—	—	—
Hextend	Hetastarch	670,000	70,000	0.7	143	124	3	5	0.9	99
Gentran 40	Dextran 40	40,000	25,000	—	154	154	—	—	—	—
Gentran 70	Dextran 70	70,000	39,000	—	154	154	—	—	—	—
Rheomacrodex	Dextran 40	40,000	25,000	—	154	154	—	—	—	—
Macrodex	Dextran 70	70,000	39,000	—	154	154	—	—	—	—

MWw, weight averaged mean molecular weight; MWn, number averaged mean molecular weight.
Reproduced with permission from Grocott et al. [21].

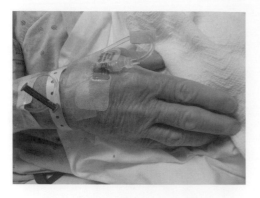

Figure 5.5. Example of an intravenous catheter.

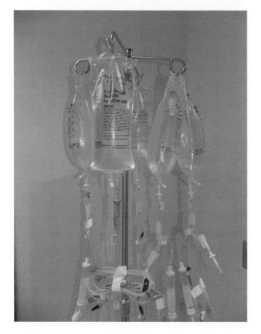

Figure 5.6. Examples of intravenous solutions in plastic containers.

Several factors may influence the selection of a vein for vascular access. The selection should be based on the surgical site, patient positioning, diagnostic procedure, post-procedure activity level, and anticipated length of time that intravenous access will be required [24] (Figure 5.5).

After placement of the intravenous catheter, the solution is adjusted to the catheter point of entry and then should easily flow from the container to the patient by means of an intravenous administration set.

Intravenous solutions have been available in plastic containers since 1971, and these offer many advantages over glass. Plastic containers do not require venting because the container will collapse as fluid flows out of it (Figure 5.6). Plastic containers are practical in the sense that they are lightweight, portable, and unbreakable. A variety of administration sets are currently available. Each facility will have its own guidelines on the proper placement of intravenous lines.

Complications of intravenous access

Complications related to intravenous peripheral access are uncommon, but problems do occur. That is why there are guidelines in each healthcare facility about how a peripheral IV line should be placed. Common complications of IV catheters and their treatments are listed below.

(1) **Phlebitis** is an acute inflammation of the blood vessel that commonly occurs after the insertion of an intravenous catheter. Multiple factors may contribute to the development of phlebitis, such as the insertion technique, the type of medication administered, or the catheter size and length. The incidence of phlebitis may vary from 2.5% to 45% or more. The inflammation causes redness, pain, and warmth at the IV insertion site. Treatment includes catheter removal and warm compresses. To prevent phlebitis, it is recommended that the catheter be removed and the IV access site changed every 48–72 hours. It is also recommended that when irritating solutions are administered, a large vein should be selected for access and strict aseptic methods followed during the insertion.

(2) **Local infection** is essentially a contamination at the IV insertion site secondary to a break in aseptic technique. Common signs include a large lump that is painful and hot to the touch, or the presence of purulent exudates at the insertion site. Treatment includes catheter removal, a culture of the catheter tip, and antibiotics, if indicated. For prevention of a local infection, infusion containers should be changed after 24 hours, accompanied by a venoset change every 48–72 hours and strict aseptic technique.

(3) **Infiltration** occurs when the catheter unintentionally enters the tissues surrounding the blood vessel. Common signs and symptoms include localized edema, decreased infusion rate, burning pain, tenderness at the IV site, and the area may be cool to the touch due to fluid accumulation. The IV infusion must be stopped, IV removed, and pressure dressing should be placed.

(4) **Hematoma** is a collection of blood caused by internal bleeding, which can occur with unsuccessful IV insertion, but can also happen when an IV is removed. Common signs and symptoms are bruising and pain at the site. Treatment consists of removal of the catheter, followed by pressure and warm soaks applied to the insertion site.

(5) **Extravasation** may occur when the vein itself ruptures, if the vein is damaged during insertion of IV access devices, or if the device is not sited correctly. Signs and symptoms include burning at the catheter insertion site, swelling, and localized tissue destruction [24].

Summary

Adequate patient monitoring is essential for successful and safe practice of sedation. Monitoring must be performed by a designated healthcare provider and should be performed during all phases of the procedure. Monitoring for sedation procedures primarily involves the observation of blood pressure, oxygenation, respiratory function, ECG and capnography tracings. Intravenous access is mandatory to allow for a safe, effective, and immediate delivery of medications and supplemental fluids to patients. Different crystalloid and colloid fluid solutions are available.

References

1. Merchant R, Bosenberg C, Brown K, *et al.* Guidelines to the practice of anesthesia revised edition 2010. *Can J Anaesth* 2010; 57: 58–87.

2. Association of Anaesthestists of Great Britain and Ireland. *Recommendations for Standards of Monitoring During Anaesthesia and Recovery*, 4th edn. London: AAGBI, 2007. www.aagbi.org/sites/default/

files/standardsofmonitoring07.pdf (accessed June 2011).

3. Kost M. Monitoring modalities. In *Manual of Conscious Sedation*. Philadelphia, PA: Saunders, 1998; 115–48.

4. De Silva A. Anesthetic monitoring. In Stoelting RK, Miller RD, eds., *Basics of Anesthesia*, 5th edn. Philadelphia, PA: Churchill Livingstone, 2007; 305–16.

5. Blitt CD. History and philosophy of monitoring. In Lake CL, Hines RL, Blitt CD, eds., *Clinical Monitoring: Practical Applications for Anesthesia and Critical Care*. Philadelphia, PA: Saunders, 2001; 3–6.

6. Bogetz MS. Outpatient surgery. In Stoelting RK, Miller RD, eds., *Basics of Anesthesia*, 5th edn. Philadelphia, PA: Churchill Livingstone, 2007; 538–49.

7. Chobanian AV, Bakris GL, Black HR, *et al*. Seventh report of the Joint National Committee on Prevention, Detection, Evaluation, and Treatment of High Blood Pressure. *Hypertension* 2003; **42**: 1206–52.

8. Bergese SD, Puente EG. Clevidipine butyrate: a promising new drug for the management of acute hypertension. *Expert Opin Pharmacother* 2010; **11**: 281–95.

9. Bryant H, Bromhead H. Intraoperative hypotension anaesthesia tutorial of the week 148 August 2009. totw. anaesthesiologists.org/wp-content/uploads/2009/08/148-Intraoperative-hypotension.pdf (accessed March 2011).

10. Williams B, Poulter NR, Brown MJ, *et al*. Guidelines for management of hypertension: report of the fourth working party of the British Hypertension Society, 2004-BHS IV. *J Hum Hypertens* 2004; **18**: 139–85.

11. Walsh JL, Small SD. Monitoring. In Hurford WE, Bailin MT, Davison KJ, Haspel KL, Rosow C, eds., *Clinical Anesthesia Procedures of the Massachusetts General Hospital*, 5th edn. Philadelphia, PA: Lippincott Williams & Wilkins, 1998.

12. Pickering TG. Principles and techniques of blood pressure measurement. *Cardiol Clin* 2002; **20**: 207–23.

13. Canzanello VJ, Jensen PL, Schwartz GL. Are aneroid sphygmomanometers accurate in hospital and clinic settings? *Arch Intern Med* 2001; **161**: 729–31.

14. American Society of Anesthesiologists Task Force on Sedation and Analgesia by Non-Anesthesiologists. Practice guidelines for sedation and analgesia by non-anesthesiologists. *Anesthesiology* 2002; **96**: 1004–17.

15. Webster A, Brady W, Morris F. Recognising signs of danger: ECG changes resulting from an abnormal serum potassium concentration. *Emerg Med J* 2002; **19**: 74–7.

16. St John RE. End-tidal carbon dioxide monitoring. *Crit Care Nurse* 2003; **23**: 83–8.

17. Galvagno SM, Kodali B. Patient monitoring. In Urman R, Gross W, Philip BK, eds., *Anesthesia Outside of the Operating Room*. Oxford: Oxford University Press, 2011; 20–7.

18. Bower AL, Ripepi A, Dilger J, *et al*. Bispectral index monitoring of sedation during endoscopy. *Gastrointest Endosc* 2000; **52**: 192–6.

19. Hrelec C, Puente E, Bergese S, Dzwonczyk R. SNAP II versus BIS VISTA monitor comparison during general anesthesia. *J Clin Monit Comput* 2010; **24**: 283–8.

20. Rosenthal MH. Intraoperative fluid management: what and how much? *Chest* 1999; **115**: 106S–112S.

21. Grocott MP, Mythe, MG, Gan TJ. Perioperative fluid management and clinical outcomes in adults. *Anesth Analg* 2005; **100**: 1093–106.

22. Kleespies A, Thiel M, Jauch KW, Hartl WH. Perioperative fluid retention and clinical outcome in elective, high-risk colorectal surgery. *Int J Colorectal Dis* 2009; **24**: 699–709.

23. Barron ME, Wilkes MM, Navickis RJ. A systematic review of the comparative safety of colloids. *Arch Surg* 2004; **139**: 552–63.

24. Kost M. Intravenous insertion techniques. In *Manual of Conscious Sedation*. Philadelphia, PA: Saunders, 1998; 162–75.

Chapter 6

Credentialing, competency, and education

Ellen K. Bergeron

Introduction

The safe transition of patients through procedures performed under moderate or deep sedation is a complex and challenging clinical situation. In recognition of the safety risks involved in caring for patients requiring any level of sedation, in the USA the Joint Commission has set specific standards around credentialing, competency assessment, and education [1].

Credentialing

The Joint Commission standard MS.06.01.01 requires US organizations to collect, verify, and evaluate a provider's valid state license, current federal Drug Enforcement Administration (DEA) number, and appropriate education and training prior to granting privileges [1]. When privileges involving procedural sedation are requested, the Joint Commission standard PC.03.01 further requires that individuals "permitted" to administer sedation are able to rescue patients at whatever level of sedation or anesthesia is achieved [1]. Specific education and certification around the administration of procedural sedation and management of possible complications may be added as a requirement for credentialing. There is no consensus among professional organizations and regulatory agencies around education and training requirements for those caring for patients undergoing procedural sedation. Defining specific elements for credentialing is left to the institution's credentialing body, based on their assessment of what is required for safe practice at the local level.

Minimally, most organizations require successful completion of institutionally developed programs specific to the management of moderate procedural sedation. Certification by an established educational provider such as the American Heart

Moderate and Deep Sedation in Clinical Practice, ed. Richard D. Urman and Alan D. Kaye.
Published by Cambridge University Press. © Cambridge University Press 2012.

Table 6.1. ACGME Outcome Project (1999): six general competencies for medical practice [3]

Patient care
Medical/clinical knowledge
Practice-based learning and improvement
Interpersonal and communication skills
Professionalism
Systems-based practice

Association or the American College of Surgeons Committee on Trauma is standard for providers of deep sedation. Board certification in anesthesiology, critical care, or emergency medicine may be the minimum requirement for providers of deep sedation in some organizations.

Credentials must be renewed every 2 years, a practice which often coincides with license and certification expiration and renewal. The organization is responsible for determining and reviewing required elements for credentialing. Individuals are responsible for maintaining professional, legal, and organizational credentials on a current basis.

General competencies

Competence to perform is assessed as an element of the initial credentialing process. Epstein and Hundert, while emphasizing the multidimensional aspects of competency, highlight the importance of basic clinical skills, scientific knowledge, and moral development as the foundations of competency in practice [2]. The six general competencies identified by the Accreditation Council for Graduate Medical Education and the American Board of Medical Specialties [3] are cited by the Joint Commission [1] as a framework for credentialing and ongoing competency assessment (Table 6.1).

Developing programs that identify and assess knowledge, skill, behavior, and commitment in the context of complex medical treatments and unpredictable patient response is challenging. An initial review of institutional procedures and practice settings should be conducted to define both general and specific competencies. Orientation programs address the minimal requirements and standards for safe practice. Subsequently, the organization must be vigilant and responsive to the need for ongoing competency development as new procedures, medications, and equipment are introduced into practice settings. Annual or biannual competency programs provide an opportunity not only for practitioner competency validation but also for program evaluation. Current quality reports and safety data provide evidence that existing programs incorporate competencies relevant to practice within the organization.

Sedation-specific competencies

The primary goal of procedural sedation is to manage the pain and anxiety of patients undergoing invasive or unpleasant procedures [4]. Pharmacologic agents induce a depressed level of consciousness while allowing the patient to maintain stable cardiorespiratory function and the ability to respond to verbal and/or tactile stimulation [5].

Patient response to pharmaceutical agents is unpredictable and requires that providers "be qualified to manage the patient at whatever level of sedation is achieved either intentionally or unintentionally" [1]. The opinion of the American Society of Anesthesiologists (ASA) Task Force is that the primary causes of morbidity associated with sedation/analgesia are drug-induced respiratory depression and airway obstruction [5]. Therefore, competency programs for providers of moderate and deep sedation must focus on specific knowledge, skills, and behaviors that prevent these complications.

Managing levels of sedation

The ability to identify varying levels along the sedation continuum enables providers to successfully intervene when intended levels of sedation are not successfully achieved or inadvertently exceeded. Skillful application of a validated and reliable sedation assessment tool provides an objective measure of when providers should intervene [6].

Medication management competencies

Comprehensive knowledge of the pharmacologic agents of procedural sedation, and accuracy in the choice of the right combination of agents for specific patient populations, is an essential competency. The ability to safely administer the medication, monitor for intended and unintended effects, and appropriately use reversal agents provides behavioral evidence of competence in the management of procedural sedation medications.

Hemodynamic and cardiac monitoring

An understanding of the effects of pharmacologic agents on hemodynamic and cardiac function is required to safely manage procedural sedation. Skillful initiation and management of hemodynamic and cardiac monitoring equipment and interpretation of the changes in the patient's baseline status are required to anticipate and prevent complications. Knowledge of normal cardiac rhythm, skill in ECG interpretation, identification of and response to potentially serious dysrhythmias are minimal requirements of providers and monitors of procedural sedation.

Airway management

Basic and advanced competence in the assessment and management of the patient's airway is required before, during, and following the procedure. Knowledge of normal anatomy and physiology, and skilled assessment of the oral cavity to evaluate need for anesthesia consultation, should be part of the pre-procedure evaluation.

Skills required to maintain a patent airway can range from basic repositioning and manipulation of the airway with chin-lift and jaw-thrust maneuvers to the more sophisticated implementation of respiratory adjuncts such as oropharyngeal airways and bag-valve mask devices.

Oxygenation and ventilation

An understanding of the mechanics of breathing and the physiology of oxygenation and ventilation is required to anticipate, intervene in, and prevent the more serious respiratory and cardiac complications associated with procedural sedation. The use of continuous oxygen saturation monitoring as a reliable tool to supplement the clinical observation and auscultation of breathing and to detect changes in oxygenation has long been supported in clinical practice and strongly recommended by the consultants to the ASA [5].

More recently, the standards for basic anesthetic monitoring approved by the ASA House of Delegates in October 2010 state that "during moderate or deep sedation the adequacy of ventilation shall be evaluated by continual observation of qualitative clinical signs and monitoring for the presence of exhaled carbon dioxide unless precluded or invalidated by the nature of the patient, procedure or equipment" [7].

A recent clinical study demonstrating that the addition of capnography to standard monitoring assisted in early identification of hypoxic events supports this recommendation. [8].

Therefore, providers must demonstrate skill in the application and management of both the oximetry and capnography devices to assure the adequacy of the pleth or waveform. The provider must also be competent in the interpretation of the various waveforms and digital readouts and correlate this data to clinical changes in the patient's condition.

Education

The intended audience of educational programs around procedural sedation is the professional healthcare provider. As adult learners, these individuals must be recognized as highly motivated learners who accept responsibility for learning and approach new knowledge and skill acquisition as an extension of previous knowledge and practice experience [9].

The intent of procedural sedation education is to develop and validate knowledge, skills, and behavioral competency in the management of patients requiring pharmacologic intervention during procedures. Traditional classroom instruction and testing is limited to addressing only the cognitive aspects of learning and does not validate competency. The addition of flexible and experiential learning strategies should be considered to address other modalities of learning and skill acquisition.

Significant advances in technology over the past few decades have created opportunity for organizations to meet the challenges of competency development and validation for healthcare practitioners. Through computer-based tutorials and web-based learning environments healthcare practitioners can acquire the core cognitive knowledge required for certification in basic and advanced cardiac life support, basic ECG analysis, and airway management. Knowledge acquisition occurs at the individual learner's own pace, at times and in places convenient for the learner.

Knowles et al. emphasize the importance of experiential learning for adult learners [9]. Teaching the skills required to translate knowledge into clinical practice is best accomplished in environments that recreate real-life clinical situations. The high-risk, high-stakes practice environment of modern healthcare organizations has forced a shift from knowledge-based to outcomes-based education [10]. The competent application of knowledge and skills in the context of unpredictable patient response must be accomplished using sound clinical reasoning and expert communication skills.

Management of procedural sedation is a complex clinical situation. More than merely knowing (cognitive) or knowing how (psychomotor), the clinician must demonstrate high-level clinical reasoning and decision-making behaviors (affective) around knowing why and when certain actions must be initiated in response to specific patient needs. Such decision making is accomplished within the context of the integrated team. All team members must have the interpersonal and communication skills to clearly articulate the goals of sedation and analgesia, and the confidence and ability to clearly communicate their clinical concerns.

Simulation-based education is an emerging learning and assessment modality that educates, provides practice experience, and validates the competencies required to manage procedural sedation (see Chapter 13). In simulated clinical environments all learning domains (cognitive, psychomotor, and behavioral) can be assessed in controlled settings where immediate feedback is provided to change or reinforce behaviors. Table 6.2 lists common educational strategies and outcomes that address domains of learning.

The Association of periOperative Registered Nurses (AORN) has published *Recommended practices for managing the patient receiving moderate sedation/analgesia* [11]. These practice guidelines were developed by the AORN Recommended Practices Committee and have been approved by the AORN Board of Directors, effective January 1, 2002. As the practice guidelines state, "these recommended practices are intended as achievable recommendations representing what is believed to be an optimal level of practice. Policies and procedures will reflect variations in practice settings and/or clinical situations that determine the degree to which the recommended practices can be implemented."

In 2009 the ASA released an updated *Statement on safe use of propofol* [12]. The statement emphasizes that sedation is a continuum and that moderate sedation can inadvertently evolve into deep sedation or general anesthesia. When propofol is used, the patient should "receive care consistent with that required for deep sedation."

In 2010, the American Association of Nurse Anesthetists (AANA) published *Considerations for policy development number 4.2: registered nurses engaged in the administration of sedation and analgesia* [13]. These considerations are intended to provide registered nurses (RNs) with the definitions of sedation and analgesia, to establish suggested qualifications, and to provide suggestions for patient management and monitoring practices.

The ASA recently published two guideline statements, one addressing educational and competency standards for the practitioner (an MD or DO physician, dentist, or podiatrist) supervising or directly administering moderate sedation, and the other for practitioners participating in deep sedation [14,15]. Each healthcare facility should establish its own educational standards and guidelines, but may choose to incorporate some or all of the elements of moderate and/or deep sedation privileging process as outlined by the ASA, and use the guideline information as the basis for the healthcare facility's sedation policy.

The first statement, originally introduced in 2005, is the *Statement on granting privileges for administration of **moderate sedation** to practitioners who are not anesthesia professionals* [14]. This statement is intended to offer "a framework for granting privileges that will help ensure competence of individuals who administer or supervise the administration of moderate sedation." This statement is intended as a guide for any type of facility "in which an internal or external credentialing process is required for administration of sedative and analgesic drugs to establish a level of moderate sedation."

The second guideline statement, introduced in 2010, is the *Statement on granting privileges for **deep sedation** to non-anesthesiologist sedation practitioners* [15]. It helps provide a "framework to identify those physicians, dentists, oral surgeons, or podiatrists who may potentially qualify to administer or supervise the administration of deep sedation." The entire guideline statement addresses education, training, licensure, performance evaluation, and improvement.

Table 6.2. Procedural sedation competencies: learning and assessment modalities

Learning domain	Educational strategies	Outcome and measurement
Cognitive (knowledge)		

1. Levels of sedation
2. Pharmacology of sedation/analgesia
3. Airway assessment
4. Basic hemodynamics and ECG analysis
5. Oxygenation/ ventilation
	Traditional classroom
	Computer-based tutorial
	Interactive web-based module
	Case study
	Standardized patient
		1. (a) Accurately identifies levels of sedation
		  (b) Applies valid sedation assessment tool
		2. (a) Identifies intended/unintended medication effects
		  (b) Initiates use of reversal agents
		3. (a) Pre-procedure assessment using Mallampati
		  (b) Appropriate request for anesthesia consult
		4. (a) Appropriately identifies changes in patient status
		  (b) Intervenes in response to changes
		5. (a) Identifies changes from patient baseline
		  (b) Initiates airway management techniques

Psychomotor (skills)		

1. Levels of sedation
2. IV and medication skills
3. ECG/hemodynamic skills
4. Airway management
5. Oxygenation management
6. Ventilation management
	Traditional classroom
	Computer-based tutorial
	Simulation training
	• low-fidelity simulation
	• task trainer
	• virtual reality trainers
	• high-fidelity simulation
		1. Responds therapeutically to intended/ unintended levels of sedation
		2. (a) Establishes and maintains IV access
		  (b) Responds to intended/unintended side effects
		  (c) Appropriately administers reversal agents
		3. (a) Effectively troubleshoots monitoring equipment
		  (b) Initiates appropriate intervention in response to changes in patient status
		4. (a) Stimulates/repositions patient to maintain airway
		  (b) Effectively uses respiratory adjuncts as needed
		5. (a) Identifies normal O_2 sat pleth
		  (b) Troubleshoots oximetry device
		  (c) Applies supplemental oxygen as needed
		6. (a) Identifies normal/abnormal CO_2 wave form
		  (b) Troubleshoots capnography device
		  (c) Initiates use of bag-valve mask device to support ventilation when indicated

Affective (behavioral)		
1. Clinical decision making 2. Interpersonal relationships	Case study/role play Group discussion Standardized patient Human patient simulation	1. Appropriate response to variations in patient response 2. (a) Identifies role/responsibilities of team members (b) Understands and functions within scope of practice

Table 6.2. (cont.)

Learning domain	Educational strategies	Outcome and measurement
3. Communication skills	Simulation technology • moderate-fidelity • high-fidelity	3. (a) Effectively communicates as member of the team (b) Timely/clearly articulates changes in patient status (c) Uses closed-loop communication within team

Summary

Care of patients undergoing procedural sedation is predicated on compliance with state and federal laws governing practice and educational programs that ensure positive outcomes for patients undergoing procedural sedation. It is an organizational and individual commitment to ensure that credentialing, competency, and education requirements are consistently met.

References

1. Joint Commission (2010) *Joint Commission E-dition*: Standards: HR 01.06.01, PC 03.01.01–07 and MS 06.01.01. e-dition. jcrinc.com (accessed June 2011).

2. Epstein RM, Hundert EM. Defining and assessing professional competence. *JAMA* 2002; **287**: 226–35.

3. Accreditation Council for Graduate Medical Education. Outcome Project. www.acgme.org/outcome (accessed June 2011).

4. American Association of Nurse Anesthetists (AANA). Position statement: qualified providers of sedation and analgesia; considerations for policy guidelines for registered nurses engaged in the administration of sedation and analgesia. Park Ridge, IL: AANA, 2003.

5. American Society of Anesthesiologists Task Force on Sedation and Analgesia by Non-Anesthesiologists. Practice guidelines for sedation and analgesia by non-anesthesiologists. *Anesthesiology* 2002; **96**: 1004–17.

6. Rassin M, Sruyah R, Kahakon A, *et al.* "Between the fixed and the changing": examining and comparing reliability and validity of 3 sedation–agitation measuring scales. *Dimens Crit Care Nurs* 2007; **26**(2): 76–82.

7. American Society of Anesthesiologists (ASA). Standards for basic anesthetic monitoring (effective July 1, 2011). Park Ridge, IL: ASA, 2010. www.asahq.org/For-Healthcare-Professionals/Standards-Guidelines-and-Statements (accessed August 2011).

8. Deitch K, Miner J, Chudnosfsky C, Dominici P, Latta D. Does end tidal CO_2 monitoring during emergency department procedural sedation and analgesia with proprofol decrease the incidence of hypoxic events? A randomized controlled trial. *Ann Emerg Med* 2010; **55**: 258–64.

9. Knowles M, Holton E, Swanson R. *The Adult Learner*, 5th edn. Woburn: Butterworth-Heinemann, 1998.

10. Michelson J, Manning L. Competency assessment in simulation-based procedural education. *Am J Surg* 2008; **196**: 609–15.

11. Association of periOperative Registered Nurses (AORN). Recommended practices for managing the patient receiving moderate sedation/analgesia. *AORN J* 2002; **75**: 642–6, 649–52.

12. American Society of Anesthesiologists (ASA). Statement on safe use of propofol. Park Ridge, IL: ASA, 2009. www.asahq.org/For-Healthcare-Professionals/Standards-Guidelines-and-Statements.aspx (accessed June 2011).

13. American Association of Nurse Anesthetists (AANA). Considerations for policy development number 4.2: registered nurses engaged in the administration of sedation and analgesia. Park Ridge, IL: AANA, 2010.

14. American Society of Anesthesiologists (ASA). Statement on granting privileges for administration of moderate sedation to practitioners who are not anesthesia professionals. Park Ridge, IL: ASA, 2006. www.asahq.org/For-Healthcare-Professionals/Standards-Guidelines-and-Statements.aspx (accessed June 2011).

15. American Society of Anesthesiologists (ASA). Statement on granting privileges for deep sedation to non-anesthesiologist sedation practitioners. Park Ridge, IL: ASA, 2010.

Further reading

American Association of Critical-Care Nurses. Position statement on the role of the RN in the management of patients receiving IV moderate sedation for short-term therapeutic, diagnostic, or surgical procedures. www.aacn.org/WD/ Practice/Docs/Sedation.doc (accessed June 2011).

American Society of Anesthesiologists (ASA). Statement on granting privileges to nonanesthesiologist practitioners for personally administering deep sedation or supervising deep sedation by individuals who are not anesthesia professionals. Park Ridge, IL: ASA, 2006. www.asahq.org/For-Healthcare-Professionals/Standards-Guidelines-and-Statements.aspx (accessed June 2011).

Eichorn V, Henzler D, Murphy M. Standardizing care and monitoring for anesthesia or procedural sedation delivered outside the operating room. *Curr Opin Anaesthesiol* 2010; **23**: 494–9.

Godwin SA, Caro DA, Wolf SJ, *et al.* American College of Emergency Physicians. Clinical policy: procedural sedation and analgesia in the emergency department. *Ann Emerg Med* 2005; **45**: 177–96.

Levine A, Swartz M. Standardized patients: the "other" simulation. *J Crit Care* 2008; **23**: 179–84.

Tetzlaff J. Assessment of competence in anesthesiology. *Curr Opin Anaesthesiol* 2009; **22**: 809–13.

Quality, legal, and risk management considerations: ensuring program excellence

Mary T. Antonelli and David E. Seaver

The policy

The overall goal of a procedural sedation program is to provide the best standard of care, yielding the best outcome for the patient. This ambition starts with the development of a comprehensive, practical policy that provides an institutional philosophy as a basis for sedation care standards, followed by the clinical and technical requirements that provide the infrastructure to successfully meet the institutional goal. It is the policy that establishes the foundation for the program and for excellence in practice (Figure 7.1).

Though the clinical and technical requirements may have similarities between organizations, it is unwise to adapt a policy directly from one organization to another. Policies are generally organizationally specific since the document is expressing a care approach which addresses specific patient populations, scope of services offered, professional mix, and educational requirements needed. Since all of these may vary from institution to institution, practice may vary. Since policy sets the framework for practice, each hospital needs to develop its own policy.

Policy development

Policy development begins with the establishment of a multidisciplinary team encompassing all professions and expertise which have a role in the underlying processes of procedural sedation (Figure 7.1). This team should include, but not be limited to, anesthesia, nursing, surgery, physician assistants, emergency department, quality, risk management, pharmacy, and other representatives from areas performing moderate or deep sedation by non-anesthesiologists. Chair selection for the team should be based on the demonstration of strong leadership skills and the ability to move a team towards successful outcomes. It is also essential that the chair holds a position within the organization that is recognized as expert within the field of sedation practice, as he/she will need to provide feedback to practitioners to reinforce the standard set by the policy. One suggestion is to

Moderate and Deep Sedation in Clinical Practice, ed. Richard D. Urman and Alan D. Kaye.
Published by Cambridge University Press. © Cambridge University Press 2012.

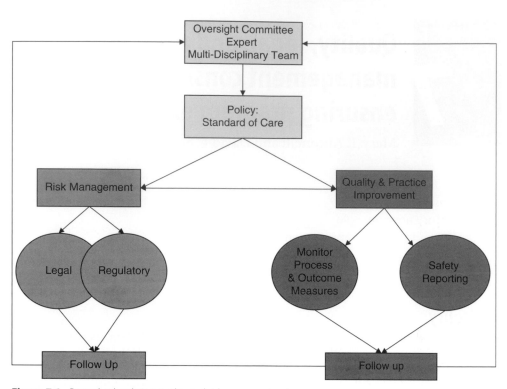

Figure 7.1. Procedural sedation quality and risk program structure.

have members from the departments of anesthesia and nursing co-chair, since regulatory bodies hold anesthesia accountable over this domain, and nursing is usually involved in most sedation procedures.

Once the team is established, a review and evaluation of current nationally endorsed position statements, practice guidelines, research, and regulatory requirements, and an analysis of "community" standards, should be conducted to establish the evidence-based foundation of the care practices within the policy (Table 7.1). An analysis of all the information should be completed to determine the mandatory elements required to establish best practice. The mandatory elements and mission concepts are then built into the body of the policy.

The format of the policies varies and is determined by the specific institution. The following, however, is an example of such a format:

- **Purpose** – intent of the policy and scope of practice.
- **Philosophy/mission statement** – a framework for the development of practice processes.
- **Definitions** – a list of key definitions that provides a basis for interpretation and application of the policy. Examples: procedural sedation, levels of sedation, what is meant by a rescue. It is suggested to use the American Society of Anesthesiologists (ASA) definitions, since the definitions are endorsed by most regulatory agencies.
- **Governance** – structure for overall accountability.
- **Personnel/education/competency** – expectations for education and competency for the healthcare professionals involved in the moderate/deep sedation procedure and recovery.

Table 7.1. Professional and regulatory organizations and their representative practice guidelines and standards for the administration of sedation

American Society of Anesthesiology	Practice guidelines for sedation and analgesia by non-anesthesiologists
American Association of Nurse Anesthetists	Position statements
American Nurses Association	Position statement on the role of the registered nurse in the management of patients receiving conscious sedation
American Academy of Pediatrics Committee on Drugs	Guidelines for monitoring and management of pediatric patients during and after sedation for diagnostic and therapeutic procedures
American College of Emergency Physicians	Clinical policy: procedural sedation and analgesia in the emergency department
Centers for Medicare and Medicaid	Condition of Participation 482.52
The Joint Commission	Sedation and anesthesia care standards Review of glossary for definitions of key words
State Boards of Medicine	Sedation policy/position statements
State Nursing Practice Acts	Scope of practice
University HealthSystem Consortium	Moderate and deep sedation best practice recommendations

- **Care elements** – required supplies and equipment, medication guidelines, assessment and monitoring requirements from pre-procedure through recovery, discharge criteria, and documentation expectations.
- **Quality assessment** – outlines the required process of monitoring and response to care practices at the point of care, based on identified criteria measures for practice or care processes.
- **References** – a list of all resources and materials that were used to support the development of the policy.
- **Addendums** – additional information which supports the application of the policy. Examples: sedation scale used; requirements for pre-procedure assessment; list of approved medications for moderate/deep sedation with dosing, clearance, and contraindications; education/competency curriculum; list of areas where moderate/deep sedation can occur; process for new site approval for procedural sedation.

When a draft of the policy is completed, the document should be reviewed by key stakeholders for feedback and input. This step will assist the flow through the administrative approval process. To assist the movement of the policy through this phase, an approval plan and an itemized timeline are helpful, to ensure all key stakeholders and committees are captured. Concurrently, the oversight committee should develop a communication and education plan regarding the policy and practice expectations. This can be accomplished in a number of ways. However, the methods should be diverse and robust, with the information easily accessible and concise. In-service training may be required, along with ongoing informational reinforcements to make sure all appropriate professionals are made aware of the policy and care standards to establish continuity of practice and to ensure patient safety.

Quality and risk-management considerations

As stated, the policy sets the framework for the practice. However, it is the presence of a strong quality and risk management structure that ensures the practices outlined in the policy are appropriately and consistently applied at the point of care (Figure 7.1). This structure has risk management focusing on the minimization of risk for adverse patient outcomes, and quality acts as a mechanism to improve practice. The work is collaborative. Therefore, every procedural sedation program must have both components in place, and they must be valued by the multidisciplinary team, to guarantee that the program structure is functional and effective.

Though most procedures with sedation occur without an adverse event or breach in care standards, there are occasions when these events do happen. It is at these times when these structures help to identify the cause and strengthen the care processes, and ensure safety.

Professional liability: malpractice/negligence

Risk management mitigates the potential legal risks associated with procedural sedation to promote safety and minimize risk of injury. A malpractice case is a type of tort, which is a civil wrong committed by one person against another that can be adjudicated in a court of law. There are four required elements to substantiate malpractice. The first is that a duty must be owed to the injured person. That duty then must be breached, and that breach must be the cause of an injury. Lastly, there must be damages from the injury [1].

Negligence is "conduct which falls below the standard established by law for the protection of others against unreasonable risk of harm" [1]. Medical negligence, in a legal sense, is the failure to act in accordance with the accepted standards of the healthcare practice.

Duty

A duty is established when the healthcare provider develops a relationship with the patient. The duty the healthcare provider owes the patient is to treat the patient within accepted healthcare standards. The provider is then held to the standard of those clinicians with similar education and training in a similar clinical situation.

Breach of duty

A duty is breached when the provider does not act according to the accepted healthcare standards. This may be a specific act that is below accepted standard of care, or a failure to act when a particular action is appropriate.

Causation

The action(s) that did not meet the standard(s) must be shown to have caused an injury. This is the most difficult element to prove. Often, it is difficult to separate a known complication from an action that would constitute a breach of duty. Expert testimony is required to establish causation.

Damages

The patient must suffer a form of damage from the injury to establish a case. Damage may take the form of economic damages (financial losses such as medical expenses, lost wages, or other economic harm) and/or noneconomic damages (physical suffering, emotional distress, and loss of enjoyment of relationship with significant other and/or family). Some states may permit punitive damages on top of economic and noneconomic damages when it can be shown the clinician acted with willful recklessness, gross negligence, malice, or deceit.

Each element needs to be proved by a preponderance of the evidence. A preponderance of the evidence is a reasonable medical probability (typically, a 51% chance) that the element has been proved. Therefore, as an example of a successful case, the plaintiff is required to establish that the patient was under the care of the provider (*duty*), the provider responsible for the administration of procedural sedation did not act according to the standard of care (*breach*), the failure to act according to the standard of care was directly responsible for the patient's injury (*cause*), and the patient's injury was the cause of some sort of economic or noneconomic harm (*damage*).

In addition, the courts may look to state statutes and regulations when evaluating the breach element. Should it be shown that the clinician defendant was in violation of an applicable statute or regulation, the court may find either that the plaintiff automatically proved this element, or that the violation of the statute or regulation is strong evidence of proof of a breach of the standard of care. As state boards promulgate regulation in the area of procedural sedation, it is wise to review your state regulations to assure all regulatory compliance requirements are met when administering procedural sedation. The courts will also give great weight to the adopted policies on procedural sedation of state boards.

As noted above, the most difficult element to prove in a medical malpractice case is causation. In almost all medical malpractice cases, expert opinion is needed to prove causation. Expert opinion is required because the subject matter is not within the common knowledge of the average juror. The expert should be "expert" in the particular subspecialty at issue in the lawsuit. The expert does not need to practice in that arena, but must be familiar with that arena. As applicable to procedural sedation, the clinician expert would not necessarily have to be an anesthesiologist, but would typically have to be familiar with procedural sedation practices, policies, and procedures. The expert would have to show that the clinician's failure to meet the standard of care directly harmed the patient.

Mitigating the risk of malpractice lawsuit: documentation

Since it is often difficult to distinguish a complication of care from a tortuous act, the best defense to a claim of malpractice is good documentation that maps the decision making. It has often been said, "If it was not documented, it did not occur." Even absence of relevant findings should be documented. Failure to document the absent findings may indicate that the clinician failed to elucidate the findings.

A key documentation requirement is the informed consent prior to the procedure. Since the patient must consent to the administration of procedural sedation, the clinician must have a conversation with the patient noting the risks and benefits of procedural sedation (or with the patient's representative, for patients who cannot make their own decisions). The patient or representative must sign an informed consent form documenting the conversation. A note in the medical record detailing the conversation and the patient's or representative's understanding of the conversation is equally important. The consent process permits the clinician to understand and manage the patient's expectations, and to individualize the plan of care. A patient who has unreasonable expectations about the success of a procedure may be more likely to initiate a lawsuit should a complication of care occur. Having an open and frank conversation with the patient, addressing all material complications and their likelihood, may dissuade the patient from litigation. Documenting that conversation protects the clinician from allegations that the patient did not understand the nature of the procedure and the likelihood of complications.

Other key documentation requirements include a history and physical (H&P) documented prior to the procedure. During the procedure, the patient's response to the sedation must be documented, and post-procedure the patient's status must be documented, including that all discharge criteria are met before the patient leaves or is transferred.

Regulatory agencies

In the USA, several regulatory bodies have promulgated regulations or developed guidelines regarding the administration of procedural sedation, both at state and federal levels. The major regulatory bodies include the State Boards of Medicine and Nursing, the Centers for Medicare and Medicaid (federal government agencies), and The Joint Commission (a healthcare facility accreditation organization).

State boards

State professional boards are charged with licensing and regulating healthcare professionals including physicians, nurses, pharmacists, and in some states anesthesia assistants practicing within hospitals and at other standalone locations such as clinics and professional offices. State legislatures pass statutes that authorize the state boards to promulgate regulation enforceable upon professionals licensed by that board. The boards also adopt policies that, while lacking the authority of a regulation or statute, are evidence of appropriate practice. For example, the Massachusetts Board of Medicine has a policy entitled *Patient Care Assessment Guidelines for Intravenous Conscious Sedation* [2]. These guidelines are applicable to both anesthesia and non-anesthesia providers, and note that physicians practicing in compliance with the guidelines do not need to provide any further justification of their practice regarding the administration of procedural sedation. Boards of medicine may provide guidance for developing a policy, in collaboration with the anesthesia department; citing the evidence used to develop the sedation policy; identifying clinicians administering procedural sedation and the necessary credentialing requirements, medications, patient selection, and equipment; and establishing appropriate patient assessment and monitoring frequency [3]. Boards also may establish appropriate resource allocation for sedation procedures, ongoing education requirements for competence, and requirements for anesthetic care performed in the office setting.

Boards of medicine may also be more prescriptive and require specific compliance measures. One example is dentistry, where procedural sedation is administered in an office setting, which may be considered high risk, if rescue is required.

The Centers for Medicare and Medicaid Services

The Centers for Medicare and Medicaid Services (CMS) promulgates regulations that are enforceable upon hospitals. The CMS also mandates hospital compliance with all applicable state laws [4]. The Condition of Participation 482.52 states, "If the hospital furnishes anesthesia services, they must be provided in a well-organized manner under the direction of a qualified doctor of medicine or osteopathy. The service is responsible for all anesthesia administered in the hospital." Within a facility, the anesthesia service is responsible for all anesthesia administered, including procedural sedation administered by both anesthesia and non-anesthesia providers, including physicians, dentists, certified registered nurse anesthetists, and anesthesiologist assistants (if permissible by state law).

The CMS also requires appropriate anesthesia care throughout the process [4]. The preanesthesia process requires a patient assessment within 48 hours before the administration of anesthesia. Intraoperatively, the responsible clinician is required to monitor the patient and document the key elements that are outlined. Postoperatively, the CMS does not require an evaluation. However, it is stated that appropriate postoperative anesthesia evaluation is required. Therefore, current practice dictates that the patient receiving procedural sedation be monitored and evaluated before, during, and after the procedure by trained practitioners.

The CMS only allows anesthesia professionals (anesthesiologist, nurse anesthetist, and anesthesiologist assistant) or other qualified non-anesthesiologist physicians (as well as dentist, oral surgeon, or podiatrist who is qualified to administer anesthesia under state law) are permitted to administer deep sedation [3]. Registered nurses, advanced practice registered nurses, or physician assistants may not administer deep sedation per CMS. The 2010 ASA *Statement on granting privileges for deep sedation to non-anesthesiologist sedation practitioners* was created to "assist healthcare facilities in developing a program" for the delineation of procedure-specific clinical privileges for non-anesthesiologist physicians to administer or supervise the administration of sedative and analgesic drugs to establish a level of deep sedation [5]. The statement outlines recommendations for education, training, licensure, performance evaluation, and performance improvement.

In contrast, mild to moderate sedation usually can be administered safely by non-anesthesia practitioners who have had specialized training, as outlined in the ASA *Statement on granting privileges for administration of moderate sedation to practitioners who are not anesthesia professionals* [6]. Knowledge of the pharmacologic profiles of sedation agents is necessary to maximize the likelihood that the intended level of sedation is targeted accurately [7]. If cardiorespiratory compromise occurs, the non-anesthesia practitioners should possess the skills necessary to "rescue" a patient whose level of sedation is deeper than planned, and return the patient to the intended level. Therefore, one person must be available whose only responsibility is to monitor the patient, identify cardiorespiratory compromise, and institute bag-mask ventilation and cardiopulmonary resuscitation if necessary. Backup emergency services, including protocols for summoning emergency medical services, must be established and maintained [7].

The Joint Commission

The Joint Commission (TJC) is an independent, not-for-profit organization. It accredits and certifies more than 18,000 healthcare organizations and programs in the United States. The Joint Commission is the "auditor" for CMS and recently aligned their care standards with the CMS's conditions of participation, which makes it easier to track compliance. Currently TJC standards for sedation and anesthesia care apply when the administration of analgesia or sedative medication to an individual, in any setting, for any purpose, by any route, induces a partial or total loss of sensation for the purpose of conducting an operative or other procedure [8]. The definitions of four levels of sedation and anesthesia include the following:

(1) Minimal sedation (anxiolysis) is a drug-induced state during which patients respond normally to verbal commands. Although cognitive function and coordination may be impaired, ventilatory and cardiovascular functions are unaffected.

(2) Moderate sedation/analgesia ("conscious sedation") is a drug-induced depression of consciousness during which patients respond purposefully to verbal commands, either alone or accompanied by light tactile stimulation. Reflex withdrawal from a painful stimulus is not considered a purposeful response. No interventions are required to maintain a patent airway, and spontaneous ventilation is adequate. Cardiovascular function is usually maintained.

(3) Deep sedation/analgesia is a drug-induced depression of consciousness during which patients cannot be easily aroused, but respond purposefully following repeated or painful stimulation. The ability to independently maintain ventilatory function may be impaired. Patients may require assistance in maintaining a patent airway, and spontaneous ventilation may be inadequate. Cardiovascular function is usually maintained.

(4) Anesthesia consists of general anesthesia and spinal or major regional anesthesia. It does not include local anesthesia. General anesthesia is a drug-induced loss of consciousness during which patients are not arousable, even by painful stimulation. The ability to independently maintain ventilatory function is often impaired. Patients often require assistance in maintaining a patent airway, and positive-pressure ventilation may be required because of depressed spontaneous ventilation or drug-induced depression of neuromuscular function. Cardiovascular function may be impaired.

These definitions are based upon the ASA practice guidelines for sedation and analgesia by non-anesthesiologists, and are generally accepted by most organizations.

These definitions are used as the foundation for a number of TJC standards related to procedural sedation that address clinician credentials and patient assessment, monitoring, and treatment before, during, and after the administration of procedural sedation (Table 7.2). Recognizing the risks involved with sedation and analgesia, TJC mandates that sedation practices throughout the institution be monitored and evaluated by the department of anesthesia.

Joint Commission sedation and analgesia standards

There are additional TJC standards that apply to procedural sedation events located within the Universal Protocol for preventing wrong-site, wrong-procedure, and wrong-person surgeries or procedures (UP.01.01.01–UP.01.03.01) [8]. This protocol applies to all surgical and nonsurgical invasive procedures, and is required to reinforce the need for teamwork to

Table 7.2. Summary of The Joint Commission (TJC) standards for procedural sedation

Standard number	Standard	Requirement	Compliance
PC.03.01.01	Procedural sedation must be administered by a qualified provider	Plan for procedures requiring procedural sedation	Personnel credentialed, sufficient personnel available, nurse supervising perioperative care, appropriate equipment available to administer medications/blood, resuscitation equipment available
PC.03.01.03	Patients must be assessed prior to sedation/procedure Provider must discuss risks/options with the patient/family prior to sedation/procedure Provider must reassess the patient immediately before sedation is initiated	Provide patient with care prior to the administration of sedation	Pre-procedure assessment conducted and reassessment performed just prior to sedation administration, evidence of post-procedure patient needs planning, pre-procedure education complete and based on plan of care, and clinician responsible for patient concurs with sedation plan
PC.03.01.05	Mandatory monitoring of the patient's oxygenation, ventilation, and circulation during sedation	Monitor patient during the administration of procedural sedation	Documentation of evidence for continuous monitoring of patients during the procedure including oxygenation, ventilation and circulation measures
PC.03.01.07	Post-sedation assessment in the recovery area is necessary before the patient is discharged A qualified provider must discharge the patient from the post-sedation recovery area, or discharge must be based on established criteria	Provide care after the administration of procedural sedation	Assessment of the patient's physiological status, mental status, and pain is complete immediately post procedure and then at determined frequencies, discharge is conducted by a qualified provider based on established criteria, and outpatients are discharged with a responsible individual
PC.02.01.03	Documentation of the use of procedural sedation	Medical record documents the use of procedural sedation	Documentation contains provisional diagnosis, pre-procedure history and physical exam, administration of sedation with patient's response, a procedure note, patient discharged by a qualified provider according to established criteria, and any unanticipated events/complications followed by how they were managed

ensure and protect patient safety. The protocol specifies three standards: pre-procedure verification, site marking, and a time-out immediately before the procedure.

- First, the pre-procedure verification is an ongoing process to obtain and confirm information to ensure all relevant documents, equipment, and information are known and present. The organization, within the policy, should dictate the frequency and location for this process. It may need to occur more than once prior to the procedure, and it is best if the patient can be involved.
- Site marking is the second component of the Universal Protocol, and is required to prevent wrong-site procedures. This standard is most successful when a consistent site-marking process is developed within the organization's policy. The markings should be used when the procedure is to be done on those areas that have various sides, limbs, or spine or organ levels. Site marking is not required when the provider doing the procedure is continuously with the patient until the procedure is performed.
- A *time-out* or *safety pause* is to be conducted just prior to the procedure to ensure the identification of the patient, and to check for the correct site and the correct procedure. It is ideal to conduct the time-out before sedation is administered to the patient, so that the patient can be involved. A member of the procedure team is to initiate the time-out, which includes active communication from all members of the team. The procedure is not started until all members confirm the information. A standardized process is required throughout the organization.

There are other associated TJC standards which apply generally to a number of other care events that might occur in connection with procedural sedation. These standards, MS.06.01.03, MM.03.01.03, RC.02.01.01, and PI.01.01.01, are denoted within the body of the sedation and analgesia standards and should be evaluated to ensure compliance. The standards for the administration of procedural sedation continue to evolve. The ASA amended the Standards for Basic Anesthetic Monitoring, effective July 1, 2011 (Standard 3.2.4). The updated standard calls for continuous patient monitoring for the presence of expired carbon dioxide. The downstream effect of the change will be that all patients administered moderate or deep sedation must have their expired carbon dioxide monitored by capnography.

The foregoing statutes, regulations, and standards function together to provide a framework for both the individual clinician and the practice site. They demonstrate a strong public interest in providing safe and effective care of the patient undergoing a procedure. The boards regulate the individual clinicians and their office-based practice. CMS and TJC regulate procedural sedation practice in the institutional setting. CMS and TJC each have regulations and standards that govern the clinician, the practice site, and the quality of the program. When TJC surveys a facility, it is also with the eyes of the CMS, since the CMS deems TJC to be the enforcer of their own Conditions of Participation. Therefore, if an institution has passed a TJC survey and has been fully accredited by TJC, that institution is deemed an accredited CMS organization and is permitted to participate in Medicare and Medicaid programs.

Quality and practice improvement

The purpose of the quality and practice improvement program is to ensure best practice at the point of care through the review and evaluation of key care processes and patient outcomes, along with the oversight committee, to provide a systematic approach to safe, consistent practice. It is through these dynamics that the standards of care and the mission of the policy are actualized, and consistency of care is assured.

Monitoring practice

A systematic data collection process is required at the departmental and physician level to capture each key regulatory standard and any other identified important care processes impacting practice at the local level. The oversight committee is accountable for this process and for the review of the results at regular intervals to ensure adherence to the policy and to evaluate patient outcomes. Depending on the resources available at an institution or facility, the structure of this system may vary. However, the priority is for all areas performing procedural sedation to complete a select volume of random chart reviews monthly or, better, concurrently. The Joint Commission requires the percentage of records audited to be based upon the number of procedures performed within that area. For example, if the yearly number of procedures performed is between 1 and 30, then 100% of those records need to be audited, 31–100 procedures, 30% audited, and for 101–500 procedures 70 audits per month need to be conducted. The best way to track and organize these data for review and analysis is to record the data via a hospital database, allowing access to area leadership. The results are then presented at the oversight committee for discussion and development of an action plan, if needed. This information loop is important as a means of providing feedback to the oversight committee so that any potential areas of risk can be addressed or practice improvement initiatives enacted. Figure 7.2 depicts an example of a procedural sedation monitoring tool.

Outcome measures

The monitoring tool is a collection of process and patient outcome measures. The tool design reflects all mandatory regulatory requirements that need to be measured as well as any identified processes that the oversight committee wants to follow. The tool should be reviewed on a yearly basis and revised as needed by the oversight committee.

The University HealthSystem Consortium (UHC), an alliance of academic medical centers and affiliated hospitals that focuses on excellence in quality, safety, and cost-effectiveness, recommends the following process measures and patient outcomes [9,10]:

- Process measures:
  - informed consent for procedure
  - nil by mouth (NPO) status
  - history obtained
  - physical and airway exam completed
  - requirements for anesthesia consult identified
  - operator credentialed
  - adherence to required patient monitoring
- Patient outcomes:
  - deaths
  - aspirations
  - reversal agent used
  - unplanned transfer to higher level of care
  - cardiac/respiratory arrest

PROCEDURAL SEDATION AUDIT

MRN: _____   Type of sedation   ☐ Deep sedation

Patient Name _____   ☐ Moderate sedation

Auditor Name _____

Pod / Area _____

Procedure Date: _____

Was PS administered in an outpatient area   ☐ Yes   ☐ No

    If yes, patient discharged with designated adult   ☐ Yes   ☐ No

LIP credentials   ☐ Verified   ☐ Not credentialed   ☐ Unable to locate

All sections of pre-sedation assessment completed   ☐ Yes   ☐ No

Consent for sedation signed   ☐ Yes   ☐ No

NPO status confirmed   ☐ Yes   ☐ No

Anesthesia consult obtained   ☐ Yes   ☐ No

Safety pause process completed (time out)   ☐ Yes   ☐ No

Prior to Procedure

○ Yes	○ No	Vital Signs
○ Yes	○ No	Sedation Level
○ Yes	○ No	Pain Level

During Procedure (at least every 5 minutes)

○ Yes	○ No	Vital Signs
○ Yes	○ No	Sedation Level
○ Yes	○ No	Pain Level

Post Procedure (every 10 mins for first 30 mins; then every 15 mins until post sedation score is greater/equal to 8)

○ Yes	○ No	Vital Signs
○ Yes	○ No	Sedation Level
○ Yes	○ No	Pain Level

COMPLICATIONS

☐ Acute coronary syndrome

☐ Adverse drug reaction

☐ Aspiration

☐ Cardiac/Respiratory Arrest

☐ Death

☐ Greater than 5 minutes of mask/bag ventilation

☐ Inability to complete the procedure as planned

☐ Intubation required

☐ Medications used other than those approved

☐ Unplanned hospital admission

☐ Unplanned transfer to ICU

☐ Use of reversal agent

Figure 7.2. Procedural sedation audit reporting form. Courtesy of Vineeta Vaidya, Brigham and Women's Hospital Center for Clinical Excellence.

- medications administered other than those approved
- inability to complete procedure as planned
- emergency procedures without a licensed independent practitioner present

The Joint Commission has a number of measures that concur with the UHC list. However, there are differences, and these should be reviewed. TJC requires the collection of three measures that are located in the *Provision of care* chapter [8]:

- pre-procedural patient education based on plan of care (PC.03.01.03)
- monitoring of the patient's physiological status, mental status, and pain level at a frequency and intensity consistent with the potential effect of the sedation provided (PC.03.01.07)
- outpatients discharged in the company of an individual who accepts responsibility for the patient (PC.03.01.07).

There are other TJC standards (noted in the *Provision of care* chapter) requiring data to support compliance. These standards should be reviewed to verify that the information is collected via another data collection process, and, if not, evaluated to be added to the procedural sedation tool. In addition to the regulatory measurement requirements, the oversight committee may add additional measures to target specific care processes of interest.

Safety/incident reporting

A safety reporting system, paper or electronic, is an additional tool required to reinforce a culture of safety and provide a direct source of feedback regarding practice by the practitioners at the point of care. These reports are used by those responsible for both risk management and quality to bring forth practice issues or gaps in care for resolution. The important aspect in creating a successful reporting system is an understanding that the report will be used in a nonpunitive fashion, and the information will lend itself to the correction of the causation of the event or a change in the system to prevent further occurrences [11]. The system should also have a feedback loop to the reporting authors as to the follow-up and outcome of the event. Once these components are well established, the goal of robust use by differing practitioners will be achieved.

For procedural sedation, complications occurring from the start of the procedure through recovery can be documented within the safety reporting system as well as any breach in policy, or concern regarding the processes surrounding the procedure. These reports are closely monitored by local leadership, risk management, and quality depending on the hospital structure. Trending of care events or process issues is conducted, with an immediate response to any adverse event occurrences.

Responding to risk or potential risk events

The response to potential risk or actual risk events is a collaborative effort by local-level leadership, risk and quality managers, with the oversight committee acting as the final review for recommendations. The early identification of such events through the active monitoring of practice creates the ability to respond proactively and immediately when needed. (Table 7.3). Though the immediacy of a response varies, depending on the severity of the event, the process for the review remains the same, to make certain all possible causation is addressed and not overlooked [11].

Table 7.3. Elements to reduce risk

The director of the anesthesia services assures that all clinicians providing anesthesia, including procedural sedation, in all settings, are doing so in a safe and compliant manner
Each clinician involved in the administration of procedural sedation is competent to do so, and all records are up to date
Each procedural sedation area has required equipment immediately available for the safe administration of the sedating agent, as well as for resuscitation of the patient from oversedation and/or respiratory depression
A strong informed consent process is established
Pre-procedure assessment is complete and detailed, especially airway, to identify any risk and possible need for anesthesia consult
Patient monitoring is conducted pre-procedure through recovery
Discharge criteria are established and documented
A process is created to approve sites where procedural sedation is performed
A systematic data collection process is developed at the departmental and physician level to assess compliance with policy and evaluate practice

Risk management and quality are involved to varying degrees with most responses, working closely with local leadership and other expert practitioners. This activity of review, analysis, and evaluation is the cornerstone to developing and ensuring a clinically excellent and safe sedation program. It provides an opportunity to make sure all policy and procedure steps are followed, ultimately resulting in a reevaluation of practice and care process points. This activity should never be short-changed, and it should be a regular item on the oversight committee's agenda.

The initial communication of an event or concern can occur in various ways depending on the severity of the situation and the hospital structure. For a severe event, local-level leadership notifies risk and quality immediately. An investigation is initiated to gather additional facts and information, including discussions with the practitioners involved. In other situations risk, quality, or care providers may identify an event or a trend in practice. At that point, leadership is contacted to report on the situation and to support further inquiry. The investigation phase is very important, since it establishes the "what, how, and why" of the incident to clearly articulate the issues [11]. A standardized analysis to review an incident should be utilized to capture all possible areas of causation and to identify improvement areas. One such framework is proposed by Vincent and colleagues [12] (Table 7.4). The event should be reviewed by all those involved as well as interested hospital forums that can add to the strength of the overall action plan. Examples of such are morbidity and mortality rounds, nursing departmental practice committees, and quality forums.

The oversight committee chair is notified as well, and the incident is reviewed at the next committee meeting to review the findings from the investigation with all stakeholders in attendance for analysis and resolution, or development of next steps. The action plans are carried out and the final findings are documented and reported up through the hospital's committee structure. The oversight committee is responsible for closing the loop, making certain the action plan is completed and continuing monitoring as appropriate.

Table 7.4. Event follow-up framework

Main factors	Contributory factors
Institutional	Economic pressures, regulatory requirements, hospital mission/priorities
Organizational	Financial priorities, structure, policies, standards, safety culture
Work environment	Staffing, skill mix, workload, shift patterns, design, equipment availability and maintenance, support
Team factors	Communication, supervision, team culture
Individual	Knowledge, skills, competence, health
Task factors	Task design, availability and use of protocols, test results, accuracy and availability of patient notes
Patient factors	Complexity and seriousness, language, communication, personality, special factors

Modified with permission from Vincent et al. [12].

Reportable events

There are specific events which require a response to regulatory agencies. These events, sentinel or serious reportable, are those mandated by regulatory bodies – CMS, state, Department of Public Health (DPH), or TJC – and they may require a root-cause analysis to identify causation and an action plan for correction. TJC requires a review of a sentinel event by the institution, and leaves it to each institution whether to report it to TJC. Some sentinel events that may involve the administration of procedural sedation include [8]:

- unanticipated death or major permanent loss of function not related to the natural course of the patient's illness or underlying condition
- death or major permanent loss of function associated with a medical error
- hemolytic transfusion reaction involving administration of blood or blood products having major blood group incompatibilities
- procedure on the wrong patient or wrong body part
- death resulting from nosocomial infection
- unintended retention of a foreign object in a patient after the procedure

State regulatory agencies such as the professional boards and departments of public health may also require specific reporting. For example, the Massachusetts Department of Public Health requires reporting of all serious reportable events. Serious reportable events (SREs), once known as "never events," are those on a list of events compiled by the National Quality Forum (NQF) [13,14]. Some states require an institution to report the SRE to the DPH, the third-party insurer, and the patient. Further, a preventability analysis of each event must be made by the institution. Should the event be found to be preventable, the institution cannot bill out any charges for care that flows from the event. In a vertically integrated care organization, should the patient be discharged to the care of a sister institution within the organization, the sister institution may not bill for care associated with the event as well. The DPH may also require reporting of other events not captured by SRE reporting requirements. All reports submitted to DPH are available for public review.

State professional boards may also have particular reporting requirements. For example, the Massachusetts Board of Medicine requires reporting of all SREs, in addition to the following that may be associated with sedation procedures:

- deaths related to elective ambulatory procedures
- any invasive diagnostic procedure or surgical intervention performed on the wrong organ, extremity, or body part
- all deaths or major or permanent impairments of bodily functions that are not ordinarily expected as a result of the patient's condition on presentation

State board reports are likely to be de-identified and peer-review protected. Therefore, they are not available for public review. Each state will have different review and reporting requirements. The trend in the states is toward more disclosure of adverse events. A review of your own state's regulations will be required to discern your own reporting requirements.

By using a two-pronged approach-evaluating patient outcomes and care processes, improvement can be identified resulting in changes to treatment algorithms, care processes, and environmental issues. These changes must be evaluated after implementation to ensure they have created a safer patient care environment.

Summary

A successful procedural sedation program is built with a collaborative team of experts who clearly articulate the goal and standards of care through an institutional policy. This policy is based upon national and state recognized practice requirements and guidelines which lay the foundation for patient safety and clinical excellence. A robust risk and quality structure built within the program ensures best practice at the point of care. It is through this framework that procedural sedation program excellence is attained.

References

1. Restatement (Second) of Torts, §282. 1965.

2. Massachusetts Board of Registration in Medicine. Policy 94–04. *Patient Care Assessment Guidelines for Intravenous Conscious Sedation.*

3. Massachusetts Board of Registration in Medicine regulation 243 CMR 3.00.

4. Centers for Medicare and Medicaid Services (CMS). Conditions of participation: regulations at 42 CFR 482.

5. American Society of Anesthesiologists (ASA). Statement on granting privileges for deep sedation to non-anesthesiologist sedation practitioners. Park Ridge, IL: ASA, 2010.

6. American Society of Anesthesiologists (ASA). Statement on granting privileges for administration of moderate sedation to practitioners who are not anesthesia professionals. Park Ridge, IL: ASA, 2006. www.asahq.org/For-Healthcare-Professionals/Standards-Guidelines-and-Statements.aspx (accessed June 2011).

7. Metzner J, Domino KB. Procedural sedation by nonanesthesia providers. In Urman R, Gross W, Philip BK, eds., *Anesthesia Outside of the Operating Room.* Oxford: Oxford University Press, 2011; 49–61.

8. Joint Commission. Provision of care, treatment and services standards, record of care, and improving organizational performance. In *Comprehensive Accreditation Manual for Hospitals.* Oakbrook Terrace, IL: Joint Commission, 2011.

9. University HealthSystem Consortium Consensus Group on Moderate Sedation. *Moderate Sedation Best Practice Recommendations.* Oak Brook, IL: UHC, 2005.

10. University HealthSystem Consortium Consensus Group on Deep Sedation. *Deep Sedation Best Practice Recommendations.* Oak Brook, IL: UHC, 2006.

11. Mahajan RP. Critical incident reporting and learning. *Br J Anaesth* 2010; **105**: 69–75.

12. Vincent C, Taylor-Adams S, Stanhope N. Framework for analysing risk and safety in clinical medicine. *BMJ* 1998; **316**: 1154–7.

13. Massachusetts Department of Public Health regulation 105 CMR 130.332, Serious reportable events.

14. Massachusetts Department of Public Health regulation 105 CMR 130.331, Serious incident and accident reports.

Chapter

8

Nursing considerations for sedation

Louise Caperelli-White

Introduction

Previous chapters of this book have defined moderate and deep sedation, and have presented a range of clinical situations and patient populations in which these types of sedation may be used. In the past, procedural sedation was administered and managed primarily by an anesthesiologist. Today, the nurse is an active participant in the management of patients receiving all levels of sedation. As a result of a multitude of scenarios and increased patient acuity, most institutions have developed a strict policy for safe administration and monitoring of patients in relation to moderate and deep procedural sedation. This policy serves as a guideline to follow regardless of location or procedure type. This chapter will focus on the key role of the nurse.

Training

Regardless of the location where procedural sedation is being provided, all patients should receive comparable levels of care by qualified professionals. In the Joint Commission regulation 03.01.01, it states that "In addition to the individual performing the procedure, a sufficient number of qualified staff are present to evaluate the patient, to provide the sedation and/or anesthesia, to help with the procedure, and to monitor and recover the patient" [1]. In most institutions the standard is that there is a minimum of two qualified professionals attending to the patient: the "operator" and the "monitor." The role of the nurse is to act as a "monitor." The monitor can be defined as a licensed and credentialed healthcare professional (physician, dentist, physician assistant, nurse practitioner, or registered nurse) who will monitor appropriate physiologic parameters as well as the patient's response to the drugs administered and the procedure itself. According to the American Society of Anesthesiologists (ASA) *Statement*

Moderate and Deep Sedation in Clinical Practice, ed. Richard D. Urman and Alan D. Kaye.
Published by Cambridge University Press. © Cambridge University Press 2012.

on granting privileges for administration of moderate sedation to practitioners who are not anesthesia professionals, certain educational and training requirements must be met [2]. The following information should be included in a formal training program:

(1) Practice guidelines for sedation and analgesia by non-anesthesiologists.
(2) Definition of general anesthesia, levels of sedation/analgesia, and continuum of depth of sedation.
(3) The pharmacology and safe administration of sedatives and analgesics used to establish a level of moderate sedation, and the pharmacology and safe administration of their antagonists.
(4) Airway management with facemask and self-inflating bag-valve mask device.
(5) Oxygen delivery with oral and nasal equipment.
(6) Monitoring and documentation of patient's physiologic parameters during sedation at regular intervals. These parameters include, but are not limited to, blood pressure, respiratory rate, oxygen saturation by pulse oximetry, ECG monitoring, depth of sedation, and capnography if in a setting where ventilatory function cannot be directly assessed. Appropriately set audible alarms on all physiologic parameters should be stressed.
(7) Recognition of common complications that can occur, and the appropriate intervention.

All practitioners who are the designated "monitors" must also be competent in CPR skills.

These educational requirements are part of an institution wide process and should be consistent across the institution. In addition to this initial education, a formal re-credentialing process must be in place for all "monitors." Evaluation and documentation of competence occurs on a periodic basis according to each institution's guidelines.

Nursing responsibilities

The nurse has a number of important duties to accomplish before the procedure can proceed. The nurse's primary responsibility during procedural sedation is exclusively to that patient. The American Association of Nurse Anesthetists (AANA) suggests that the registered nurse managing and monitoring the patient receiving sedation and analgesia should have no other responsibilities during the procedure [3].

Pre-procedure
Equipment

All necessary equipment must be present and in working order. Examples of such equipment include:

- oxygen – a source and means for providing supplemental oxygen
- an airway and a self-inflating oxygen delivery system capable of delivering 100% oxygen
- a source of suction with Yankauer-type suction catheters
- a pulse oximeter with audible alarms
- a cardiac monitor with audible alarms
- a blood pressure device and stethoscope
- capnography (if necessary)
- an emergency cart and defibrillator

- pharmaceutical agents to be used for the procedure, and their reversal agents
- liter bags of 0.9% normal saline or Lactated Ringer's solution

Documentation

It is usually the responsibility of the individual who is performing the procedure to obtain the procedural sedation documentation. It is, however, the responsibility of the monitor/ nurse to review this documentation and ensure that it is present and complete (Figure 8.1). The following should be completed prior to the procedure:

- Informed consent – which includes risk, benefits, and alternatives. This needs to be accomplished before any procedural sedation drugs are given.
- Physical examination and medical history review – which assesses for risks and comorbidities. The exam should include a thorough airway assessment to aid in the recognition of potential difficult airway management. The ASA classification of physical status and the Mallampati classification system have been described elsewhere in this book (see Chapters 3 and 4).
- Recording of weight and height is important for medication dosing and BMI calculation.
- Review of pre-procedure labs or tests.

It is the responsibility of the team members to identify those patients who, based on the information obtained in the documents above, are deemed at higher risk for complications, and whether an anesthesia consult should be called.

Patient education

Patient education is one of the nurse's chief responsibilities. As the monitor during procedural sedation, the nurse is in constant communication with the patient. Nurses are the ones who keep patients "safe" by continous monitoring, while the proceduralist is performing the procedure. The procedure should be thoroughly explained before any drugs are given to the patient. Prior to the procedure, the nurse should describe any sensations that the patient might feel – e.g., burning, pulling, pressure, etc. This will help allay anxiety if and when these sensations are felt. The nurse needs to explain to the patient what positions he or she will be in during the procedure. The patient also needs to know that you will keep him or her as pain-free as possible. Agree on a method of communication for patients to let you know if and when they need something, perhaps by holding up a finger or making eye contact. Instruct them to let you know if they experience any problems. Let them know that the medications will make them feel "sleepy" and that they may not remember much, although individual response to sedative medications varies widely. You should explain to them that you will be monitoring their progress constantly during the procedure. Allow time for clarifying any questions the patient may have.

Patients should be made aware of what will happen post-procedure and during discharge. They should also be aware that a "responsible adult" should be available to accompany them home when the recovery from the procedure is complete. This is in accordance with the Joint Commission regulation 03.01.03, which states, "Patients who have received sedation or anesthesia as outpatients are discharged in the company of an individual who accepts responsibility for the patient" [1].

REGIONAL MEDICAL
CENTER

PATIENT IDENTIFICATION PLATE

Moderate / Deep Procedural Sedation
Pre-Procedure Evaluation

Planned Procedure:		Diagnosis:	

Wt.	Kg	Ht.	

State of Consciousness: ☐ Alert ☐ Oriented ☐ Disoriented ☐ Relaxed ☐ Anxious ☐ Agitated
☐ Intubated ☐ Responds only to pain ☐ Medicated ☐ Non-Medicated

☐ Interpreter Services Needed

Pertinent Laboratory Studies:

Pertinent
Diagnostic Studies:

WBC ⟩ Hgb / Hct ⟨ Plt ⟩ Glu ⟨ Bun / Cr ∣ Cl / CO₂ ∣ Na / K

LMP ___
PT ___
PTT ___
INR ___

Current
Medications: ☐ Current medication list reviewed with patient

Allergies or
Adverse Drug Reactions: Contrast Hx:

Pertinent Medical History & Current Physical Exam		Consideration for anesthesia consultation:

Head / Neck   ☐ WNL

Oral: ☐ Natural Airway   ☐ Oral piercing or foreign body ☐ Tracheostomy ☐ Dentures ☐ Partial Plate

Respiratory System   ☐ WNL

Cardiovascular System ☐ WNL

Hepato/Gastrointestinal ☐ WNL

Substance Abuse   ETOH ☐ Yes ☐ No / Recreational Drug Use ☐ Yes ☐ No

Neuro/Musculoskeletal ☐ WNL

Consideration for anesthesia consultation:
• Recent post-op patient followed by POPS (post op pain service)
• Patient followed by Palliative Care Service or Chronic Pain Service
• Patient with significant chronic opioid use
• Patient with documented history of not tolerating procedural sedation
• Patient or team member request for an anesthesiologist to provide sedation
• Patient unable to either lie still for the duration of the procedure or assume certain position for the procedure given the level of sedation planned
• Patient with history of difficult intubation

Additional Comments:

Assessment / Sedation Plan:
   ☐ NPO greater than or equal to 6 hours
   ☐ Clear liquids until 2 hours before procedure   Precautions: ☐ MRSA ☐ VRE ☐ TB
   ☐ Meds with sips of clear liquids only   ☐ Neutropenia ☐ Other
   ☐ Procedure urgency outweighs aspiration risk   Other:_____
Consent Obtained: ☐ patient ☐ family ☐ BWH

Planned Medication: **Level of Sedation:** ☐ Moderate   ☐ Deep
   ☐ Diazepam ☐ Midazolam ☐ Fentanyl ☐ Morphine ☐ Hydromorphone ☐ Other
   For Deep Sedation only ☐ Ketamine ☐ Propofol ☐ Etomidate

Date _____ Time _____ _____ MD/NP/PA CID [ ][ ][ ][ ]

IF greater than or equal to 48 hours between evaluation and procedure ☐ Y ☐ N
If yes, have there been any changes in the patient status?   ☐ Y ☐ N

Date _____ Time _____ _____ MD/NP/PA CID [ ][ ][ ][ ]

WHITE - MEDICAL RECORD COPY   YELLOW - DEPARTMENT NURSING DIRECTOR   0601937 (9/10)

Figure 8.1. Sample procedural sedation pre-procedure review form.

Table 8.1. Richmond Agitation–Sedation Scale (RASS)

Score	Term	Description
+4	Combative	Overtly combative or violent; immediate danger to staff
+3	Very agitated	Pulls on or removes tube(s) or catheter(s) or has aggressive behavior toward staff
+2	Agitated	Frequent nonpurposeful movement or patient–ventilator dyssynchrony
+1	Restless	Anxious or apprehensive but movements not aggressive or vigorous
0		Alert and calm
−1	Drowsy	Not fully alert but has sustained (more than 10 seconds) awakening, with eye contact, to voice
−2	Light sedation	Briefly (less than 10 seconds) awakens with eye contact to voice
−3	Moderate sedation	Any movement (but no eye contact) to voice
−4	Deep sedation	No response to voice, but any movement to physical stimulation
−5	Unarousable	No response to voice or physical stimulation

Procedure

1. Observe patient. Is patient alert and calm (score 0)?
   Does patient have behaviour that is consistent with restlessness or agitation (score +1 to +4 using the criteria listed above under Description)?

2. If patient is not alert, in a loud speaking voice state patient's name and direct patient to open eyes and look at speaker. Repeat once if necessary. Can prompt patient to continue looking at speaker.
   Patient has eye opening and eye contact, which is maintained for more than 10 seconds (score −1).
   Patient has eye opening and eye contact, but this is not maintained for 10 seconds (score −2).
   Patient has any movement in response to voice, excluding eye contact (score −3).

3. If patient does not respond to voice, physically stimulate patient by shaking shoulder and then rubbing sternum if there is not response to shaking shoulder.
   Patient has any movement to physical stimulation (score −4).
   Patient has no response to voice or physical stimulation (score −5).

Reproduced with permission from Sessler *et al.* [4].

Immediately prior to the procedure and the administration of the sedation the nurse/monitor should:

- Verify correct identification of the patient per institution's standards. Using two patient identifiers meets The Joint Commission's National Patient Safety Goal #1.
- Obtain baseline vital signs: heart rate and rhythm, blood pressure, respiratory rate, oxygen saturation, temperature, level of consciousness, and level on a reliable and validated sedation and pain scale (Table 8.1). Include a capnography trace, if capnography is being utilized.
- Review allergies.

Table 8.2. American Society of Anesthesiologists (ASA) pre-procedure fasting guidelines [5]

Ingested material	Minimum fasting period ^{a}
Clear liquids ^{b}	2 h
Breast milk	4 h
Infant formula	6 h
Nonhuman milk ^{c}	6 h
Light meal ^{d}	6 h

These recommendations apply to healthy patients who are undergoing elective procedures. They are not intended for women in labor. Following the guidelines does not guarantee a complete gastric emptying has taken place.
^{a} The fasting periods apply to all ages.
^{b} Examples of clear liquids include water, fruit juices without pulp, carbonated beverages, clear tea, and black coffee.
^{c} Since nonhuman milk is similar to solids in gastric emptying time, the amount ingested must be considered when determining an appropriate fasting period.
^{d} A light meal typically consists of toast and clear liquids. Meals that include fried or fatty foods or meat may prolong gastric emptying time. Both the amount and type of foods ingested must be considered when determining an appropriate fasting period.

- Check NPO status (Table 8.2).
- Check that all monitoring equipment is on the patient, with audible alarms enabled.
- Review the order for benzodiazepine, opioids, and other drugs planned for sedation analgesia.
- Ensure that medications and antagonists have been obtained.
- Ensure that there is working intravenous access for medications and IV fluids, if necessary.
- Verify that the patient is tolerating the position required for the procedure.
- Undertake a last-minute assessment for patient understanding and questions.

Before starting the procedure, the whole patient care team should perform a time-out or safety pause to ensure that the correct procedure is being performed on the correct patient. This meets The Joint Commission's Universal Protocol regulation [1].

During the procedure

During this period, the nurse's primary responsibilities are to deliver moderate sedation medications and to assess and monitor the patient for anticipated and unanticipated responses to the therapy. The most common complications are respiratory depression and airway obstruction. Other common complications that can occur are cardiac arrhythmias and hemodynamic instability. According to the ASA's practice guidelines, certain measurements should be taken at regular intervals to reduce the likelihood of adverse outcomes. Most authorities agree that the following information should be assessed and documented at **a minimum of every 5 minutes** (Figure 8.2):

- vital signs – blood pressure, heart rate and rhythm, respiratory rate, oxygen saturation
- medications given – drug, dose, route, and time
- oxygen delivery – amount and the means of delivery
- airway assessment – checking of head position and patency of the airway

REGIONAL MEDICAL CENTER

PATIENT IDENTIFICATION AREA

Moderate-Deep Procedural Sedation

Date: _____ / _____ / _____   Time: _____

2 NCR Form – Use ball point pen (press hard)

Patient Identification:	Patient Status:	☐ In-patient	☐ Emergency Dept.
☐ Bracelet ☐ Verbal	☐ Out-patient ☐ Adult escort verified		

Procedure:	Procedure Status:		
	☐ Pre-Scheduled	☐ Emergency	☐ Urgent

Level of Sedation: ☐ Moderate   ☐ Deep | Procedure Location: Building_____ Floor _____ Room ____ | Recovery Location: Building _____ Floor _____ Room ____

Signed Consent   ☐ Y | NPO since: _____   _____ AM / _____ PM | Height | Weight _____ Kg

Allergies/Adverse Reactions:

Diagnosis: ☐ Pre-procedure evaluation reviewed

☐ Equipment Safety Check   ☐ Alarms Enabled   ☐ Emergency Equipment Available   ☐ Antagonist Available

☐ SAFETY PAUSE PERFORMED BY PROCEDURE TEAM
Safety pause includes: verification of correct patient name by name and date of birth, procedure, site and position, and safety precautions based on the patient's history or medication use. Also, if applicable, correct implants and equipment are available, diagnostic exams are labeled and displayed, and the need to administer antibiotics or fluid for irrigation is discussed.

Pre-Sedation Assessment: Time _____ AM/PM

Temp_____ HR_____ Cardiac Rhythm_____ BP____ / ____ mmHg Loc _____

Resp_____ O$_2$ Sat_____ % on_____ ☐ Room Air or_____ O$_2$ L/min via _____

Sedation Level:_____ Pain Level:_____ | Intravenous: Type:_____ Size:_____ Site:_____

Procedure Start _____ | Sedation Start _____ | Recovery Start _____
Time   Stop _____ | Time   Stop _____ | Time   Stop _____

TIME	OBSERVATIONS	B.P.	H.R.	R.R.	O$_2$ SAT.	CO$_2$	SEDATION LEVEL	PAIN LEVEL	DRUG, DOSE, ROUTE	TIME GIVEN	GIVEN BY	ORDERED BY

Page _____ of _____ Pages   White: Medical Records   Yellow: Department Director   0600646 (8/10)

Figure 8.2. Sample procedural sedation flow sheet.

- presence of capnography waveform, if utilized
- level of sedation on approved scale
- level of pain on approved scale
- any observations that occur during procedure (e.g., complaints of pain, treatment of hypotension with IV fluids, snoring, etc.)

One of the most important things the nurse can do to prevent complications is to avoid overmedication. Intravenous sedative and analgesic drugs should be given in small, incremental doses that are titrated to the desired end point of sedation and analgesia. Enough time between doses must be allowed for the effect of the drug to take place. A thorough knowledge of each individual drug's usual dose, its mechanism of action, and its onset and duration of action is imperative. The treatment of respiratory complications can usually be relieved by stimulating the patient, delivering oxygen, repositioning airway with chin tilt or jaw-thrust, suctioning any upper airway secretions, and withholding further medications until the issue is resolved. If necessary, temporarily assist the patient's breathing with a bag-valve mask device. If respiratory depression continues, an antagonist should be considered.

Hemodynamic problems may be resolved with administration of IV fluids, raising the patient's legs, and/or withholding further medications. Certainly, the operator should be made aware of any complications and a decision to abort the procedure would be made if all efforts to treat complications have failed. Usually, the administration of the antagonist medication remedies the situation.

Medications

The goals of moderate sedation are analgesia, sedation, and amnesia. These are usually accomplished with a combination of opioids and benzodiazepines. The ASA defines moderate sedation as "a drug-induced depression of consciousness during which patients respond purposely to verbal commands, either alone or accompanied by light tactile stimulation. No interventions are required to maintain a patent airway, and spontaneous ventilation is adequate. Cardiovascular function is usually maintained" [6]. One must remember that while this is the intended response, individuals may react differently. The nurse must strictly adhere to the institution's monitoring guidelines.

Procedural sedation is usually accomplished through intravenous drugs, but oral doses may be appropriate in some situations. The most common combination of drugs used is midazolam and fentanyl. However, no single regimen is ideal for all situations. Your institution may use other combinations for atypical patient populations or for deep sedation. The reader is referred Chapter 2 for a description of medications and their reversal agents. It is important to remember that administering these medications for procedural sedation should not be undertaken without full knowledge of this pharmacology. It is also important to be aware of specific institutional and state board of nursing guidelines regarding the administration of procedural sedation medications.

Post-procedure: recovery and discharge

Since most of the medications used in procedural sedation are not immediately metabolized, it is important to establish a post-procedure monitoring routine. The Joint Commission states that the patient receiving sedation or anesthesia must be assessed in a post-sedation recovery area before discharge. Furthermore, a qualified licensed independent practitioner must discharge the patient from the recovery area or from the hospital. In the absence of the above practitioner, patients are discharged according to criteria approved by clinical leaders. The ASA agrees that continued observation, monitoring, and predetermined discharge criteria decrease the likelihood of adverse outcomes for both moderate and deep sedation. They recommend that patients are observed in an appropriately staffed and equipped area until they are near their baseline level of consciousness and no longer at increased risk for cardiopulmonary depression. If the patient must be moved from the area where the procedure has taken place, the recovery area must have available the same monitoring and resuscitative equipment. Both the operator and the monitor must stay with the patient until they can spontaneously protect their airway and their vital signs are stable. At the conclusion of the procedure, the patient must be monitored for a specified period of time. The duration and frequency of monitoring is subject to institutional and practice standards. Many facilities will monitor the patient every 5–10 minutes for **at least 30 minutes** after the last medication is administered. Monitoring continues at this frequency until the patient reaches baseline. Parameters monitored should be the same as those observed during the procedure. If the patient received a reversal agent during the procedure, the monitoring period is generally extended to at least 2 hours after the reversal agent was administered. This is because once the reversal agent has worn off, respiratory depression can reoccur.

When this standardized time period has passed and the patient is at baseline, he or she must meet objective discharge criteria. This is true both for the patient being discharged to home and for the patient being transferred within the institution to a less intensively monitored level of care. One of the first sets of objective discharge criteria used was the Aldrete scoring system first published in 1970 [7]. This system scored the patient in five parameters: activity, respiration, oxygenation, circulation, and consciousness (see Chapter 4, Table 4.2). Since this time, many institutions have modified this scale, based on post-sedation advances. One example of post-sedation discharge criteria can be found in Figure 8.3. Each of the six criteria listed here receives anywhere from 0 to 2 points based on their absence or presence. A total of eight points must be achieved for discharge. Any patient who receives a score of seven or less must be reevaluated by a physician before discharge can occur. Within the inpatient setting, patients can be transferred back to their previous unit once they have met the discharge criteria. The nurse who has recovered the patient will provide a complete report to the receiving nurse. This hand-off communication should include, but not be limited to:

- patient name
- diagnosis
- procedure performed
- review of vital signs, oxygen saturation, pain and sedation levels
- sedation medications administered, total dose, and antagonist, if used
- fluid balance
- complications and their treatment

Those patients who will be discharged to home need to receive both verbal and written discharge instructions (Figure 8.4). It is very important that both the patient and the accompanying adult are present to receive the instructions. The patients may still be experiencing some degree of amnesia and may not remember everything they have been told. Most discharge instructions include specific limitations or requirements associated

REGIONAL MEDICAL
CENTER

PATIENT IDENTIFICATION AREA

Moderate-Deep Procedural Sedation

2 NCR Form – Use ball point pen (press hard)

Time						Total		Yes	No	Post Sedation Assessment
Intake							CIRCLE THE CORRECT ANSWER:	2	0	Vital signs within 20% of baseline
								2	0	Oxygen saturation plus or minus 2% from baseline
Output								1	0	Swallow, cough, gag reflexes present to baseline
								2	0	Alert or appropriate to baseline
Procedure Site:				☐ N/A				2	0	Able to sit/walk appropriate to baseline
Dressings:		Tubes:						1	0	Minimal nausea or dizziness
Drains:		Other:					TOTAL SCORE			Total score 8 - 10 may be discharged or transferred per established criteria
										Total score 7 or less must be evaluated by MD prior to discharge or transfer

Printed / Operator _____ Initials _____	N/A	Yes	No	Post Procedure Assessment
MD/PA/NP Signature / Operator _____ Clinical ID # _____				Hydration adequate
Printed / Operator _____ Initials _____				Dressing and/or procedure site checked if applicable
MD/PA/NP Signature / Operator _____ Clinical ID # _____				Patient and/or family given written discharge instructions
Printed / Monitor _____				Patient and/or family questions answered
RN Signature / Monitor _____ Initials _____				Patient and/or family verbalizes their understanding of instructions
Printed / Monitor _____ RN Signature / Monitor _____ Initials _____				Discharge order written

Disposition: ☐ Discharge to Home ☐ Admit ☐ Transfer to _____

Time _____ Date _____ Signed _____, R.N.

Page _____ of _____ Pages

Figure 8.3. Sample discharge criteria.

REGIONAL MEDICAL
CENTER

PATIENT IDENTIFICATION AREA

**Colonoscopy / Sigmoidoscopy
Discharge Instructions**

I.   If you have received medication, you must, for your own safety and well-being for the first 12 hours after your procedure;

   A) NOT DRIVE an automobile
   B) NOT drink any alcoholic beverages
   C) NOT make any important decisions
   D) NOT do anything that requires concentration

II. If tissue specimens have been taken for examination - you may experience a small amount of bleeding on the toilet tissue. This is normal. A large amount of blood in the toilet bowl is not normal. You must call your doctor at the number listed below or go to the Emergency Room.

III. You may experience some distention of your abdomen from air that was placed into the gastrointestinal tract by the physician during the examination. This is normal and you will pass gas. Any persistent pain or persistent abdominal distension is abnormal. Call your doctor at the number listed below.

IV. You may return to your usual diet and resume taking prescription drugs.

V.   Any questions/problems:

   Between 8 a.m. and 5 p.m. call _____ M.D.,
   _____. After 5 p.m. call 617-732-6660 to page the physician on call, ask the Page operator to page the GI Fellow on call. A physician is always available.

   If you are a member of HPHC before 5 p.m. call _____, after 5 p.m. call your center main number.

VI. Additional instructions:

   The above material has been reviewed with me, my questions have been answered and I understand the contents.

   Date: _____   _____
                                                   Patient

                                 _____
                                                   Witness

WHITE - MEDICAL RECORD   YELLOW - PATIENT   50662810 (5/10)

Figure 8.4. Sample discharge instructions.

with the procedure that has been completed. For example, with a colonoscopy, patients will be advised that they may experience abdominal distention or flatus from air that was placed in the gastrointestinal tract. Any activity or diet restrictions should also be addressed. There are certain restrictions that stem from the use of the procedural sedation medications themselves. Post-procedural sedation discharge instructions should include the following statements, which pertain to the next 12 hours:

- Do not drive an automobile.
- Do not drink any alcoholic beverages.
- Do not make any important decisions.
- Do not do anything that requires mental concentration.

Patients should be instructed to contact the healthcare provider listed on the form if they experience problems or have questions. The name and telephone number should be clearly listed. After the information has been discussed and all questions are answered, both the patient and a witness should sign. They should receive a copy, and a copy should go into the patient's medical record. On a rare occasion, despite everyone's best efforts, the patient may decide to travel home without a responsible adult to accompany him or her. This is not recommended, and the patient should be dissuaded. If, however, they insist, they should be required to sign an "against medical advice" form.

Summary
The nurse plays a very important role in administering procedural sedation and monitoring the patient receiving it. Receiving specialized training and adhering to strict institutional standards will help to keep patients safe.

References

1. Joint Commission. *Comprehensive Accreditation Manual for Hospitals.* Oakbrook Terrace, IL: Joint Commission, 2011. e-dition.jcrinc.com/frame.aspx (accessed December 2010).

2. American Society of Anesthesiologists (ASA). Statement on granting privileges for administration of moderate sedation to practitioners who are not anesthesia professionals. Park Ridge, IL: ASA, 2006. www.asahq.org/For-Healthcare-Professionals/Standards-Guidelines-and-Statements.aspx (accessed June 2011).

3. American Association of Nurse Anesthetists (AANA). Considerations for policy development number 4.2: registered nurses engaged in the administration of sedation and analgesia. Park Ridge, IL: AANA, 2010.

4. Sessler CN, Gosnell MS, Grap MJ, *et al.* The Richmond Agitation–Sedation Scale: validity and reliability in adult intensive care patients. *Am J Respir Crit Care Med* 2002; **166**: 1338–44.

5. American Society of Anesthesiologists Committee. Practice guidelines for preoperative fasting and the use of pharmacologic agents to reduce the risk of pulmonary aspiration: application to healthy patients undergoing elective procedures: an updated report by the American Society of Anesthesiologists Committee on Standards and Practice Parameters. *Anesthesiology* 2011; **114**: 495–511.

6. American Society of Anesthesiologists Task Force on Sedation and Analgesia by Non-Anesthesiologists. Practice guidelines for sedation and analgesia by non-anesthesiologists. *Anesthesiology* 2002; **96**: 1004–17.

7. Aldrete JA, Kroulik D. A postanesthetic recovery score. *Anesth Analg* 1970; **49**: 924–34.

Further reading

O'Donnell J, Bragg K, Sell S. Procedural sedation: safely navigating the twilight zone. *Nursing* 2003; **33** (4): 36–44.

Voynarovska M, Cohen LB. The role of the endoscopy nurse or assistant in endoscopic sedation. *Gastrointest Endosc Clin N Am*, 2008; **18**: 695–705.

Wiener-Kronish JP, Gropper MA. *Conscious Sedation*. Philadelphia, PA: Hanley & Belfus, 2001.

Chapter

9

Physician assistants and nurse practitioners

Heather Trafton

Introduction

Nurse practitioners (NPs) and physician assistants (PAs) are healthcare professionals committed to delivering high-quality health care, and they strive to meet the needs of their patients in an effective, caring, and efficient manner. Across the USA, there are approximately 125,000 NPs and 88,771 PAs.

NPs are licensed independent practitioners who practice in ambulatory, acute, and long-term care as primary and or specialty providers [1]. NPs are nationally certified, and their scope of practice in an "expanded role" is dictated by education and training, national certification, state law, and institutional policy. According to their practice population focus, NPs deliver nursing and medical services to individuals, families, and groups. NP education provides theoretical and evidence-based clinical knowledge and learning experiences for role development as an NP [2]. The emphasis in a graduate NP program is on the development of the clinical and professional expertise necessary for comprehensive primary and specialty care.

PAs are healthcare professionals who practice medicine as members of a team with their supervising physicians. PAs deliver a broad range of medical and surgical services to diverse populations in rural and urban settings. As part of their comprehensive responsibilities, PAs conduct physical exams, diagnose and treat illnesses, order and interpret tests, counsel on preventive health care, assist in surgery, and prescribe medications [3]. The scope of practice for a PA is defined by four parameters: state law, institutional policy, education and experience, and physician delegation. PA education and training mirrors that of physicians; rigorous coursework in medicine is followed by over 2000 hours of supervised clinical practice in diverse healthcare institutions and medical practices. PAs practice in all areas of medicine, surgery, and subspecialties.

There has been a steady growth in the utilization of NPs and PAs, and the United States Bureau of Labor Statistics projected that the number of PA jobs would increase by 27%

Moderate and Deep Sedation in Clinical Practice, ed. Richard D. Urman and Alan D. Kaye.
Published by Cambridge University Press. © Cambridge University Press 2012.

between 2006 and 2016. The Patient Protection and Affordable Care Act of 2010 included several aspects that will encourage the continued utilization of NPs and PAs to deliver health care, including the provision of financial support for PA training and the establishment of new NP-led clinics. Academic medical centers are hiring NPs and PAs to improve patient care access, to increase patient throughput, to improve continuity of care, to reduce length of stay, and to fill the workforce shortage created by restrictions placed on resident work hours.

Regulatory considerations

There are several entities that govern how NPs and PAs can practice. These include but are not limited to the Centers for Medicare and Medicaid Systems (CMS), Medicare Conditions of Participation (CoP), the Joint Commission (TJC), state law, private payor policies, established institutional polices, medical staff bylaws, and the defined scopes of practice of the NP or PA. This is important to recognize because language contained within the respective policies can be contradictory and/or interpreted differently by different institutions. The following sections provide clarification on each of the entities' policies regarding NPs and PAs providing moderate sedation and highlight the nuances of such language.

The Centers for Medicare and Medicaid Systems (CMS) and The Joint Commission (TJC)

Neither CMS nor TJC policies prohibit NPs or PAs from administering moderate sedation. The policies do prohibit NPs and PAs from administering deep sedation, as this level of sedation is classified as a type of anesthesia which requires specific medical training not obtained by NPs and PAs.

Interpretive guidelines for the anesthesia services condition of participation (Section 42 CFR 482.52) of the CMS *Manual* outlines the requirements an organization must meet if it furnishes "anesthesia services" [4]. These guidelines define what types of services are considered anesthesia and who may administer such services. Because minimal and moderate sedation are not classified as anesthesia, the guidelines covering who may administer these two types of sedation are not dictated by the guidelines for the administration of anesthesia. This is an important distinction, and it is the reason why NPs and PAs may administer minimal and moderate sedation but not deep sedation.

These same guidelines still have an impact on NP and PA practice, because they require that the organization's anesthesia department be responsible for developing policies and procedures governing the provision of all categories of "anesthesia services," including specifying the minimum qualifications for each category of practitioner who is permitted to provide "anesthesia services" that are not subject to the anesthesia administration requirements of 42 CFR 482.52(a), which would include minimal and moderate sedation.

The Joint Commission's anesthesia care standards do not define specifically who can administer sedation but require that the individuals who are permitted to administer sedation are able to rescue patients at whatever level of sedation or anesthesia achieved, either intentionally or unintentionally [5]. Each organization is tasked with defining how it will determine whether these individuals are able to perform the required types of rescue. Because sedation is a continuum, it is not always possible to predict how an individual patient will respond, and the level of sedation has the potential to become deeper than initially intended. "Rescue" from a deeper level of sedation is defined by CMS as the correction of the adverse physiologic consequences of the deeper-than-intended level of sedation that returns the patient to the originally intended level of sedation. Rescue requires that the provider administering the sedation has the ability to fulfill this responsibility, which requires advanced training and may include advanced life support, airway management, and/or courses created by an institution specifically for this purpose. For moderate sedation, rescue implies the ability to manage a compromised airway or hypoventilation. Advanced training can be successfully completed by both NPs and PAs and is often a component of training required to provide other types of care within their clinical roles.

TJC language around sedation and throughout their policies includes the term "licensed independent practitioner" (LIP). This language creates confusion because PAs as professionals are not defined as LIPs. In response to this confusion, TJC has added the following language to the definition of LIP: "When standards reference the term licensed independent practitioner, this language is not to be construed to limit the authority of a licensed independent practitioner to delegate tasks to other qualified health care personnel (for example, physician assistants and advanced practice registered nurses) to the extent authorized by state law or a state's regulatory mechanism or federal guidelines and organizational policy" [6].

State laws and regulations

Individual states have the ability to regulate anesthesia practices, which can be more restrictive than federal laws and CMS and TJC policies. In the last decade there has been a growth of professionals who administer anesthesia, such as Certified Registered Nurse Anesthetists (CRNAs) and Anesthesia Assistants (AAs). This has created a need for states to review their laws and determine the types of professionals allowed to practice within their state, the scopes of practice of those professionals, and whether or not they require professional registration or licensure. In many cases these decisions have preempted statute and regulation language changes which include a definition of what constitutes anesthesia.

Depending on how states define anesthesia determines whether the different levels of sedation are included or excluded from anesthesia regulations. In some states the definition has inadvertently prohibited NPs and PAs from administering any kind of sedation. This is problematic because a large percentage of NPs and PAs practice in procedural areas and/or provide care where pain management and patient comfort are best achieved with some form of sedation.

PA laws generally state that a physician may delegate any legal task for which the PA is appropriately trained. The problem arises when the task the physician would like to delegate is a task that is prohibited in other sections of state law. Anesthesia and sedation are typically tasks addressed in state laws outside of the ones defining physician and PA practice. When there is a discrepancy between the two languages it must be determined which law has precedence. If the reader encounters this type of discrepancy, the state regulatory body governing medical and PA practice may provide guidance and help make this determination.

Institutional policies and privileging

TJC and CMS policies drive the need to develop institutional policy for moderate and deep sedation for non-anesthesiologists and non-anesthetists. This policy may be included in the medical staff bylaws or as a separate policy. In order to comply with CMS regulations, the policy must include criteria for determining the "anesthesia services" privileges to be granted to an individual practitioner and a procedure for applying the criteria to individuals requesting the privileges. CMS policies require that "anesthesia services" includes the administration of moderate sedation even though it is not classified specifically as anesthesia. NPs and PAs need to be included in the institutional policy as types of providers allowed to administer moderate sedation. In addition, the guidelines will need to outline the training required to meet the necessary competencies to safely administer moderate sedation and a process to audit outcomes. Institutions have the option of mandating that if an institution intends to allow NPs and/or PAs to perform moderation sedation, NPs and PAs receive the same training as their non-anesthesia physician colleagues or requiring that they receive additional training.

PAs practice with a supervising physician, and NPs with a collaborating physician. State laws determine how close the supervising and collaborating physician's relationship needs to be with the PA and NP, respectively. The laws governing PA practice in general allow the supervising physician to delegate those tasks he or she determines the PA to be competent in. Because of this relationship a PA's scope of practice is determined by the supervising physician's scope of practice, and therefore if a PA is going to be privileged to administer moderate sedation the supervising physician should have equivalent privileges. In some states NPs practice independently, and equivalent privileges may not be required.

Credentialing, privileging, and education

TJC's policies address the credentialing and privileging of practitioners, including those of NPs and PAs. These policies require that privileging is competency-based, with defined criteria to meet and maintain competency. TJC does not require that moderate sedation be included as a separately delineated privilege, and it may be defined and included in procedure-based privileges. This does not preclude an institution's decision to have separate delineated privileges specifically for moderate sedation. In either scenario, the privileging must specify whatever training the institution has determined to be necessary for that practitioner to have the capacity to rescue the patient, as discussed above. NPs and PAs do not necessarily receive training in advanced life support and advanced airway management as part of their baseline education, and therefore it is important for an institution to provide such training. During the training process NPs and PAs should be made aware of any state laws that restrict their practice in the administration of moderate sedation.

Competency-based privileging requires an institution to define a process to assess a practitioner's ability to perform requested privileges competently and safely. The assessment of the ability of all practitioners, including NPs and PAs, to administer moderate sedation should include case audits and an internal review of any complications. In addition, an institution may determine that an NP or PA cannot obtain privileging unless their collaborating or supervising physician has equivalent privileging.

NP and PA educational requirements specific to the administration of moderate sedation should be at a minimum those of a non-anesthesia physician and should contain all the components outlined in Chapter 6.

Clinical practice

NPs and PAs who administer moderate sedation are responsible for the pre-procedure patient evaluation, which includes a history and physical, review of any previous adverse effects of sedation, and an airway assessment (see Chapter 4). As for a physician, there should be a process in place that allows NPs and PAs to consult anesthesia if they feel it is needed at any time.

In general, NPs and PAs spend the majority of their time as clinical care providers, which allows them to gain years of experience in the procedures they are performing. In many cases, the NPs and PAs become some of the more qualified to perform the procedures, administer the sedation, and perform the patient evaluation. All practitioners should have the ability to manage complications during moderate sedation and the ability to activate the appropriate emergency response team for that practice area.

Summary

Community and Academic Medical centers are employing nurse practitioners (NPs) and physician assistants (PAs) to improve patient care access, increase patient throughput, improve continuity of care, reduce length of stay and to fill the workforce shortage created by restrictions placed on resident work hours. NPs and PAs, in general, spend the majority of their time as clinical care providers which allows them to gain years of experience in the procedures they are performing. In many cases, the NPs and PAs are qualified to perform the procedures, administer the sedation and perform the patient evaluation. There are several entities that govern how NPs and PAs can practice. These include but are not limited to: the Centers for Medicare Systems (CMS), Medicare Conditions of Participation (CoP), The Joint Commission, state law, private payer policies, established institutional polices and medical staff bylaws and the defined scopes of practice of the NP or PA. In this chapter we attempt to provide clarification on each of the entities' policies regarding NPs and PAs administering moderate sedation and highlight the nuances of such language. All practitioners should have the ability to manage complications during moderate sedation and have the ability to activate the appropriate emergency response team for that practice area.

References

1. American Academy of Nurse Practitioners. *Quality of Nurse Practitioner Practice*. Fact sheet. Austin, TX: AANP, 2007.

2. American Academy of Nurse Practitioners. Position statement on nurse practitioner curriculum. Austin, TX: AANP, 2010.

3. American Academy of Physician Assistants. *2008 AAPA Physician Assistant Census Report*. Alexandria, VA: AAPA, 2008. www.aapa.org/images/stories/2008aapacensusnationalreport.pdf (accessed June 2011).

4. Centers for Medicare and Medicaid Systems. CMS Manual System: interpretive guidelines for the anesthesia services condition of participation, May 2010. www.cms.gov/transmittals/ downloads/R59SOMA.pdf (accessed June 2011).

5. The Joint Commission. Introduction to Standards PC.03.01.01 through PC.03.01.07, July 2010. e-dition.jcrinc.com/ Standard.aspx (accessed June 2011).

6. The Joint Commission. CAMH *Refreshed Core*, January 2010, GL-16.

Further reading

American Society of Anesthesiologists Task Force on Sedation and Analgesia by Non-Anesthesiologists. Practice guidelines for sedation and analgesia by non-anesthesiologists. *Anesthesiology* 2002; **96**: 1004–17.

Watson DS, Odom-Forren J. *Practical Guide to Moderate Sedation/Analgesia*, 2nd edn. New York, NY: Mosby, 2005.

Chapter 10

High-risk patients: sedation considerations in coexisting disease

Charles Fox, Henry Liu, Michael Yarborough,
Mary Elise Fox, and Alan D. Kaye

Introduction

Certain patient populations requiring sedation for procedures present the clinician with challenging decisions regarding their care and management. Some underlying medical disease states, airway abnormalities, or extremes of age require cautious pre-procedural assessment and planning when sedation is required to minimize the incidence of morbidity or mortality. It should be noted that some of these higher-risk patients should only be sedated by trained anesthesia providers. The following commonly encountered conditions are considered high risk and are associated with a higher rate of complications: old age, obesity, chronic obstructive pulmonary disease, coronary artery disease, and chronic renal failure. This chapter will discuss important features of these higher-risk patients and practice management when sedation is required.

The elderly

The elderly population (65 years of age or older) is a rapidly growing segment of our society. The Census Bureau predicts that by 2030 one in five Americans (71 million) will be older than 65. Currently, we have 36 million Americans who are older than 65. Although those individuals considered elderly are at higher risk for complications, the more accurate predictor of outcome may be the patient's physiologic age. This may be determined more clearly during a pre-procedure evaluation. For example, a 65-year-old patient who is wheelchair-bound may be considered higher risk than an 85-year-old marathon runner. Careful pre-procedure evaluation of the patient's coexisting diseases and medications, and a thorough physical examination, are the initial steps in risk stratification for these patients. Knowledge of the physiologic changes associated with aging is important when trying to determine a medication plan for sedation (Table 10.1).

Moderate and Deep Sedation in Clinical Practice, ed. Richard D. Urman and Alan D. Kaye.
Published by Cambridge University Press. © Cambridge University Press 2012.

Table 10.1. Physiological differences and sedation considerations in the elderly population

System	Physiological differences	Sedation considerations
Cardiovascular	Reduced tissue elasticity in arteries and veins Ventricular hypertrophy Reduced cardiac output Reduced arterial oxygenation Deterioration of the cardiac conduction system	Increased oxygen consumption Inability of the body to adjust to hemodynamic changes Higher likelihood of arrhythmias Slower cardiorespiratory response to hypercarbia and hypoxia
Body composition	Higher proportion of body fat Less intracellular fluid	Expanded distribution volume for pharmacologic agents Higher risk of oversedation with water-soluble drugs Slower recovery period for lipid-soluble drugs
Pulmonary	Decreased respiratory drive Less lung capacity Diminished response to hypoxemia or hypercarbia Increased work of breathing due to loss of chest wall elasticity	Decreased ability for the body to compensate for respiratory depression caused by sedative agents Higher incidence of transient apnea
Neurological	Loss of neuronal density Reduced levels of neurotransmitters	Increased sensitivity to CNS-depressant drugs Higher incidence of confusion and delirium with sedation
Renal	Reduced blood flow to the kidneys Decreased glomerular filtration rate	Increased risk of renal insufficiency Longer duration of action for some anesthetics and adjuvant drugs
Hepatic	Reduced blood flow to the liver Less liver enzyme activity	Increased duration of action for lipid-soluble drugs Altered metabolism of drugs
Airway	Diminished gag reflex Chronic microaspirations Loss of teeth and use of dentures Arthritis of the neck	Increases risk of aspiration Difficulty in mask ventilation Difficulty performing head-tilt, jaw-thrust maneuver of airway

Adapted from www.sedationfacts.org (accessed December 2010).

Cardiovascular system

A large portion of the elderly report participation in strenuous and frequent athletic activities, so the patient's self-reported list of daily activities and exercise tolerance provides the best initial assessment of cardiac function. This can be more accurately expressed in metabolic equivalent levels (METs). Patients achieving a level of 4 METs or higher have a significantly decreased risk of complications. If the patient has a limited exercise tolerance, then chemical stress testing, stress echocardiography, or cardiac catheterization should be considered to explore possible etiologies and degree of cardio-vascular disease before proceeding with sedation.

Elderly patients experience a reduction in exercise tolerance (maximally obtainable cardiac output, heart rate, and stroke volume) and progressive loss of vascular elasticity. This loss of elasticity commonly leads to a compensatory left ventricular hypertrophy and hypertension. Chronic elevation of blood pressure leads to decreased baroreceptor sensitivity. If this process continues, the development of congestive heart failure is common. Lastly, it should be recognized that the elderly have an increased incidence of coronary artery disease and valvular heart disease.

The majority of medications used for sedation produce a vasodilatory effect, while a smaller percentage also depress cardiac function. Typical patients with chronic hypertension have overly constricted arterioles and consequently a reduction in intravascular volume. Long-standing hypertension, valvular disease, or coronary artery disease may result in depression of ventricular function. Depending upon the type and dose of medication administered and level of sedation achieved, these patients can experience clinically signi-ficant hemodynamic changes, including drops in blood pressure. An excellent example is seen in the response to propofol, which in any population can cause significant hypotension.

Respiratory system

The respiratory system undergoes numerous changes related to aging. The upper airway protective reflexes (coughing and swallowing) are diminished in the elderly by the reduction in nerve ending of irritant receptors. This potentially results in chronic alveolar inflammation and loss of alveolar surface area from constant microaspirations. Thus, elderly patients can potentially aspirate with no or low levels of sedation, so the clinician must constantly assess the patient's level of consciousness and aggressively seek to eliminate risks for aspiration.

The elderly lose chest wall elasticity and respiratory muscle mass and see an increase in turbulent flow in airway passages as they narrow. Because of these changes, the elderly experience reductions in forced vital capacity and forced expiratory volume at 1 second, and increased air trapping, closing capacity, and respiratory residual volume. The summation of these changes is a reduction in arterial oxygenation and an increase in the work of breathing, and this is reflected in the increased incidence of shortness of breath that elderly people experience when performing their daily activities. Mean arterial oxygenation tension averages 70 mmHg at age 80, which is significantly decreased from the oxygen tension of 95 mmHg at age 20. Additionally, the elderly have a decreased responsiveness to hypercapnia and hypoxemia. Therefore, these patients are at increased risk for considerable respiratory depression when receiving sedation medications. With the epidemic of smokers worldwide, an elderly patient can easily have damaged lungs, which will be discussed later in this chapter.

Hepatic and renal systems

Hepatic and renal changes seen in the elderly primarily reflect reduction in cardiac output. This reduction decreases hepatic and renal blood flow, dramatically affecting their meta-bolic capabilities. Also, in the liver there is a reduction in protein synthesis. These two changes in liver physiology decrease drug metabolism and mandate decreased dosing with sedation medications. The reduction in renal blood flow decreases the glomerular filtration rate and prolongs the elimination half-time of drugs cleared by the kidneys. Additionally, renal parenchymal atrophy results in a 50% reduction in glomeruli by age 80, and the kidneys reduce their ability to conserve free water and concentrate urine changes as we age.

Central nervous system

Aging causes multiple changes in the central nervous system. By age 80, there is a 30% reduction in brain mass and a concomitant decrease in serotonin, dopamine, and acetyl-choline receptors. The incidence of diseases such as Parkinson's and Alzheimer's increases as one ages. For example, 3% of people aged 66 have symptoms of Parkinson's, and by age 85 that number increases to 50%. Delirium, a disturbance of consciousness that limits one's ability to focus or shift attention, affects 10–15% of elderly hospitalized patients. Patients with a history of preexisting cognitive dysfunction experience delirium and cognitive dysfunction more frequently post procedure. An understanding of the patient's baseline cognitive function should be established before sedation medications are administered.

Temperature regulation

The ability to regulate body temperature is diminished in elderly patients. Shivering does not occur until a much lower temperature, and the ability to vasoconstrict or conserve heat is impaired in this population. These factors, together with a decreased ability to generate body heat (lower metabolic rate), increase the time needed to recover from hypothermia and can dramatically increase the time required to metabolize and clear sedation medications. Forced-air warming of the patient, along with warming intravenous solutions and warming the procedure room, can help prevent hypothermia in these patients.

Obesity

The rate of obesity in the United States has increased dramatically in the last decade. In 1990, the incidence of adult obesity was less than 15%; by 2000, that percentage had increased to 27%. Some estimate that over 67% of our adult population is either overweight or obese. Annually, obesity is responsible for more than 300,000 premature deaths and more than $100 billion of related costs. The rate of obesity now affects 17% of children between the ages of 2 and 19. This rate has tripled in the last two decades.

The calculation of overweight, obesity, or morbid obesity is based on a patient's body mass index (BMI). BMI is calculated using the patient's height and weight:

$$BMI = [weight(kg)]/[height(m)]^2$$

or

$$BMI = [weight(lb)]/[height(inches)]^2 \times 703$$

A BMI > 25 is considered overweight while a BMI > 30 is considered obese. An individual with a BMI > 40 is considered morbidly obese.

These patients present a multitude of challenges for the clinician (Table 10.2). Special gowns, operating room tables, monitoring equipment, stretchers, and wheelchairs are needed to properly care for these individuals. They also have anatomical, organ-system, and pharmacokinetic changes which add complexity to their care. A subset of these patients have advanced anatomical and physiologic changes, resulting in diseases such as obstructive sleep apnea, coronary artery disease, and pulmonary hypertension, which may warrant sedation by trained anesthesia providers.

Table 10.2. Health consequences of severe obesity

High blood pressure
Diabetes
Heart disease
Joint and bone problems
Sleep apnea
Decreased self-esteem
Decreased mobility/daily function
Decreased longevity
Higher incidence of nerve injury under sedation

Table 10.3. Pulmonary and respiratory changes in the obese patient

Increased oxygen consumption due to the metabolic activity of fat
Increased energy expenditure in breathing due to increased chest and abdomen wall mass
Obese patients desaturate faster
Airway changes can make ventilation difficult

Pulmonary and airway systems

Many critical changes happen to both the pulmonary system and the airway in people who are obese (Table 10.3).

The extra weight added to the thoracic cage and abdominal cavity restricts thoracic wall and diaphragmatic movement. This process progresses to a restrictive lung disease (Figure 10.1), initially reducing functional residual capacity (FRC) and expiratory reserve volume. The functional residual capacity serves as the oxygen "storage tank," and this is reduced exponentially with increasing BMI (Figure 10.2). As BMI continues to increase, airway closure ensues when FRC equals closing capacity. Morbid obesity causes reduction in vital capacity and total lung capacity, and the added weight reduces chest wall compliance and increases airway resistance. These changes are accentuated by medications that cause respiratory depression when the obese patient is sedated in the supine position. Also, obese individuals have increases in both oxygen consumption, which can be double or triple that of lean patients, and carbon dioxide production. Therefore, the rate of desaturation is much faster in the obese patient (Figure 10.2).

Obstructive sleep apnea (OSA) is present in 5% of obese patients. OSA increases postoperative complication rates, increases the need for intensive care intervention, and prolongs hospital stays. OSA is associated with serious health consequences, such as stroke and a number of cardiovascular conditions – hypertension, coronary artery disease, and atrial fibrillation.

With sleep apnea, breathing stops and starts as one sleeps. These individuals have redundant adipose and soft tissue that narrows the airway. Pharyngeal patency and

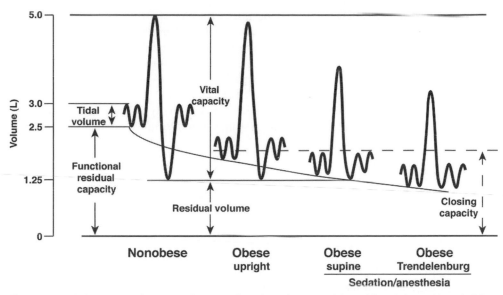

Figure 10.1. Pulmonary mechanics as a function of weight and position. Adapted from Baker and Yagiela [1].

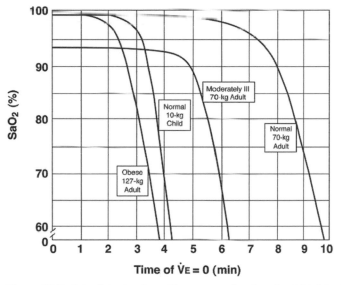

Figure 10.2. Rate of desaturation with apnea as a function of weight. Adapted from Benumof et al. [2].

prevention of airway collapse are dependent on the action of pharyngeal muscle tone. This tone is decreased during sleep or sedation, resulting in airway obstruction. As the disease advances, some patients will develop obesity hypoventilation syndrome, which can progress into "Pickwickian syndrome." This syndrome is characterized by gross obesity, somnolence, periodic breathing (when awake), hypercapnea, hypoxemia, polycythemia, and pulmonary hypertension. Patients with obstructive sleep apnea are considered high risk for obstruction when sedated and should be approached cautiously by the clinician. Because these patients are usually sedated by anesthesiologists or nurse anesthetists, they should be screened pre-procedurally by the sedation service to avoid potential mishaps. Failure to recognize OSA preoperatively is one of the major causes of post-procedural complications.

Presently, there are three commonly used screening tools for OSA: the Berlin questionnaire (Table 10.4), the American Society of Anesthesiologists (ASA) checklist (Table 10.5), and the STOP-BANG questionnaire (Table 10.6). The STOP-BANG questionnaire was developed by Dr. Frances Chung and colleagues at the University of Toronto, and currently it is the only one of the three which has been validated in a surgical population [3].

Cardiovascular system

There are many changes in the cardiovascular system of obese people (Table 10.7). Systemic hypertension, ischemic heart disease, and congestive heart failure are common cardiovascular issues found in the obese patient. Mild to moderate systemic hypertension is found in approximately 50–60% of the obese population. Obesity-induced hypertension is commonly associated with hypervolemia (increased extracellular fluid volume) and increased cardiac output. Cardiac output increases approximately 0.1 L/minute for each kilogram of weight gained related to fat tissue. Over time, this increase in systemic hypertension and cardiac output can result in cardiomegaly.

Obesity is an independent risk factor for the development of heart disease. Ischemic heart disease is commonly found in patients with a central distribution of fat. Lastly, these individuals are at higher risk for diabetes mellitus and hypercholesterolemia, which are significant risk factors for the development of ischemic heart disease.

Concentric left ventricular hypertrophy can develop over time in patients with systemic hypertension. This increase in ventricular mass eventually causes a decrease in ventricular compliance. In obese patients, coupled with hypervolemia, this increases the risk of congestive heart failure and the development of obesity-induced cardiomyopathy.

Gastrointestinal system

Obesity invokes changes in the gastrointestinal system over time. Although many believe that the increased intra-abdominal pressure, higher rate of hiatal hernias, and increased rate of gastroesophageal reflux exists in this population and leads to an increased risk for aspiration pneumonitis, it is not true. The obese population, without symptoms of gastroesophageal reflux, experiences the same gradient between the stomach and esophagus as the non-obese population. However, gastric emptying in this population may be increased when compared to the non-obese patient. The high incidence of diabetes in the obese population, this will affect how most providers administer sedation. Given that all diabetic patients have a degree of gastroparesis and therefore a risk of aspiration, NPO status should be carefully evaluated when sedation is planned. It is typical, although not uniform, practice to intravenously administer an H_2-blocker such as famotidine and a drug that will increase gastric emptying such as metoclopramide.

The changes invoked by obesity commonly invade the hepatobiliary section of the gastrointestinal system. Fatty infiltration of the liver and the development of gallbladder and biliary tract disease are the most common culprits in obese patients. This may influence the pharmacokinetics (distribution, binding, and elimination) of sedation medications. The volume of distribution is increased because of the hypervolemia and increased

Table 10.4. Berlin questionnaire for obstructive sleep apnea

Height (m) _____ Weight (kg) _____ Age_____ Male/Female

Please choose the correct response to each question

Category 1

1. Do you snore?
   - ☐ (a) Yes
   - ☐ (b) No
   - ☐ (c) Don't know

If you snore:

2. **Your snoring is:**
   - ☐ (a) Slightly louder than breathing
   - ☐ (b) As loud as talking
   - ☐ (c) Louder than talking
   - ☐ (d) Very loud – can be heard in adjacent rooms

3. **How often do you snore?**
   - ☐ (a) Nearly every day
   - ☐ (b) 3–4 times a week
   - ☐ (c) 1–2 times a week
   - ☐ (d) 1–2 times a month
   - ☐ (e) Never or nearly never

4. **Has your snoring ever bothered other people?**
   - ☐ (a) Yes
   - ☐ (b) No
   - ☐ (c) Don't Know

5. **Has anyone noticed that you quit breathing during your sleep?**
   - ☐ (a) Nearly every day
   - ☐ (b) 3–4 times a week
   - ☐ (c) 1–2 times a week
   - ☐ (d) 1–2 times a month
   - ☐ (e) Never or nearly never

Category 2

6. **How often do you feel tired or fatigued after your sleep?**
   - ☐ (a) Nearly every day
   - ☐ (b) 3–4 times a week
   - ☐ (c) 1–2 times a week
   - ☐ (d) 1–2 times a month
   - ☐ (e) Never or nearly never

7. **During your waking time, do you feel tired, fatigued, or not up to par?**
   - ☐ (a) Nearly every day
   - ☐ (b) 3–4 times a week
   - ☐ (c) 1–2 times a week
   - ☐ (d) 1–2 times a month
   - ☐ (e) Never or nearly never

Table 10.4. *(cont.)*

Height (m) _____ Weight (kg) _____ Age_____ Male/Female
Please choose the correct response to each question

8. **Have you ever nodded off or fallen asleep while driving a vehicle?**
   □ (a) Yes
   □ (b) No

If yes:

9. **How often does this occur?**
   □ (a) Nearly every day
   □ (b) 3–4 times a week
   □ (c) 1–2 times a week
   □ (d) 1–2 times a month
   □ (e) Never or nearly never

Category 3

10. **Do you have high blood pressure?**
    □ Yes
    □ No
    □ Don't know

Categories and scoring

Category 1: items 1, 2, 3, 4, 5
Item 1: if "yes," assign **1 point**
Item 2: if "c" or "d" is the response, assign **1 point**
Item 3: if "a" or "b" is the response, assign **1 point**
Item 4: if "a" is the response, assign **1 point**
Item 5: if "a" or "b" is the response, assign **2 points**

Add points. Category 1 is positive if the total score is 2 or more points

Category 2: items 6, 7, 8 (item 9 should be noted separately)
Item 6: if "a" or "b" is the response, assign **1 point**
Item 7: if "a" or "b" is the response, assign **1 point**
Item 8: if "a" is the response, assign **1 point**

Add points. Category 2 is positive if the total score is 2 or more points

Category 3 is positive if the answer to item 10 is "yes" OR if the BMI of the patient is greater than 30 kg/m^2

(BMI must be calculated. BMI is defined as weight (kg) divided by height (m) squared, i.e., kg/m^2).

High risk: if there are 2 or more categories where the score is positive

Low risk: if there is only 1 or no categories where the score is positive

Additional question: item 9 should be noted separately

Adapted from Chung *et al.* [3].

Table 10.5. American Society of Anesthesiologists (ASA) checklist for obstructive sleep apnea

Category 1: predisposing physical characteristics

  (a) BMI: 35 kg/m^2

  (b) Neck circumference: 43 cm/17 inches (men) or 40 cm/16 inches (women)

  (c) Craniofacial abnormalities affecting the airway

  (d) Anatomical nasal obstruction

  (e) Tonsils nearly touching or touching the midline

Category 2: history of apparent airway obstruction during sleep

Two or more of the following are present (if patient lives alone or sleep is not observed by another person, then only one of the following need be present)

  (a) Snoring (loud enough to be heard through closed door)

  (b) Frequent snoring

  (c) Observed pauses in breathing during sleep

  (d) Awakens from sleep with choking sensation

  (e) Frequent arousals from sleep

Category 3: somnolence

One or more of the following is present

  (a) Frequent somnolence or fatigue despite adequate "sleep"

  (b) Falls asleep easily in a nonstimulating environment (e.g., watching TV, reading, riding in or driving a car) despite adequate "sleep"

  (c) [Parent or teacher comments that child appears sleepy during the day, is easily distracted, is overly aggressive, or has difficulty concentrating] [a]

  (d) [Child often difficult to arouse at usual awakening time] [a]

Scoring:

  If two or more items in category 1 are positive, category 1 is positive

  If two or more items in category 2 are positive, category 2 is positive

  If one or more items in category 3 are positive, category 3 is positive

  High risk of OSA: two or more categories scored as positive

  Low risk of OSA: only one or no category scored as positive

Adapted from Gross *et al.* [4].
[a]Items in brackets refer to pediatric patients.

cardiac output experienced by obese patients. If liver disease exists, reductions in protein binding can occur, but the overall effects are variable. The elimination of medications can be slowed, especially in obese patients with congestive heart failure. It is not a surprise that providing sedation to this group of patients results in higher morbidity and mortality (Table 10.8).

Table 10.6. STOP-BANG screening for obstructive sleep apnea

STOP		
S (snore)	Have you been told that you snore?	YES/NO
T (tired)	Are you often tired during the day?	YES/NO
O (obstruction)	Do you know if you stop breathing or has anyone witnessed you stop breathing while you are asleep?	YES/NO
P (pressure)	Do you have high blood pressure or on medication to control high blood pressure?	YES/NO
If you answered YES to two or more questions on the STOP portion you are at risk for obstructive sleep apnea.		
To find out if you are at moderate to severe risk of obstructive sleep apnea, complete the BANG questions below.		
BANG		
B (BMI)	Is your body mass index greater than 28?	YES/NO
A (age)	Are you 50 years old or older?	YES/NO
N (neck)	Are you a male with a neck circumference greater than 17 inches, or a female with a neck circumference greater than 16 inches?	YES/NO
G (gender)	Are you a male?	YES/NO
The more questions you answer YES to on the BANG portion, the greater your risk of having moderate to severe obstructive sleep apnea		
≥ 3 yes answers: high risk for OSA		
< 3 yes answers: low risk for OSA		

Adapted from Chung *et al.* [3].

Table 10.7. Cardiovascular changes in the obese patient

Hypertension, congestive heart failure, and pulmonary hypertension are more likely in these patients, adding to the challenge of managing safe anesthesia delivery

Framingham study demonstrated direct link between blood pressure and weight
    ↑blood volume with obesity
    ↑stroke volume with obesity
    ↑cardiac output with obesity

↑Pulmonary wedge pressures
    pulmonary hypertension
    especially when aggravated by perioperative hypoxic vasoconstriction in the lung

Moderate hypertension is seen in 50%
Risk of ischemic heart disease is doubled in the obese patient

Table 10.8. Sedation issues with overweight patients

Increased risk of complications

Difficulty with maintaining and recovering the airway

Increased risk of positioning injuries

Increased comorbidities (e.g., diabetes, coronary artery disease, obstructive sleep apnea)

Chronic obstructive pulmonary disease

Chronic obstructive pulmonary disease (COPD) is a common pulmonary disorder that affects millions of people worldwide. COPD is frequently found in patients with chronic bronchitis or emphysema. It is characterized as a progressive inflammatory process and/or parenchymal destruction of small airways resulting in increased resistance to expiratory gas flow. These patients need a prolonged period of time for lung emptying. The process may be fixed or variable (reversible with medications), and some patients have features of both.

Because of increased airway resistance and/or parenchymal destruction, patients with COPD have an inefficient gas exchange. The muscles of respiration must generate a significantly greater negative pressure to overcome the increased airway resistance and over time become dysfunctional. This dysfunction ultimately leads to hypoxemia and hypercapnia. Chronic hypercarbia resets the central receptor, thus blunting the ventilatory response to carbon dioxide. Most sedation medications compromise this response and, in the patient with COPD, can result in severe respiratory depression and significant complications if the patient is oversedated. Lastly, most procedures are performed in the supine position, which impairs chest wall muscle function, further reducing functional residual capacity and oxygenation.

Patients with COPD should have a thorough pre-procedural evaluation to ensure that any reversible component to their disease (e.g., bronchospasm, infection) is maximally treated with appropriate drugs (e.g., bronchodilators, antibiotics, or corticosteroids) before proceeding. Bronchodilators should be administered before initiation of sedation, and supplemental oxygen and airway management equipment must be readily available. Sedation medication should be slowly titrated in smaller doses and used sparingly. If possible, local anesthetics should be used in combination with sedation medication to reduce dosing of the latter.

Common procedural complications in this patient population include hypoventilation (hypoxemia and hypercapnia) and bronchospasm. Bronchospasm manifests as wheezing, and it is commonly caused by an exacerbation of the patient's COPD, but an anaphylactoid reaction to a sedation medication should be ruled out.

Coronary artery disease

Patients with coronary artery disease (CAD) present a multitude of challenges for the clinician. This disease presents with various symptoms or conditions, and regardless of the "indicator" (chest pain, exercise intolerance, hypertension, congestive heart failure, or valvular heart disease), the patient presenting with any of the above should be explored meticulously before receiving sedation. There are several issues in these patients that should be cleared up before proceeding.

Frequently, patients presenting for sedation have a history of angina. In the pre-procedure evaluation, the clinician needs to identify if the condition is stable or unstable. Unstable angina is characterized by a change in frequency, intensity, or duration from the "usual" pattern of angina or if it does not recede with rest or the use of angina medication. Any angina patient classified as unstable should be evaluated by a cardiologist before proceeding with sedation.

Exercise tolerance is a central element of any pre-procedure evaluation. This serves as a rough estimate of the patient's left ventricular ejection fraction and correlates with the heart's ability to function during stressful events. Since patients with coronary artery disease struggle with both oversedation and undersedation, this serves as a useful predictive guide. Anesthesiologists commonly ask patients if they can climb two flights of stairs without chest pain or shortness of breath. This approximates 4 METs and is the amount of cardiac reserve needed by a patient when starting or concluding an anesthetic for surgery.

Striking the balance between adequate sedation and maximal cardiac functioning can be difficult. Patients with known CAD who become oversedated experience cardiac complications related to hypotension and/or hypoxemia. On the other hand, the undersedated patient experiences an increase in anxiety and pain, which stimulates the release of catecholamines, and increases the demands on the heart. Because of this, all cardiac medications, especially beta-blockers and statins, should be taken on the day of the procedure. Oxygen is always advised for these patients, and the "MONA" (morphine, oxygen, nitroglycerin, and aspirin) protocol should serve as an initial treatment plan if cardiac ischemia occurs.

Chronic renal failure

Chronic renal failure is a progressive permanent loss of renal function, and it is caused by a multitude of diseases. Hypertension and diabetes mellitus are the two leading causes. These patients ultimately lose significant renal function and require dialysis or transplantation. The manifestations of chronic renal failure are summarized in Table 10.9.

When these patients present for their pre-procedure evaluation, a thorough medication list, post-dialysis labs, and exploration of other comorbidities should be undertaken before

Table 10.9. Manifestations of chronic renal failure

Electrolyte imbalance	Hyperkalemia, hypermagnesemia, hypocalcemia
Metabolic acidosis	
Unpredictable intravascular fluid status	
Anemia	Increased cardiac output, and oxyhemoglobin dissociation curve shifted to the right
Uremic coagulopathies	Platelet dysfunction
Neurologic changes	Encephalopathy
Cardiovascular changes	Systemic hypertension, congestive heart failure, attenuated sympathetic nervous system activity due to antihypertensive drugs

proceeding with the case. All antihypertensive medication should be taken on the day that the procedure is to be performed, and because many of these patients are diabetics there should be a mechanism in place for glucose management. Ideally these patients should undergo dialysis within 24 hours of the planned procedure. Knowledge of the pre- and post-dialysis weight will help the clinician better understand the fluid status of the individual. Lastly, the post-dialysis potassium level should not exceed 5.5 mEq/L.

Medication used for sedation should be titrated in slowly, carefully watching hemodynamic response to the medication. These patients are commonly hypertensive and have a decreased intravascular volume or they may respond as if they were hypovolemic because of the central nervous system effects of the antihypertensive medication when combined with the sedation medication. Because of this, they should always be treated as if they were hypovolemic.

Many pharmacokinetic changes occur in these patients. Hypoalbuminemia and acidosis are usually present, and this can increase the free drug availability of medications that are highly protein-bound. Benzodiazepine dosing should therefore be reduced in this patient population. Most post-dialysis patients have a decreased volume of distribution, and therefore reduced dosing requirements.

Certain sedation medications should be avoided or used very cautiously in patients with chronic renal failure. Meperidine should be avoided because it produces a metabolite, normeperidine, which accumulates in these patients, increasing the risk of seizures. Also, morphine produces a neurotoxic metabolite that is nondialyzable, so it should be avoided in this patient population. Fentanyl is an attractive option, because it produces no active metabolites, but it should be slowly titrated to avoid complications.

Summary

Certain patient populations provide challenging clinical situations for the sedation provider. Patients with cardiovascular disease, chronic obstructive pulmonary disease, chronic renal failure, obesity, or advanced age are considered high risk and possess a higher rate of procedural complications. Because of this, they should have a thorough pre-procedural assessment and sedation plan before proceeding, in order to minimize morbidity and mortality.

References

1. Baker S, Yagiela JA. Obesity: a complicating factor for sedation in children. *Pediatr Dent* 2006; **26**: 487–93.

2. Benumof JL, Dagg R, Benumof R. Critical hemoglobin desaturation will occur before return to an unparalyzed state following 1 mg/kg intravenous succinylcholine. *Anesthesiology* 1997; **87**: 979–82.

3. Chung F, Yegneswaran B, Liao P, *et al.* STOP questionnaire: a tool to screen patients for obstructive sleep apnea. *Anesthesiology* 2008; **108**: 812–21.

4. Gross JB, Bachenberg KL, Benumof JL, *et al.* Practice guidelines for the perioperative management of patients with obstructive sleep apnea: a report by the American Society of Anesthesiologists Task Force on Perioperative Management of Patients with Obstructive Sleep Apnea. *Anesthesiology* 2006; **104**: 1081–93.

Further reading

Adams JP, Murphy PG. Obesity in anaesthesia and intensive care. *Br J Anaesth* 2000; **85**: 91–108.

Chambers EJ, Germain M, Brown E, eds. *Supportive Care for the Renal Patient*. New York, NY: Oxford University Press, 2004.

Hevesi Z. Geriatric disorders. In Hines R, Marschall K, eds., *Anesthesia and Co-Existing*

Diseases, 5th edn. Philadelphia, PA: Churchill Livingstone, 2008; 639–49.

Kalarickal P, Fox C, Tsai J, Kaye AD. Perioperative statin use: an update. *Anesthesiol Clin* 2010; **28**: 739–51.

Kost M. Administration of conscious sedation/analgesia. *Nursing Spectrum* 2003. nsweb.nursingspectrum.com/ce/ce159.htm (accessed December 2010).

Maddali MM. Chronic obstructive pulmonary disease: perioperative management. *Middle East J Anesthesiol* 2008; **19**: 1219–40.

Martin ML, Lennox PH. Sedation and analgesia in the interventional radiology department. *J Vasc Interv Radiol* 2003; **14**: 1119–28.

Murphy EJ. Acute pain management pharmacology for the patient with concurrent renal or hepatic disease. *Anaesth Intensive Care* 2005; **33**: 311–22.

National Institutes of Health (NIH). Monitoring of patients undergoing conscious sedation. Critical care medicine department: critical care therapy and respiratory section. Bethesda, MD: NIH, 2000. www.cc.nih.gov/ccmd/cctrcs/pdf_docs/Clinical%20Monitoring/09-conscious%20Sedation.pdf (accessed December 2010).

Older P, Hall A, Hader R. Cardiopulmonary exercise testing as a screening test for perioprative management of major surgery in the elderly. *Chest* 1999; **116**: 355–62.

Vaughan S, McConachie I, Imasogie N. The elderly patient. In McConachie I, ed., *Anesthesia for the High Risk Patient*, 2nd edn. Cambridge: Cambridge University Press, 2009.

Chapter 11

Management of complications of moderate and deep sedation

Henry Liu, Charles Fox, Philip Kalarickal,
Theodore Strickland, and Alan D. Kaye

Introduction

Intravenous pharmacological sedation is widely used for various surgical and nonsurgical procedures by anesthesia providers or other trained professionals. In general, the use of intravenous sedation offers patients undergoing diagnostic and therapeutic procedures a positive experience, reducing or eliminating the fear, anxiety, pain, and discomfort associated with these procedures. There are also added benefits of reducing stress on the cardiovascular system. Sedation is described as a continuum, and it is often categorized according to the patient's level of consciousness as minimal, moderate, and deep sedation (Figure 11.1). This categorization is very subjective, with no objective cutoff line between the categories, and it does not take the sedative/hypnotic dosing strategies into account. There are overlapping zones between categories. In clinical practice, there is a gray area between deep sedation and general anesthesia; many so called "deep sedations" are virtually general anesthesia.

Intravenous sedation can potentially cause numerous complications. The clinicians should therefore have a thorough knowledge of these possible complications and understand their management strategies. In many respects, moderate and deep sedations could potentially be more challenging for anesthesia providers than general endotracheal anesthesia. There are several reasons: (1) sedation procedures are usually done outside of operating rooms, so equipment availability for anesthesia and airway management can be limited; (2) the plethora of equipment/machines in some procedure rooms can place anesthesia machines far away from the patient, and anesthesia providers may have to contend with physical distance from the patient; (3) the patient's airway is well secured during general anesthesia, but must be actively managed and protected during the procedure by the clinician providing sedation. In this regard, Boynes *et al.* reported that in dental procedures airway obstruction occurred in 18

Moderate and Deep Sedation in Clinical Practice, ed. Richard D. Urman and Alan D. Kaye.
Published by Cambridge University Press. © Cambridge University Press 2012.

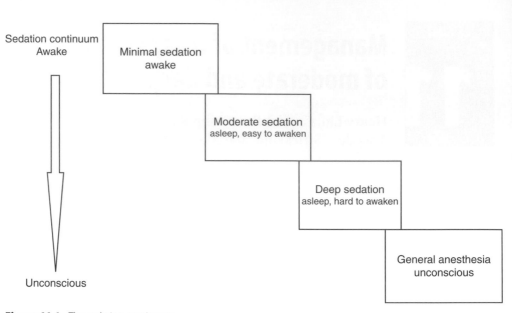

Figure 11.1. The sedation continuum.

Table 11.1. Inova Health System Sedation Scale (ISS)

Level	Description
1	Alert
2	Occasionally drowsy
3	Dozing intermittently
4	Asleep, easy to waken
5	Difficult to awaken
6	Unresponsive

Source: Nisbet et al. [3].

out of 286 patients, and nausea/vomiting in 12 out of 286 patients, although no severe complications occurred [1].

Sedation scoring scales

There are several scoring systems used to document the patient's mental status and depth of sedation, such as the Richmond Agitation–Sedation Scale (RASS) [2] (see Tables 4.1 and 8.1) and the Inova Health System Sedation Scale (ISS) [3] (Table 11.1). ISS levels 1 and 2 appear equivalent to minimal sedation, levels 3 and 4 are equivalent to moderate sedation, level 5 is probably deep sedation, and level 6 is general anesthesia.

RASS is a logical, easily administered, and readily recalled evaluation system. It has high reliability and validity in medical and surgical, ventilated and nonventilated, and sedated and nonsedated adult ICU patients [2]. However, RASS is a less favored evaluation technique for procedural sedation.

Preoperative risk assessment

Prevention of complications starts with a thorough pre-procedural patient assessment. Knowledge of a patient's coexisting diseases gives the clinician insight into possible medications or equipment necessary to alleviate potential complications or successfully manage them if they occur. Further details of some of the patient-related risk factors discussed below can be found in Chapter 10.

Patient-related factors

Age

Advanced age is a factor for developing complications for the patient having intravenous sedation. Closing capacity becomes equal to functional residual capacity (FRC) at the age of 66. Older edentulous patients have a higher probability of having loose oropharyngeal tissue, which potentially narrows or obstructs the airway when in the supine position. The elderly experience changes in bioavailability and biochemical metabolism of sedation medications, which predisposes older patients to sedative, hypnotic, and analgesic complications. Older patients also tend to have more coexisting medical conditions, which may complicate the anesthetic management. When approaching these patients, one should decrease the initial dose and incremental dosing. Additionally, the clinician should attempt to minimize the use of multiple sedatives, because of their potential synergistic effects.

A recent study of endoscopic retrograde cholangiopancreatography (ERCP) performed under propofol sedation in 450 patients (126 patients $\geq$ 65 years of age, 324 patients < 65 years, with a higher incidence of comorbid conditions in those $\geq$ 65 years, $p < 0.001$) reported anesthetic complications in 6% of patients, but found no statistical significance among American Society of Anesthesiologists (ASA) groups ($p = 0.7$) or age groups ($p = 0.1$). No procedure-related mortality was documented. The authors concluded that deep intravenous propofol sedation is safe in elderly patients and has a low anesthetic complication rate [4]. Another study of procedural sedations in elderly patients in the emergency department found no statistically significant difference in complication rates for patients 65 years or older; although there was a significant decrease in mean sedation dosing with increased age and ASA score [5].

In pediatric patients, airway obstruction and respiratory depression are the most common complications, with children aged 1–5 years at the most risk [6]. For those pediatric patients with reactive airway (asthma), bronchodilator therapy should be continued until the procedure commences. Airway irritants and histamine-releasing agents should be avoided if at all possible. The patient's neurologic status should be evaluated before surgery, and any intracranial pressure (ICP)-increasing medication should be avoided if the patient has increased ICP. In general, a majority of pediatric patients will not be good candidates for sedation in clinical practice; most procedures in pediatric patients will be done under general anesthesia (Chapter 19).

Body weight

Morbid obesity increases the risk for moderate and deep sedation, including both ventilatory and circulatory risks. However, there are some relatively "non-obese-looking" patients who may have unrecognized increased risks. It is these endomorphic patients who cause unexpected intraoperative ventilatory problems. Obese patients usually have a short, thick neck and a large tongue. Bulk of soft tissues and large tongue can cause supraglottic obstruction during sedation [7].

NPO status

All patients should be fasted as required for general anesthesia. A full stomach presents more risks in moderate and deep sedation than in general anesthesia, in which the airway is secured and aspiration during the procedure is less of a concern. If a patient has a full stomach and is a high risk for aspiration, sedation should be avoided, and the scheduled procedure should be done under general anesthesia with a secured airway.

Airway anatomy

The following anatomic features predispose patients to a high risk of difficult airway and ventilator problems, if sedated [7]:

- micrognathia (or retrognathia): e.g., Treacher–Collins syndrome, Goldenhar syndrome, Hallermann–Streiff–François syndrome, Crouzon syndrome
- prognathic (protruding) upper jaw
- deviated trachea
- macroglossia (large tongue) and glossoptosis (abnormal downward displacement of the tongue)
- short, thick, and firm neck
- protruding teeth
- high arched palate

Pregnancy

Pregnancy induces airway edema, which increases the risk of airway complications. Airway edema may be related to the increased level of progesterone during pregnancy. The increased abdominal pressure during pregnancy pushes the diaphragm up, significantly decreasing functional residual capacity (FRC), hence drastically decreasing the patient's tolerance to hypoventilation. Pregnant patients always have increased risk of aspiration due to constant full stomach, and aspiration prophylaxis is necessary before anesthesia or sedative/hypnotic administration. If general anesthesia is needed, rapid sequence induction and intubation is mandatory. The practitioner needs to be aware which drugs are safe during pregnancy and in breastfeeding patients.

Drug addiction

Sedation of drug addicts for diagnostic or therapeutic procedures can be challenging. The key issue is to figure out the appropriate dose of sedatives and hypnotics to be administered. These patients have usually developed high tolerance to sedatives and very low tolerance to pain and discomfort, and they may require significant amounts of analgesics and sedatives. Post-procedural pain management in the recovery period can pose significant challenges.

Coexisting pulmonary diseases

Any pulmonary disease compromising the oxygen-delivering pathway and/or oxygenating function will increase the risk of airway complications when a patient undergoes intravenous sedation. The risk increases in parallel with the severity of the underlining pulmonary pathology. Chronic obstructive pulmonary disease (COPD) patients have a blunted ventilatory response to CO_2, and commonly used sedatives further decrease the ventilatory response to CO_2. When a patient with COPD is undergoing a procedure with intravenous sedation, consider applying a bronchodilator before initiation of sedation in order to minimize potential pulmonary complications, and the total dose of sedatives should be decreased. Smokers are at increased risk for developing procedural hypoventilation and hypoxemia, especially when they have COPD and decreased pulmonary function. Smokers usually have increased airway secretions, and smokers are more prone to coughing, bronchospasm, and laryngospasm.

Coexisting cardiovascular diseases

Coronary artery disease (CAD) presents risks during sedation in case of both undersedation and oversedation [8]. Oversedation can lead to cardiac complications due to hypoxemia and hypotension. Undersedation will be accompanied by increased catecholamine plasma level, pain, anxiety, potential hypertension, tachycardia, etc., which will increase cardiac workload and oxygen demand. Anesthesia/sedation providers therefore need to achieve a balance by offering adequate sedation so that the patient does not have a high catecholamine level and the surgeons have a calm patient, and at the same time avoiding oversedating the patient and causing both hypoventilation- and hypotension-related problems.

Coexisting liver diseases

Hepatic dysfunction may lead to decreased metabolism, elimination, and excretion of multiple sedatives and hypnotics. Also, liver disease may change the volume of distribution of many sedatives and hypnotics. Dosing adjustments are necessary for patients with liver dysfunction for most sedatives/hypnotics.

Other coexisting diseases

Anterior mediastinal mass, post-radiation therapy for cancer in the head and neck, thyroid diseases and associated tracheomalacia could present serious airway problems during intravenous sedatives and/or hypnotics when the patient is in a supine position. Maintaining spontaneous breathing is crucial, and keeping the patient in the beach-chair position usually helps if there are problems maintaining the airway in the supine position.

Procedure-related factors
Position

The supine position usually used for most procedures reduces FRC by almost 30% compared with an upright position. When the patient is in the supine position, closing lung capacity becomes equal to FRC when the patient reaches his or her mid 40s. The lateral position is often used for gastroenterological endoscopic procedures. This induces ventilation/perfusion (V/Q) mismatch and causes a pulmonary shunting phenomenon, which means that unoxygenated blood bypasses the pulmonary oxygenating unit. All these positioning-related factors (decreased FRC, V/Q mismatch, pulmonary shunt) will, in the presence of other coexisting negative conditions, cause intraoperative problems if the patient is sedated.

Special procedures

When patients are having ERCP or gastroscopy, gastroenterologists insert a gastroscope through the patient's mouth and esophagus, and the patient's head is usually not close to the anesthesia/sedation provider. Airway management is a challenging task if the procedure is performed under moderate or deep sedation. It is critically important to identify those at high risk of intraoperative issues preoperatively (morbidly obese, full stomach, difficult airway, history of difficult monitored anesthesia care [MAC], intraoperative vomiting, etc.). For those at high risk, it is probably safer to proceed with general endotracheal anesthesia, thereby ensuring that the airway is secured before the procedure starts.

Potential complications and their management

Respiratory system complications

Among all the complications induced by intravenous sedation, respiratory complications are the most common. Respiratory complications may manifest a myriad of symptoms including respiratory depression, hypoventilation, hypoxemia, hypercapnia, laryngospasm, bronchospasm, and complete airway obstruction [8]. These are usually caused by over-sedations or an untoward response to the commonly used sedatives/medications and/or airway maneuvers. Laryngospasm and bronchospasm often occur in a patient who has difficulty managing airway secretions and/or a patient who is undergoing a procedure that involves stimulation of the airway system.

Hypoventilation and hypoxemia

Hypoventilation and hypoxemia may be the most common complication for a patient under sedation, especially deeper sedation. There are multiple mechanisms for the hypo-ventilation, such as relaxed laryngeal tissue obstructing the airway and decreased respiratory drive caused by opioids and other sedatives; the pharmacokinetics and pharmacodynamics of the sedative may be altered in critically ill patients, so that a sedative that normally does not cause hypoventilation or hypotension may cause cardiopulmonary complications even with reduced dosing. Benzodiazepines and opioids are synergistic in their respiratory depressant effects when used in combination. This respiratory depressant effect is dose-dependent and can compromise the pulmonary function by inhibiting respiratory drive in response to hypoventilation, hypoxemia, and decreased response to hypercapnia. Benzodiazepines and opioids can also decrease the muscle tone, which will lead to weaker ventilatory efforts, resulting in a V/Q mismatch [8].

Oversedation can be effectively prevented by applying the following strategies:

(1) Slowly titrate in smaller doses of sedatives over a period of time to achieve the sedative end point.

(2) Avoid giving multiple sedatives simultaneously. If you intend to give several sedatives/ hypnotics, administer the different sedatives over a period of time.

(3) Adjust dosage according to the patient's physiological status. In elderly patients, dehydrated patients, and critically ill patients, the dosage needs to be reduced.

For procedures such as esophagogastroduodenoscopy (EGD), sometimes it is not easy to provide adequate FiO_2 if the patient is mouth-breathing. A nasal cannula is not the best option, because the patient is mouth-breathing, and a regular facemask cannot be used

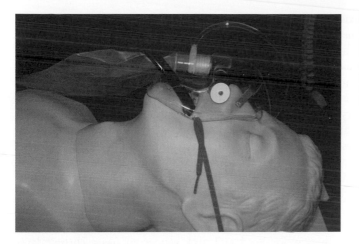

Figure 11.2. A modified 100% non-rebreather mask for gastroscopy, EGD, transesophageal echocardiography, etc., with a hole cut in the lower part of the mask for the endoscope/probe to go through. Photograph by Henry Liu, MD.

because the endoscope has to pass through the mouth. One option is to modify the regular facemask/non-rebreather by cutting a hole in the lower part of the facemask, and to supply increased FiO_2 without compromising the proceduralist's performance of the procedure (Figure 11.2).

Airway obstruction

Airway obstruction can be caused by a relaxed tongue and oropharynx, closed epiglottis, laryngospasm, bronchospasm, airway mass, airway foreign body, compression, or secretions. The tongue and oropharynx are two very common places where airway obstruction develops. It is the submandibular muscle tone that maintains the patency of the upper airway and indirectly supports the epiglottis [9]. Obesity, older age, and a history of sleep apnea are risk factors for airway obstruction.

Laryngospasm is a form of airway obstruction caused when tonic contraction of glottic muscles, including the true and false vocal cords, occurs. This obstruction may be partial or total. With total obstruction, the vocal cords are stringently closed and no air exchange is possible despite chest wall movement. In partial laryngospasm, the laryngeal opening is narrowed, but some air exchange is possible. The usual precipitants of laryngospasm are airway manipulation with oral or nasal airway placement, excessive secretions, vomitus, preexisting upper respiratory infection, or mechanical irritation caused by frequent suctioning. Laryngospasm occurs relatively more frequently in patients under general anesthesia; it is recognizable without too much difficulty and can usually be managed with positive airway pressure. However, it has the potential to cause perioperative morbidity and mortality, especially if managed poorly. Fortunately laryngospasm is significantly less common in sedation cases than following general anesthesia.

Bronchospasm is a lower airway obstruction due to an increase in bronchial smooth muscle tone. Although it is a complication less frequently experienced than laryngospasm, it can lead to morbidity and mortality if left undiagnosed and untreated. Presenting symptoms are directly related to the degree of bronchospasm. Mild bronchospasm involving a small number of bronchioles presents as mild wheezing, only detectable with a stethoscope. Chest tightness, audible wheezing, chest retractions, and accessory muscle usually signify a substantial airway obstruction requiring immediate attention. Risk factors for developing bronchospasm include preexisting bronchospastic disease, histamine release, upper respiratory or pulmonary infection, excessive airway secretions, aspiration, and bronchial irritation from suctioning. Propofol has been reported to induce bronchospasm [10].

Negative-pressure pulmonary edema (NPPE) is a rare pulmonary complication that occurs when the patient attempts to breathe against an acute upper airway obstruction. This results in significant generation of negative intrathoracic pressure, which pulls fluid from the pulmonary capillary bed and into the alveoli, resulting in significant ventilation and perfusion defects. Patients with a history of sleep apnea, laryngospasm, foreign body aspiration, opioid use, or obesity, and young healthy males, are at risk for developing NPPE.

Complete airway obstruction is a clinical emergency that may arise in several scenarios, such as a patient with preexisting obstructive airway, a patient with a neck mass and/or mediastinal mass, a patient who has had radiation therapy for a neck malignancy, a patient with acute epiglottitis or severe reactive airway, or a patient who is oversedated and has completely lost respiratory drive. If a patient has a history of sleep apnea, or has undergone multiple episodes of radiation therapy for head and neck cancer, or has a chronic large thyroid mass that might have caused tracheomalacia, sedation providers should be highly alert to the risk of loss of airway. If a patient has an obstructive airway, or a difficult airway plus sedative-induced decreased respiratory drive and muscle relaxation, the sedation provider may be at risk of losing the patient's airway. These patients may be better candidates for general anesthesia rather than moderate or deep sedation, and advanced airway management techniques (e.g., fiberoptic intubation) may be required to secure the airway. It may be too risky to proceed with sedation.

In the clinical emergency of complete airway obstruction, sedation/anesthesia providers need to immediately identify whether the patient can be ventilated with a bag-valve mask. If the patient is not ventilatable with a bag-valve mask, immediate establishment of airway patency is necessary, either by endotracheal intubation or with a laryngeal mask airway (LMA). If the anesthesia provider is still unable to intubate the patient or ventilate the patient with the LMA, for whatever reason, immediate cricothyrotomy or tracheostomy may be needed.

Several maneuvers can be used to help ventilate a patient with a facemask:

(1) Insert oral airway and/or nasal trumpet.
(2) Jaw-thrust: lift the mandibular angle perpendicularly away from the patient's vertical plane while using the thumbs to push open the mouth and apply forward pressure, as shown in Figure 11.3; this maneuver opens up the airway by upward and potentially forward forces; it is better than chin-lifting, which helps to open the airway by upward and backward forces (Figure 11.4): the backward force may not be beneficial to maintaining the patency of the airway.
(3) Positioning the patient in a semi-sitting or beach-chair position will help open up the airway, especially in a patient with neck mass, mediastinal mass, thyroid mass and neck radiation, etc.

On many occasions during intravenous sedation, inadequate ventilation and hypoxemia is caused by a combination of decreased respiratory drive, decreased muscle strength of the respiratory system, and partial airway obstruction.

Pulmonary aspiration of gastric contents

Pulmonary aspiration is the entry of gastric content into the lungs and trachea. Pulmonary aspiration can produce a variety of hazardous sequelae, depending upon the nature of the

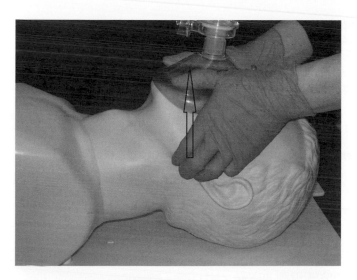

Figure 11.3. Jaw thrust by lifting mandibular angle perpendicularly away from the vertical plane and pushing the mandibular body to open the patient's mouth with both thumbs. Note the direction of the lifting force, as shown by the arrow. Photograph by Henry Liu, MD.

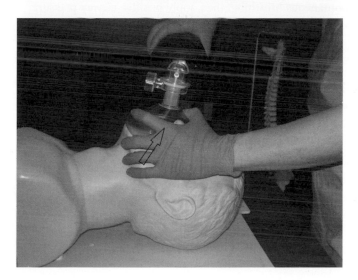

Figure 11.4. The routine chin-lift technique. Note the direction of the lifting force, as shown by the arrow. Photograph by Henry Liu, MD.

aspirate, which may include large food fragments (obstructing airway), small particles (causing granulomatous inflammation), gastric acid (causing chemical pneumonitis), blood and digestive enzymes (causing irritation and chemical reaction) [11]. Signs and symptoms of pulmonary aspiration include rales and rhonchi, wheezing, dyspnea, tachypnea, and tachycardia, and oxygen desaturation. Prophylactic strategies include head elevation/reverse Trendelenberg position, cricoid pressure, suctioning the stomach before the procedure, and administering the following medications: nonparticulate antiacids, H_2-receptor antagonists (cimetidine), and gastrokinetic drugs (metoclopramide). Patients predisposed to aspiration are those with increased intra-abdominal pressure, poor gastric emptying, or gastroesophageal reflux. Increases in intra-abdominal pressure are commonly seen in pregnant patients, in patients with ascites, and in patients with intra-abdominal masses. Poor gastric emptying is related to mechanical obstruction or poor gastric muscular contraction. The sedatives/hypnotics used for sedation have multiple effects that leave patients vulnerable to aspiration. Opioid medications commonly cause nausea and vomiting as a side effect. Protective reflexes, which guard against aspiration, are obtunded by many of the medications used for sedation. If the patient has a full stomach and has pyloric stenosis or other gastrointestinal obstruction, suctioning of the stomach can be effective in reducing the gastric volume, and this patient should then proceed with general anesthesia with rapid sequence induction and intubation.

Hypoventilation/hypoxemia summary

General rules of thumb in managing patients with hypoventilation/hypoxemia during moderate/deep sedation are outlined below:

(1) If the patient has decreased respiratory drive and compromised airway, and decreased pulse oximetry readings, immediately inform the proceduralist to pause the procedure and have you or the proceduralist apply chin-lift and jaw-thrust, to attempt to open the airway. If these maneuvers do not work, or fail to work adequately, insert an oral and/or nasal airway.

(2) If the patient maintains spontaneous breathing, then apply positive airway pressure and assist patient breathing. If the patient has no spontaneous breathing, gentle positive pressure mask ventilation should be started immediately with 100% FiO_2.

(3) Suspending the procedure or switching to general endotracheal intubation can be a hard decision to make. If the patient is not expected to resume spontaneous breathing quickly, sedation should be converted to general anesthesia with endotracheal intubation or LMA. If ventilation can be established, the procedure can be resumed.

Cardiovascular system complications

Generally, minimal sedation has a minimal effect on the cardiovascular system. Moderate and deep sedation may have varying degrees of depressive effects on cardiovascular function, depending on the patient's physiological status and the dosage of sedatives administered. Excessive sedative dosages in addition to a large dose of local anesthetics with vasoconstrictors and the procedural influences may induce significant cardiovascular changes during sedation, such as hypotension, hypertension, tachycardia, bradycardia, and dysrhythmias.

Hypotension

There are many potential causes of hypotension during sedation. Intravenous sedatives can lower systemic blood pressure, especially when the patient is overdosed with sedatives [6]. The mechanisms are the decreased sympathetic tone, leading to vasodilation, decreased venous return, and direct myocardial-depressant effects of the sedatives. Hypotension can also be procedural, arising from dehydration, vasovagal response, hemorrhage, sepsis, and anaphylaxis [8]. Patients with preexisting cardiovascular disease may have prescription drugs that act synergistically with sedative medications, or they may have depressed ventricular function and less "reserve," so that minimal doses of sedative medications cause exaggerated responses. If sedatives such as midazolam, opioids, and intravenous induction agents are administered simultaneously, they will have synergistic effects, which may present as hypotension. Hypotension during sedation is not rare. It can be managed by intravenous hydration and/or small doses of sympathomimetic agents to increase vascular tone.

Hypertension

An elevation in blood pressure is not uncommon during procedural sedation. It usually reflects inadequate intravenous sedation, procedural stimulation, or epinephrine added to local anesthetics. Stress and pain experienced by these patients directly results in an increased autonomic response. This increase in catecholamine release is manifested in tachycardia and hypertension. If given in large quantities, epinephrine-containing local anesthetic agents can be an additional risk factor, as in dental procedures. In patients with preexisting hypertension, some may develop a hypertensive crisis during the procedure, and this will require immediate and controlled reduction of blood pressure. Medications commonly used to treat these perioperative hypertensions include nicardipine, sodium nitropruside, nitroglycerin, and beta-blockers.

Tachycardia

Just like hypertension, tachycardia is usually caused by undersedation and/or procedural stimulation. An undersedated patient is likely to remain very nervous about the procedure, and if the patient can feel any procedural stimulation he/she will very likely develop tachycardia and hypertension. Tachycardia can also be a reflex response to hypoxia or hypotension, and these should be considered during patient assessment before treatment. Once these possibilities have been attended to, persistent tachycardia may cause the patient to complain of palpitations. In this case, intravenous fluids should be administered to support blood pressure if the patient's heart rate rises to help sustain cardiac output. If the episode continues, a selective beta-1-receptor antagonist such as esmolol (Brevibloc) can be titrated intravenously in an appropriate dose range to gradually decrease sympathetic stimulation to the heart. Esmolol has a short duration, so if the heart rate drops too precipitously it should recover within a few minutes.

Syncope

Syncope is one of the most common cardiac complications during sedation [12]. The mechanism for the pathogenesis of syncope is mostly cardiovascular in nature and commonly associated with hypoxemia, hypotension, or other cardiac rhythmic abnormalities. Syncope needs to be recognized immediately when it occurs, to avoid or decrease morbidity and mortality.

Other dysrhythmias

Other dysrhythmias may include premature ventricular contractions (PVCs), bigeminy, and premature atrial contractions (PACs). The majority of these complications are likely associated with hypotension and hypoxemia. These cardiac dysrhythmias should be promptly recognized and managed aggressively with appropriate therapeutic interventions.

Gastroenterological complications

Nausea and vomiting

Postoperative nausea and vomiting (PONV) is a very common "small" problem. In the ambulatory surgery group, the incidence is estimated to be 35%, while in high-risk groups the incidence is as high as 70% [13]. The incidence of PONV in patients who received intravenous sedation medications is not clear; it should be lower than after general anesthesia. Opioids used in intravenous sedation can potentially cause intraoperative nausea and vomiting (IONV) and PONV. Certain patient characteristics are associated with a higher risk of IONV and PONV: younger age, female gender, large body habitus, history of PONV or motion sickness, and anxiety. Prophylaxis for high-risk patients is necessary, and scopolamine patches and intravenous serotonin receptor antagonists have been successfully used for this purpose.

Constipation

Chronic use of opioids for the purpose of sedating patients in the ICU setting can potentially lead to constipation, although opioids used for procedural sedation are very unlikely to cause this complication.

Other complications

Urine retention

Some opioids used for procedural sedations can potentially cause urine retention. Morphine is more likely to cause this complication. Urinary catheter placement to drain the bladder may be necessary.

Delirium

Delirium is a state in which the patient has altered consciousness, orientation, memory, perception, and behavior. A patient's reaction to hypoxemia, hypercarbia, and airway obstruction can sometimes mimic delirium, so thorough examination of the patient to rule out life-threatening events is critical. Risk factors for delirium are preoperative (advanced age, cerebrovascular disease, alcohol or sedative withdrawal, endocrine and metabolic disorders), intraoperative (administration of multiple sedatives, hypotension/hypoperfusion, ophthalmic procedures, anticholinergic agents, barbiturates, and benzodiazepines) and postoperative (hypoxia, sepsis). Delirium can be managed by treating the underlying causes. Haloperidol is the drug usually used for the patient with delirium. It can be used orally, intramuscularly, or intravenously. Droperidol and chlorpromazine are also being used. However, the use of physostigmine for the management of delirium is controversial [14].

Propofol infusion syndrome

The term "propofol infusion syndrome" (PRIS) was first used by Bray in 1998 to describe a clinical state associated with propofol infusion in children [15]. PRIS is defined by FDA investigators as metabolic acidosis with or without rhabdomyolysis with progressive myocardial dysfunction [16]. The presentation of PRIS varies considerably from unexplained lactic acidosis, lipemic serum, and cardiac dysfunction or Brugada-like electrocardiogram changes, to cardiac failure, tachyarrhythmias or heart block, ventricular fibrillation or ventricular tachycardia, rhabdomyolysis (manifesting as elevated creatine kinase and myoglobinuria), hyperkalemia, renal failure, and fatty degeneration of the liver [17]. The risk factors include severe head injury, airway infection, young age, large total cumulative dose, high catecholamine and serum glucocorticoid levels, low carbohydrate intake/high fat intake, critical illness, or inborn errors of fatty acid oxidation. Infusion rate and duration of infusion are particularly important risk factors for the development of PRIS. The mortality rate is as high as 83% [15]. It is recommended that infusions of 0.4 mg/kg/h for longer than 48 hours be avoided. Early PRIS, however, has been shown to develop during high-dose, short-term infusions. Special care should be taken when such patients have factors that may increase the likelihood of development of PRIS (such as mitochondrial disease or fatty acid oxidation defects, young age, critical illness of CNS or respiratory origin, exogenous catecholamine or glucocorticoid administration, or inadequate carbohydrate intake). The monitoring of pH, lactate, and creatine kinase is recommended when unusually high doses or long infusion periods are unavoidable. If prolonged or high-dose propofol administration is necessary, supplemental sedatives can be used to decrease the amount of propofol necessary for the desired level of sedation [17]. Lactate-to-pyruvate ratio has been reported as a marker for the diagnosis of PRIS [18]. There is a report of successfully using extracorporeal membrane oxygenation (ECMO) to treat a patient with PRIS [19].

Methemoglobinemia

When benzocaine [20] or prilocaine [21] is used as a local anesthetic agent for some sedated endoscopic or echocardiographic procedures, methemoglobinemia can occur. The clinical manifestations include cyanosis, low SpO_2 reading, and normal arterial PaO_2 values. Kane et al. reported 28,478 patients who underwent transesophageal echocardiography (TEE), all of whom had topical benzocaine to the area for its local anesthetic effects. Nineteen patients (0.07%) developed methemoglobinemia (with a mean methemoglobin level of 32%). Eighteen of these 19 patients were treated with methylene blue [20]. The American Society for Gastrointestinal Endoscopy (ASGE) *Guidelines for conscious sedation and monitoring during gastrointestinal endoscopy* recommend against the routine use of topical pharyngeal anesthetics in most patients [22]. However, pharyngeal anesthesia before upper endoscopy or TEE may improve the conduction of these procedures and also improves patient tolerance and comfort. Therefore applying local anesthetics may be acceptable under certain conditions, especially if light or no sedation is administered. Methemoglobinemia can be treated with methylene blue or ascorbic acid, but methylene blue may be dangerous in patients who have or may be at risk for a blood disease called G6PD deficiency, and methylene blue should not be used in this group of patients.

Paradoxical sedative excitement

A state of excitement can occur in some patients as a reaction to sedation with benzodiazepines or propofol. This can affect the performance of the procedure, and sometimes the procedure has to be stopped so that the sedation providers can manage the patient. These paradoxical reactions can include uncooperativeness, excessive talkativeness, violent movement, and emotional release. Certain factors predispose a patient to a paradoxical reaction: young and advanced age, genetic predisposition, alcoholism or drug abuse, psychiatric and/or personality disorders. These reactions are relatively uncommon, occurring in less than 1% of cases [23]. There are reports of using physostigmine to treat these paradoxical reactions. The therapeutic effect occurs by two mechanisms: physostigmine reestablishes CNS homeostasis via augmented cholinergic pathways, with the net result being thalamacortical excitation, and a cholinergically mediated increase in cerebral blood flow increases the rate of redistribution of the intravenous sedative agents [24].

Summary

For those patients at high risk for gastric content aspiration, general endotracheal anesthesia is likely a safer choice. For those who are morbidly obese or have a potentially difficult airway, general anesthesia is the option, in order to ensure that the patient's airway is secured. However, patients who are borderline risk for aspiration, or who have a borderline difficult airway, pose a dilemma to the sedation provider. To proceed with intravenous sedation and complete the procedure is the ideal clinical course. But this approach runs the risk of intraoperative loss of airway or aspiration. Some would suggest that these borderline patients warrant a consultation with an anesthesiologist and possibly should be managed by means of endotracheal intubation and general anesthesia, thereby securing the airway and preventing aspiration.

References

1. Boynes SG, Lewis CL, Moore PA, Zovko J, Close J. Complications associated with anesthesia administered for dental treatment. *Gen Dent* 2010; **58**: e20–5.

2. Sessler CN, Gosnell MS, Grap MJ, *et al.* The Richmond Agitation–Sedation Scale: validity and reliability in adult intensive care unit patients. *Am J Respir Crit Care Med* 2002; **166**: 1338–44.

3. Nisbet AT, Mooney-Cotter F. Comparison of selected sedation scales for reporting opioid-induced sedation assessment. *Pain Manag Nurs* 2009; **10**: 154–64.

4. Güitrón-Cantú A, Adalid-Martínez R, Gutiérrez-Bermúdez J, Segura-López F, García-Vázquez A. [Endoscopic retrograde cholangiopancreatography in the elderly: a prospective and comparative study in Northern Mexico.] *Rev Gastroenterol Mex* 2010; **75**: 267–72.

5. Weaver CS, Terrell KM, Bassett R, *et al.* ED procedural sedation of elderly patients: is it safe? *Am J Emerg Med* 2011; **29**: 541–4.

6. Martin MI, Lennox PH. Sedation and analgesia in the interventional radiology department. *J Vasc Interv Radiol* 2003; **14**: 1119–28

7. Norton ML, Kyff J. Key medical considerations in the difficult airway: sleep apnea, obesity, and burns. In Norton ML, Brown ACD, eds., *Atlas of the Difficult Airway.* St Louis, MO: Mosby Yearbook, 1991; 118–28.

8. Watson DS, Odom-Forren J. Management of complications. In *Practical Guide to Moderate Sedation/Analgesia,* 2nd edn. New York, NY: Mosby, 2005; 71–96.

9. Hotchkiss MA, Drain CB. Assessment and management of the airway. In Drain CB, ed., *Perianesthesia Nursing: a Critical Care Approach.* St Louis, MO: Saunders, 2003; 409–21.

10. Takahashi S, Uemura A, Nakayama S, Miyabe M, Toyooka H. Bronchospasms and wheezing after induction of anesthesia with propofol in patients with a history of asthma. *J Anesth* 2002; **16**: 360–1.

11. Tasch MD. Pulmonary aspiration. In Atlee JL, ed., *Complications in Anesthesia,* 2nd edn. Philadelphia, PA: Saunders/ Elsevier, 2007; 186–8

12. D'Eramo EM, Bookless SJ, Howard JB. Adverse events with outpatient anesthesia in Massachusetts. *J Oral Maxillofac Surg* 2003; **61**: 793–800.

13. Post-operative nausea and vomiting (PONV): an overview. *Anesthesiology Info.* anesthesiologyinfo.com/articles/04252004. php (accessed June 2011).

14. Levin P. Postoperative delirium. In Atlee JL, ed., *Complications in Anesthesia,* 2nd edn. Philadelphia, PA: Saunders/ Elsevier, 2007; 888–9.

15. Bray RJ. Propofol infusion syndrome in children. *Paediatr Anaesth* 1998; **8**: 491–9.

16. Wysowski D, Pollock M. Reports of death with use of propofol (Diprivan) for nonprocedural (long-term) sedation and literature review. *Anesthesiology* 2006; **105**: 1047–51.

17. Wong JM. Propofol infusion syndrome. *Am J Ther* 2010; **17**: 487–91.

18. Pisapia JM, Wendell LC, Kumar MA, Zager EL, Levine JM. Lactate-to-pyruvate ratio as a marker of propofol infusion syndrome after subarachnoid hemorrhage. *Neurocrit Care* 2010 Nov 10 [Epub ahead of print].

19. Guitton C, Gabillet L, Latour P, *et al.* Propofol infusion syndrome during refractory status epilepticus in a young adult: successful ECMO resuscitation. *Neurocrit Care* 2010 May 25 [Epub ahead of print].

20. Kane GC, Hoehn SM, Behrenbeck TR, Mulvagh SL. Benzocaine-induced methemoglobinemia based on the Mayo Clinic experience from 28 478 transesophageal echocardiograms: incidence, outcomes, and predisposing factors. *Arch Intern Med* 2007; **167**: 1977–82.

21. Adams V, Marley J, McCarroll C. Prilocaine induced methaemoglobinaemia in a medically compromised patient: was this an inevitable consequence of the dose administered? *Br Dent J* 2007; **203**: 585–7.

22. Waring JP, Baron TH, Hirota WK, *et al.* American Society for Gastrointestinal Endoscopy, Standards of Practice Committee. Guidelines for conscious sedation and monitoring during gastrointestinal endoscopy. *Gastrointest Endosc* 2003; **58**: 317–22.

23. Mancuso CE, Tanzi MG, Gabay M. Paradoxical reactions to benzodiazepines: literature review and treatment options. *Pharmacotherapy* 2004; **24**: 1177–85.

24. Milam SB, Bennett CR. Physostigmine reversal of drug-induced paradoxical excitement. *Int J Oral Maxillofac Surg* 1987; **16**: 190–3.

Outcomes, controversies, and future trends

Julia Metzner and Karen B. Domino

Outcomes of procedural sedation

Sedation complications

The incidence of sedation-related complications for procedures is unknown, as mandatory reporting of outcomes is lacking. However, two sources of information are available that can shed light on the risks of sedation encountered in non-operating-room locations.

The Pediatric Sedation Research Consortium (PSRC) is a multi-institutional group that maintains a database of more than 40,000 cases and collects pediatric sedation-related adverse events. It collects outcomes for a variety of diagnostic and therapeutic procedures at different locations, delivered by anesthesiologists, emergency department specialists, intensive care physicians, pediatricians, and trained nurses [1]. Regardless of the sedation protocols and types of drugs used, the most commonly observed complications were of respiratory origin, and they included stridor, laryngospasm, airway obstruction, and apnea. One in every 200 sedations required airway and ventilation interventions ranging from bag-mask ventilation to oral airway placement to emergency intubation. No deaths occurred (Table 12.1) [1,2].

Despite the relative safety of sedation when administered by trained personnel, severe adverse events, including brain damage and death, can occur. The American Society of Anesthesiologists (ASA) Closed Claims Project collects and analyses anesthesia malpractice claims to study in detail rare adverse events and improve patient safety. Recently, the claims associated with sedation and monitored anesthesia care (MAC) [3] and care by anesthesiologists in non-operating-room locations [4,5] have been reviewed (Table 12.2). Respiratory depression from sedative agents was the leading cause of severe patient injury (death or severe brain damage) during sedation/MAC. Propofol, often administered with an opioid or benzodiazepine, increased the incidence of oversedation and respiratory depression. Complications occurred at a higher rate at extremes of age. The anesthetic care was

Table 12.1. Complications

	Incidence per 10,000	n	95% CI
Adverse events			
Death	0.0	0	0.0–0.0
Cardiac arrest	0.3	1	0.0–1.9
Aspiration	0.3	1	0.0–1.9
Hypothermia	1.3	4	0.4–3.4
Seizure (unanticipated) during sedation	2.7	8	1.1–5.2
Stridor	4.3	11	1.8–6.6
Laryngospasm	4.3	13	2.3–7.4
Wheeze (new onset during sedation)	4.7	14	2.5–7.8
Allergic reaction (rash)	5.7	17	3.3–9.1
Intravenous-related problems/complication	11.0	33	7.6–15.4
Prolonged sedation	13.6	41	9.8–18.5
Prolonged recovery	22.3	67	17.3–28.3
Apnea (unexpected)	24.3	73	19.1–30.5
Secretions (requiring suction)	41.6	125	34.7–49.6
Vomiting during procedure (nongastrointestinal)	47.2	142	39.8–55.7
Desaturation below 90%	156.5	470	142.7–171.2
Total adverse events	339.6 (1 per 29)	1020	308.1–371.5
Unplanned treatments			
Reversal agent required (unanticipated)	1.7	5	0.6–3.9
Emergency anesthesia consult for airway	2.0	6	0.7–4.3
Admission to hospital (unanticipated; sedation related)	7.0	21	4.3–10.7
Intubation required (unanticipated)	9.7	29	6.5–13.9
Airway (oral; unexpected requirement)	27.6	83	22.0–34.2
Bag-mask ventilation (unanticipated)	63.9	192	55.2–73.6
Total unplanned treatments	111.9 (1 per 89)	336	85.3–130.2
Conditions present during procedure			
Inadequate sedation, could not complete	88.9 (1 per 338)	267	78.6–100.2

Reproduced with permission from Cravero et al. [2]. Copyright 2006 American Academy of Pediatrics. This table includes adverse events and other complications reported to the Pediatric Sedation Research Consortium database.

Table 12.2. Adverse events and mechanisms of injury associated with claims from anesthesia in remote locations compared with claims from operating room procedures

	Non-operating room; $n = 87$; n (%)	Operating room; $n = 3287$; n (%)
Adverse events		
Death	47 (54)*	949 (29)*
Permanent brain damage	12 (14)	321 (10)
Airway injury	10 (11)	309 (9)
Aspiration pneumonitis	6 (7)	117 (4)
Burn injury	5 (6)	141 (4)
Stroke	3 (3)	118 (4)
Eye injury	2 (2)	183 (6)
Myocardial infarction	1 (1)	123 (4)
Mechanism of injury		
Respiratory event	38 (44)*	671 (20)*
Inadequate oxygenation/ventilation	18 (21)*	94 (3)*
Cardiovascular event	9 (10)	526 (16)
Equipment failure	12 (14)	438 (13)
Medication-related	5 (6)	256 (8)
Other events[a]	21 (24)	1113 (34)

Adapted from Metzner et al. [4].
[a]Other events include surgical technique/patient condition, patient fell, wrong operation/location, positioning, failure to diagnose, other known damaging events, no damaging event, and unknown.
*$p < 0.001$ remote location vs. operating room claims (z test).

considered substandard in most of these claims, and errors were judged as preventable by better respiratory monitoring, especially capnography, in two-thirds of claims. As a result of these findings, the ASA changed the standards for monitoring of ventilation during moderate or deep sedation to require capnography to measure exhaled carbon dioxide unless precluded or invalidated by the nature of the patient, procedure, or equipment [6].

Pino reviewed sedation outcomes outside the operating room in a single large institution (over 63,000 cases) [7]. The incidence of adverse events was comparable to that in other reports and involved respiratory mishaps caused by inadequate monitoring, drug overdose, and lack of vigilance. Although rare, sedation-induced respiratory depression may cause brain damage and/or death.

Influence of monitoring modalities on outcomes
Capnography
As respiratory depression is the most important side effect of the commonly used sedatives, early recognition and rapid intervention to avoid potentially serious complications is

paramount. Pulse oximetry is the standard monitor for detection of desaturation and hypoxemia during sedation/analgesia; however, it is inadequate to detect ventilatory compromise, e.g., hypoventilation, airway obstruction, or apnea. Significant respiratory compromise can occur despite normal oxygen saturation, particularly when supplemental oxygen is administered. Clinical monitoring of ventilation (chest excursion, respiratory rate, breath sounds) may provide some information, but only monitoring for the presence of carbon dioxide (CO_2) exhaled by the patient (capnography) is capable of detecting subtle hypoventilation before it is evident on clinical examination.

Although capnography is now a standard requirement for monitoring of ventilation during moderate or deep sedation by anesthesia providers (ASA standard) [6], it is often not employed by non-anesthesia providers. However, its use in detecting adverse respiratory events associated with procedure sedation has been the focus of studies in both anesthesiology [8] and non-anesthesiology literature [9–12]. One study reported that a quarter of patients developed 20 seconds of apnea missed by clinical signs and pulse oximetry, but detected by capnography [8]. An emergency medicine group studied sedation with propofol with and without capnography. Continuous end-tidal CO_2 monitoring decreased the incidence of desaturation ($SpO_2 < 93\%$) from 42% to 25%; the capnographic evidence of respiratory depression always occurred before the onset of hypoxia [11]. Similar findings were reported in gastroenterology [12]. In summary, use of capnography with rapid intervention to treat respiratory depression can efficiently prevent adverse respiratory events during sedation.

Brain function monitoring

Brain function monitoring, such as use of the Bispectral Index (BIS; Aspect Medical Systems, Norwood, MA, USA), uses a processed electroencephalogram signal to estimate anesthetic or sedation depth. A BIS value of 100 (unit-less scale) is considered complete wakefulness, 0 is cortical silence, 80–90 is associated with sedation, and the range of 40–60 is believed to be consistent with general anesthesia. BIS is validated for use during general anesthesia in the operating room and in the ambulatory setting, and its popularity for procedural sedation is rising. It is widely believed that brain function monitoring may be beneficial in preventing oversedation and in facilitating fast-track recovery. However, the role of brain function monitoring for sedation targeted to the moderate level has not been established. BIS monitoring has shown low accuracy to discriminate between mild to moderate and moderate to deep levels of sedation during endoscopy [13] and various emergency department procedures [14,15]. In summary, brain function monitoring may have a beneficial role for procedural sedation in the future, but requires more investigation.

Controversies of procedural sedation

The major controversies in procedural sedation are the choice of sedative agents and the administration of propofol by non-anesthesia providers.

Traditionally, moderate sedation in the gastrointestinal suite was provided with a benzodiazepine (midazolam or diazepam) used either alone or in combination with an opioid (fentanyl or meperidine). However, during the last few years, there has been increasing use of propofol, a general anesthetic agent. There is to date no demonstrated difference in endoscopic safety or efficacy with propofol sedation compared to sedation with a benzodiazepine with or without an opioid, although the studies failed to critically measure adverse respiratory effects. However, there is a trend towards higher levels of satisfaction and cost-effectiveness for the use of propofol during colonoscopies, and higher levels of patient satisfaction and improved efficacy may be expected by using propofol during upper gastrointestinal endoscopies.

For routine endoscopic procedures (e.g., colonoscopies and upper endoscopies), the safety of propofol administered by non-anesthesia providers is controversial. Most endoscopy-oriented specialty societies support propofol procedural sedation by non-anesthesia providers. However, the healthcare practitioners (e.g., anesthesia providers) who have the most experience with propofol are largely against the administration of propofol by sedation nurses and other non-anesthesia providers. While economic concerns may underlie the debate, the major concern is one of patient safety, as propofol has variable patient responses, resulting in a quick progression of moderate sedation into deep sedation.

Two major types of administration of propofol by non-anesthesia providers have been studied: nurse-administered propofol (NAPS) and proceduralist direction (Table 12.3) [16–21]. While the safety results in healthy, non-obese patients are encouraging, these studies do not thoroughly investigate respiratory depression or hemodynamic compromise, and instead focus only on extremely rare severe adverse outcomes, and therefore lack adequate power to detect differences. In a review of more than 36,000 endoscopies performed under NAPS, the rate of clinically important adverse events (defined as an episode of apnea or other airway compromise requiring bag-mask ventilation) ranged from approximately one event per 500 endoscopies to 1 per 1000 [22]. A recent multinational study of 646,000 endoscopist-directed propofol administrations for gastrointestinal procedures reported a relatively low overall risk of cardiopulmonary complications [20]. Only 0.1% of patients needed bag-mask ventilation, and only 11 patients required endotracheal intubation; no patients sustained permanent neurologic injury, and four patients with underlying severe disabling diseases died (Table 12.3). However, the magnitude and duration of oxygen desaturations, respiratory obstruction, hypoventilation, apnea, or adverse hemodynamic effects were generally not examined in these sedation studies.

Future trends
New drugs
Fospropofol

Fospropofol disodium (Eisai, Woodcliff Lake, NJ, USA), a prodrug of propofol, has recently been approved by the Food and Drug Administration (FDA) for intravenous sedation of adult patients undergoing diagnostic/therapeutic procedures. Fospropofol is water-soluble and is metabolized by alkaline phosphatase to liberate propofol (the active compound), formaldehyde, and phosphate. Propofol-derived from fospropofol has a slower onset and offset and a longer time to reach peak concentration, properties that theoretically could minimize oversedation-related risks [23]. However, pharmacokinetic data concerning fospropofol are lacking as pharmacokinetic phase I and II studies of fospropofol were recently retracted due to an analytical propofol assay inaccuracy [24]. Based on the few available studies, fospropofol seems to be an effective drug for procedural sedation, although its sedative and respiratory effects may be difficult to titrate.

Table 12.3. Selected series of administration of propofol by various providers

Author/year	Study design	Number of patients	ASA	Procedure	Provider	Drug(s)	Complications
Schilling 2009 [16]	Prospective	151	3–4	ERCP, EUS	Nurse	Propofol vs. Midaz/meper	SpO$_2$ < 90% in 11.8% vs. 9.3% Hypotension: 5.2% vs. 2.6%
McQuaid 2008 [17]	Meta-analysis	3918 (36 studies)	N/A	EGD, colonoscopy	Endoscopist	Regimens 1. BDZ 2. BDZ + opioid 3. Propofol	SpO$_2$ < 90% Hypotension 18% 0% 6% 7% 11% 5%
Cote 2010 [18]	Prospective case series	799	6% > 3	ERCP, EUS	Anesthesiologist	Propofol alone Propofol combined	SpO$_2$ < 90%: 12.8% Hypotension: 0.5%
Fatima 2008 [19]	Retrospective case series	806	N/A	EUS	Nurse	Propofol	SpO$_2$ < 90%: 0.7% PPV: 4 BMV: 1 Hypotension: 13%
Rex 2009 [20]	Retrospective review	646,080	N/A	EGD, colonoscopy	Endoscopist	Propofol	BMV: 489 patients (0.1%) ETT: 11 patients Death: 4 patients
Singh 2008 [21]	Cochrane meta-analysis	267 studies	1	Colonoscopy	Endoscopist, nurse, PCS	Propofol alone Propofol combined	SpO$_2$, apnea, and respiratory depression comparable

ASA, American Society of Anesthesiologists physical status; BDZ, benzodiazepine; BMV, bag-mask ventilation; EGD, esophagogastroduodenoscopy; ERCP, endoscopic retrograde cholangiography; ETT, endotracheal tube; EUS, esophageal sonographies; N/A, not available; PCS, patient-controlled sedation; PPV, positive-pressure ventilation. Adapted from Metzner and Domino [5].

Dexmedetomidine

Dexmedetomidine is a selective alpha-2-adrenoceptor agonist that provides cooperative sedation, anxiolysis, analgesia, a reduction of sympathetic outflow, and an increase in vagal tone. The major advantage of dexmedetomidine over other sedatives is that despite deeper levels of sedation, respiratory function remains preserved. Because of these qualities, dexmedetomidine has been proven useful in the sedation of both adult and pediatric patients in the operating room, in intensive care, and in out-of-operating-room locations [25,26]. Dexmedetomidine is most often delivered as an initial bolus of 0.5–1 µg/kg over 10–20 minutes, followed by a continuous infusion of 0.2–0.7 µg/kg/hour. As it may cause significant bradycardia and hypotension, careful hemodynamic monitoring is advisable and lower rates of administration may be required in elderly, sicker, or hypovolemic patients (such as after a bowel prep). The recovery time may also be longer than for propofol.

New drug delivery methods

Patient-controlled sedation/analgesia (PCSA)

This innovative technique allows the patient to directly control and adjust the sedation level as needed. The PCSA system resembles a conventional patient-controlled analgesia (PCA) machine and consists of an infusion pump and a patient-controlled handset (push-button). In order to avoid oversedation, lockout intervals (usually 3–5 minutes), bolus doses, and maximum infusion rates are predetermined. Patients may trigger intermittent drug boluses or control a variable-rate infusion. In clinical practice, propofol is the drug most often used, either alone or combined with an opioid. Mandel and colleagues found that colonoscopy could be performed well with PCSA with different drug regimens (midazolam–fentanyl or propofol–remifentanil) [27]. It appears that PCSA is comparable with physician-conducted traditional sedation; generally patients use lower doses, the recovery is faster, and patient satisfaction is high [28].

Computer-assisted personalized sedation (CAPS)

Computer-assisted personalized sedation is designed to deliver propofol safely and effectively when used by a trained physician/nurse team. CAPS is a procedure that uses an investigational device called SEDASYS (Ethicon Endo-Surgery, Cincinnati, OH, USA) that combines target-controlled infusion (TCI) of propofol and a physiologic monitoring unit. The device interfaces continuous monitoring of patient vital signs, including ECG, pulse oximetry, capnography, blood pressure, and patient responsiveness with computer-controlled propofol delivery to facilitate precise control of sedation. With signs of oversedation, it automatically decreases or stops the propofol infusion rate, while simultaneously increasing oxygen delivery through the nasal cannula attached to the patient. The device is programmed to reduce or stop an infusion in response to either a clinical (unresponsiveness to audible/tactile stimuli) or physiologic (oxygen desaturation, hypoventilation) indication of oversedation.

A recent study conducted in the United States and Belgium demonstrated the feasibility of SEDASYS in administering minimal to moderate propofol sedation for endoscopic procedures [29]. The results were consistent with a low mean propofol dosage (65 mg) and a very rapid recovery time (29 seconds). Oxygen desaturation lasting less than 30 seconds occurred in 6% of patients and 18 (38%) had at least one episode of apnea lasting more than 30 seconds. There was no need for airway support and there were no device-related adverse events [29]. While these results are encouraging, the FDA has not yet approved this device, because of safety concerns.

Summary

Sedation provided by trained personnel is generally safe, with the most frequent adverse effect being respiratory depression. When not detected and treated, severe brain damage or death may result. Use of end-tidal capnography improves early detection of respiratory depression and airway obstruction. Brain function monitoring may also help achieve desired sedation levels, although more studies are required. Controversies include the optimal choice of sedative agents and whether propofol can be safely administered by non-anesthesia providers. Future drugs include potential use of fospropofol and dexmedetomidine for sedation, patient-controlled sedation, and computer-assisted personalized sedation.

References

1. Cravero JP. Risk and safety of pediatric sedation/anesthesia for procedures outside the operating room. *Curr Opin Anaesthesiol* 2009; **22**: 509–13.

2. Cravero JP, Blike GT, Beach M, *et al.* Incidence and nature of adverse events during pediatric sedation/anesthesia for procedures outside the operating room: report from the Pediatric Sedation Research Consortium. *Pediatrics* 2006; **118**: 1087–96.

3. Bhananker SM, Posner KL, Cheney FW, *et al.* Injury and liability associated with monitored anesthesia care: a closed claims analysis. *Anesthesiology* 2006; **104**: 228–34.

4. Metzner J, Posner KL, Domino KB. The risk and safety of anesthesia in remote locations: the US closed claims analysis. *Curr Opin Anaesthesiol* 2009; **22**: 502–8.

5. Metzner J, Domino KB. Risks of anesthesia or sedation outside the operating room: the role of the anesthesia care provider. *Curr Opin Anaesthesiol* 2010; **23**: 523–31.

6. American Society of Anesthesiologists (ASA). Standards for basic anesthetic monitoring. Park Ridge, IL: ASA, 2010. www.asahq.org/For-Healthcare-Professionals/Standards-Guidelines-and-Statements.aspx (accessed June 2011).

7. Pino RM. The nature of anesthesia and procedural sedation outside of the operating room. *Curr Opin Anaesthesiol* 2007; **20**: 347–51.

8. Soto RG, Fu ES, Vila H, Miguel RV. Capnography accurately detects apnea during monitored anesthesia care. *Anesth Analg* 2004; **99**: 379–82.

9. Krauss B, Hess DR. Capnography for procedural sedation and analgesia in the emergency department. *Ann Emerg Med* 2007; **50**: 172–81.

10. Anderson JL, Junkins E, Pribble C, Guenther E. Capnography and depth of sedation during propofol sedation in children. *Ann Emerg Med* 2007; **49**: 9–13.

11. Deitch K, Miner J, Chudnofsky CR, *et al.* Does end tidal CO_2 monitoring during emergency department procedural sedation and analgesia with propofol decrease the incidence of hypoxic events? A randomized, controlled trial. *Ann Emerg Med* 2010; **55**: 258–64.

12. Qadeer M, Vargo JJ, Dumot JA, *et al.* Capnographic monitoring of respiratory activity improves safety of sedation for endoscopic cholangiopancreatography and ultrasonography. *Gastroenterology* 2009; **136**: 1568–76.

13. Qadeer MA, Vargo JJ, Patel S, *et al.* Bispectral index monitoring of conscious sedation with the combination of meperidine and midazolam during endoscopy. *Clin Gastroenterol Hepatol* 2008; **6**: 102–8.

14. Agrawal D, Feldman HA, Krauss B, Waltzman ML. Bispectral index monitoring quantifies depth of sedation during emergency department procedural

sedation and analgesia in children. *Ann Emerg Med* 2004; **43**: 247–55.

15. Dominguez TE, Helfaer MA. Review of bispectral index monitoring in the emergency department and pediatric intensive care unit. *Pediatr Emerg Care* 2006; **22**: 815–21.

16. Schilling D, Rosenbaum A, Schweizer S, *et al.* Sedation with propofol for interventional endoscopy by trained nurses in high-risk octogenarians: a prospective, randomized, controlled study. *Endoscopy* 2009; **41**: 295–8.

17. McQuaid KR, Laine L. A systematic review and meta-analysis of randomized, controlled trials of moderate sedation for routine endoscopic procedures. *Gastrointest Endosc* 2008; **67**: 910–23.

18. Cote GA, Hovis RM, Ansstas MA, *et al.* Incidence of sedation-related complications with propofol use during advanced endoscopic procedures. *Clin Gastroenterol Hepatol* 2010; **8**: 137–42.

19. Fatima H, DeWitt J, LeBlanc J, *et al.* Nurse-administered propofol sedation for upper endoscopic ultrasonography. *Am J Gastroenterol* 2008; **103**: 1649–56.

20. Rex DK, Deenadayalu VP, Eid E, *et al.* Endoscopist-directed administration of propofol: a worldwide safety experience. *Gastroenterology* 2009; **137**: 1229–37.

21. Singh H, Poluha W, Cheung M, *et al.* Propofol for sedation during colonoscopy. *Cochrane Database Syst Rev* 2008; (4): CD006268.

22. Rex DK, Heuss LT, Walker JA, Qi R. Trained registered nurses/endoscopy teams can administer propofol safely for endoscopy. *Gastroenterology* 2005; **129**: 1384–91.

23. Moore GD, Walker AM, MacLaren R. Fospropofol: a new sedative-hypnotic agent for monitored anesthesia care. *Ann Pharmacother* 2009; **43**: 1802–8.

24. Struys MM, Fechner J, Schuttler J, Schwilden H. Erroneously published fospropofol pharmacokinetic-pharmacodynamic data and retraction of the affected publications. *Anesthesiology* 2010; **112**: 1056–7.

25. Dere K, Sucullu I, Budak ET, *et al.* A comparison of dexmedetomidine versus midazolam for sedation, pain and hemodynamic control, during colonoscopy under conscious sedation. *Eur J Anaesthesiol* 2010; **27**: 648–52.

26. Arain SR, Ebert TJ. The efficacy, side effects, and recovery characteristics of dexmedetomidine versus propofol when used for intraoperative sedation. *Anesth Analg* 2002; **95**: 461–6.

27. Mandel JE, Tanner JW, Lichtenstein GR, *et al.* A randomized, controlled, double-blind trial of patient-controlled sedation with propofol/remifentanil versus midazolam/fentanyl for colonoscopy. *Anesth Analg* 2008; **106**: 434–9.

28. Rodrigo MR, Irwin MG, Tong CK, Yan SY. A randomised crossover comparison of patient-controlled sedation and patient-maintained sedation using propofol. *Anaesthesia* 2003; **58**: 333–8.

29. Pambianco DJ, Whitten CJ, Moerman A, *et al.* An assessment of computer-assisted personalized sedation: a sedation delivery system to administer propofol for gastrointestinal endoscopy. *Gastrointest Endosc* 2008; **68**: 542–7.

Chapter 13

Simulation training for sedation

Valeriy Kozmenko, James Riopelle, Alan D. Kaye,
and Lyubov Kozmenko

Introduction

During the past two decades, simulation has been extensively used in military and aviation training. In 2003, the Louisiana State University Health Sciences Center developed and successfully implemented a required simulation curriculum, one of the first of its kind in the United States. Since then, this practice has been widely accepted by many other medical schools, both in the USA and abroad. Simulation has been used for teaching medical students and residents, nursing students and practicing nurses, as well as clinical physicians in many fields of patient care. Simulation is one of the tools that can be effectively used to teach sedation to both anesthesiologists and non-anesthesiologists.

The purpose of simulation is "knowledge application that is an observable behavior based on understanding specific concepts and principles and executed in specific context" [1]. Multiple studies have shown that the best acquisition of new knowledge and skills occurs in the environments that are very similar or identical to the conditions in which those skills will be used – this is called situated, or immersive, teaching and learning. Simulation can create highly realistic immersive environments that can greatly enhance learning. In a real clinical setting, all patients undergoing sedation differ in gender, body weight, coexisting medical conditions, distinctive attributes of anatomy of the upper airways, reaction to medications, etc., which makes providing the same teaching experience to all trainees difficult. In contrast, simulation can deliver standardized experiences to any number of trainees an unlimited number of times by using realistic preprogrammed case scenarios. Reducing the level of anxiety associated with learning new skills, which can potentially harm a patient when the skill is learned on a real patient, significantly enhances the clinical value of the simulation experience. Simulation is an ideal tool for learning how to manage both rare clinical events and conditions which a trainee might experience on a routine basis. "Perhaps the best and most valid use of simulation training is to shorten the traditional learning curve and reduce risks" [1].

Moderate and Deep Sedation in Clinical Practice, ed. Richard D. Urman and Alan D. Kaye.
Published by Cambridge University Press. © Cambridge University Press 2012.

Simulator types

There are several classifications of simulators. One of them is based on the media used in simulation. This classification divides all simulators into two major categories:

(1) computer screen-based simulators
(2) mannequin-based simulators

Each category has its advantages and disadvantages.

Computer screen-based simulators

Screen-based simulators have several obvious positives, such as:

(1) Cost of technology – for example, one copy of Sedation Simulator, produced by Anesoft Corporation, costs about $99, while an institutional license that allows for unlimited installations of the software costs under $1000. Therefore, computer screen-based simulators are much less expensive than a mannequin-based simulator. This software has a built-in performance assessment tool that can evaluate the quality of virtual patient care. Figure 13.1 demonstrates the quality of this technology.

(2) Low cost of maintenance – no lab space is required, and there is no need to purchase an expensive hardware maintenance warranty, which is usually required in the case of mannequin-based simulators.

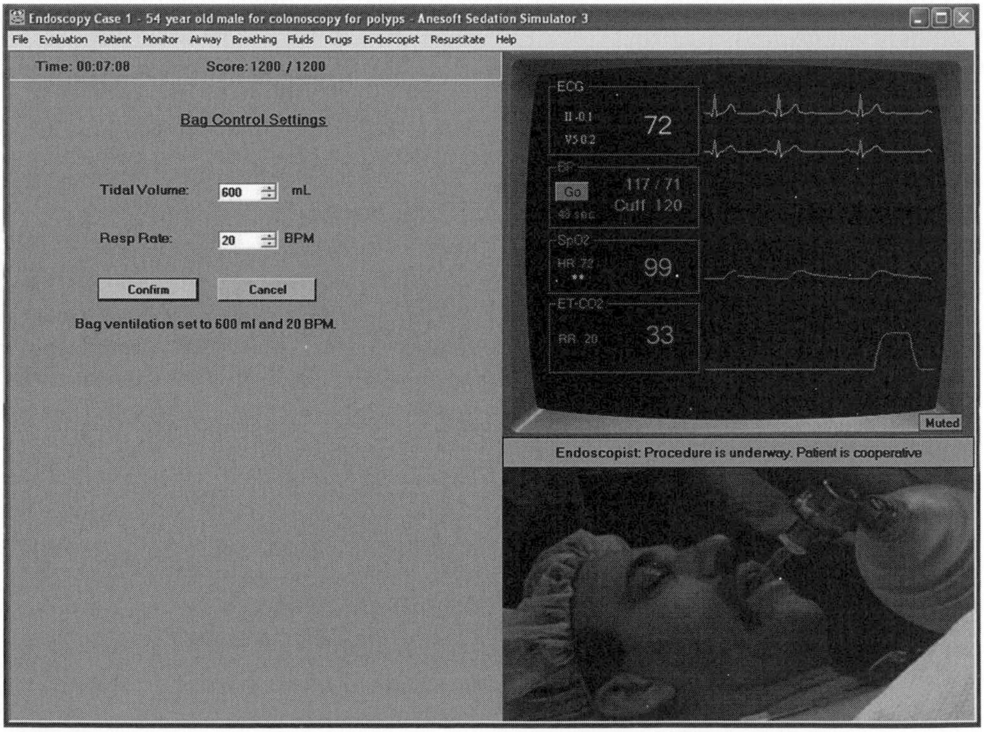

Figure 13.1. Sedation Simulator by Anesoft Corporation. Screenshot used with the permission of the manufacturer.

(3) No need for a full-time or part-time instructor to operate the simulator – in 2010, an average simulator instructor's salary was $60,000–$80,000 per year in the United States, based on the instructor's experience and qualifications.

(4) Convenience and flexibility – the trainees can run the simulator at the convenience of their own homes. This is an especially attractive feature for practicing healthcare personnel, whose schedule is usually too busy to allocate time for attending a simulation center.

Negatives of the screen-based simulators are:

(1) Lower level of physical realism in comparison to presently available mannequin-based simulators.

(2) Simulation sessions are not supervised by an instructor who can debrief the session.

(3) Efficacy of learning might be affected by the trainee's computer skills.

Mannequin-based simulators

Mannequin-based simulators have many positives, such as:

(1) Higher level of fidelity (e.g., measure of the realism of a model or simulator).

(2) Possibility of use with real clinical equipment – infusion pumps, laryngoscopes, lung ventilators, etc.

(3) They can be used for in-situ training in a real clinical environment – operating room, emergency room, radiology lab, etc.

(4) Can be used for team training in conjunction with the other simulators – for example, one can use a Medical Education Technologies (METI) Human Patient Simulator side by side with a Simbionix simulator for interventional intravascular procedures.

(5) Performing procedures on a mannequin-based simulator does not require advanced computer skills.

Negatives of the mannequin-based simulators are:

(1) Cost of the simulator, which can vary between $19,000 and $250,000, depending on the vendor and the type of simulator.

(2) Usually, a designated laboratory space is required.

(3) Frequent use of the simulator is associated with extensive wear and tear damage, which may require replacing parts and purchasing expensive maintenance warranties from the manufacturer.

(4) An interaction between the trainees and the simulator is usually performed via an instructor, which adds to the cost of operating the simulator.

(5) As technology advances, upgrades are usually expensive.

All mannequin-based simulators can be divided into three groups, based on the level of fidelity that they provide:

(1) low-fidelity simulators and part task trainers

(2) intermediate-fidelity simulators

(3) high-fidelity simulators

The difference between intermediate- and high-fidelity simulators can be subjective, and sometimes it is difficult to determine to which category a simulator belongs.

Simulators in sedation education

Appropriate airway management, which should include endotracheal intubation, is part of teaching the safe administration of sedation. An intubating head, such as a Nasco "Airway Larry" Adult Airway Management Trainer (around $1000), can be used to teach non-anesthesiologists the basic principles of maintaining patency of the patient's airway and endotracheal intubation (Figure 13.2).

Examples of a combined low-fidelity simulator and a simple vital signs simulator include the UNI-Sim (Rigel Medical: Figure 13.3) and the VitalSim (Laerdal: Figure 13.4). The Vital Signs Simulator, produced by Channing Bete Company, could be used at a fraction of the cost of a high-fidelity mannequin-based computer-driven simulator.

Louisiana State University Health Sciences Center has developed and successfully implemented a three-dimensional (3D) avatar-based simulator (Figure 13.5). A similar simulator could be used as a valuable addition to any simulation system or combination of several simulators. A 3D animated patient is the core of the avatar-based simulator. An avatar can be remotely controlled by an operator, who can trigger different verbal responses from the avatar as well as facial expressions and body movements. An avatar-based simulation can be used for pre-procedural evaluation of the patient as well as for the assessment of the level of sedation/analgesia during or after the procedure.

High-fidelity mannequin-based simulators

Currently, the following are the main high-fidelity mannequin-based computer-driven simulators utilized for teaching procedural sedation and analgesia:

(1) Laerdal SimMan simulator (www.laerdal.com)

(2) Medical Education Technologies simulators (www.meti.com)

    (a) Human Patient Simulator

    (b) Emergency Case Simulator

    (c) iStan

(3) Gaumard simulators (www.gaumard.com)

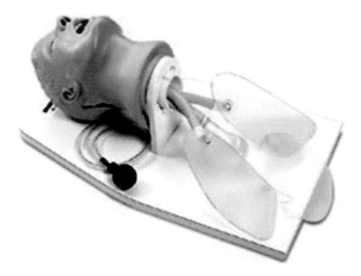

Figure 13.2. Nasco "Airway Larry" Adult Airway Management Trainer. Photo from the manufacturer's website, www.enasco.com. Reproduced with permission.

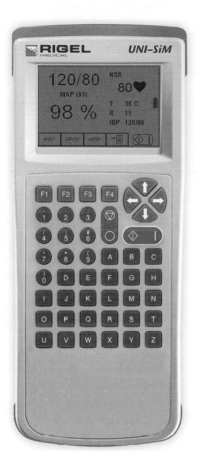

Figure 13.3. UNI-Sim vital signs simulator. Photo from the manufacturer's website, www.rigelmedical.com. Reproduced with permission.

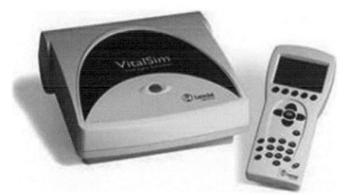

Figure 13.4. VitalSim vital signs simulator. Photo from the manufacturer's website, www. laerdal.com. Reproduced with permission.

These simulators share some common features, such as being capable of generating the patient's vital signs, including pulse oximetry, cardiac rhythm tracing, pulses, etc., but they also have unique distinctive properties. For example, the Gaumard simulator is completely tetherless (there are no wires connecting the computer to the mannequin) and is very easy to use on the fly (manually changing vital signs parameters rather than using preprogrammed scenarios). Also, the Gaumard simulator has the lowest retail price of the three above-mentioned brands.

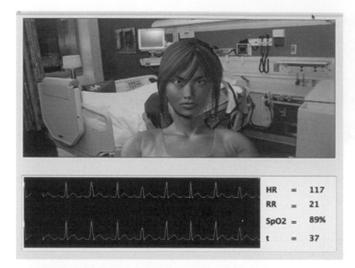

Figure 13.5. Three-dimensional avatar-based simulator developed by Louisiana State University Health Sciences Center.

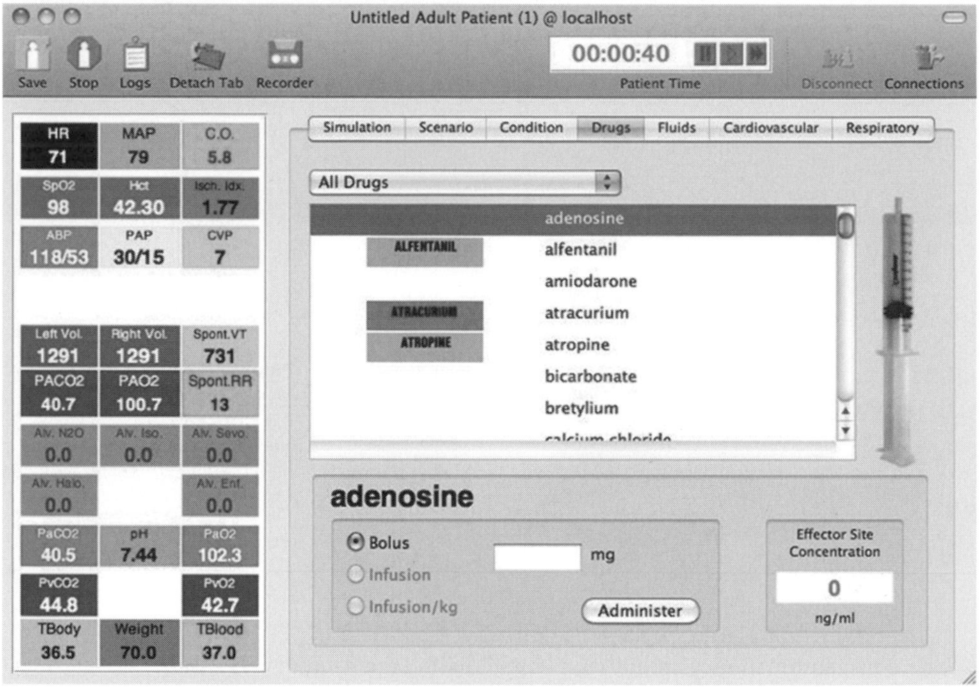

Figure 13.6. METI Human Patient Simulator (HPS Version 6.4) instructor's user interface. © 2011 METI. Used with permission.

In general, METI simulators have the most elaborate design, with built-in physiologic and pharmacologic systems that can be used for modeling different clinical conditions, and they have a sophisticated scenario editor/player (Figures 13.6 and 13.7). The METI Human Patient Simulator, the most advanced in the METI family of simulators, has an automated drug recognition system that uses barcode-labeled syringes to detect the type and amount of

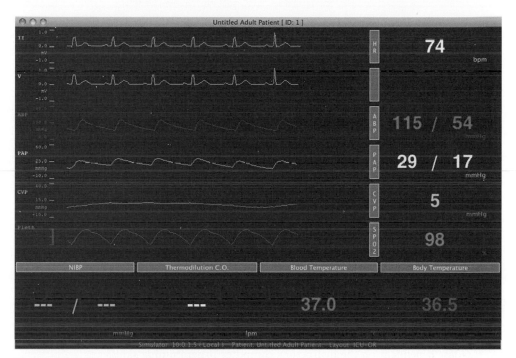

Figure 13.7. METI patient's waveform display. © 2011 METI. Used with permission.

drug injected. When the simulator detects what drug and how much has been administered to the virtual patient, its pharmacologic model will automatically generate an appropriate pharmacodynamic response.

Louisiana State University Health Sciences Center has developed a new technology that advances the automation capabilities of METI simulators even further. This technology, called "Clinical Model," enables the simulator to analyze the interventions that the trainees make and compare their appropriateness with the best practice protocols for a given medical condition. Further, it can generate an appropriate response in the form of the patient's voice response, changes of vital signs or laboratory values (e.g., changes in coagulation studies), or generate appropriate imaging studies (e.g., blood clot in a heart chamber, pneumothorax, etc.). An intuitive and user-friendly graphic user interface (GUI) of the "Clinical Model" makes using METI simulators much easier (Figures 13.6 and 13.7).

The most recent METI simulator, iStan, also runs wirelessly. All METI simulators have tremendous automation capabilities, which makes them extremely useful if the same scenarios are used on a daily basis.

Laerdal SimMan simulators also have advanced programming features that allow them to run preprogrammed scenarios as well as to be used on the fly. In its latest model, SimMan 3G, Laerdal has implemented the proximity sensors in the syringes and the mannequin, making automatic drug recognition possible.

There are two main ways to run mannequin-based simulators – on the fly and using preprogrammed scenarios. Which one is better? Again, each method has its own pros and cons' as outlined below.

Running preprogrammed scenarios

(1) Developing scenarios is time-consuming.

(2) It requires some scripting or programming skills.

(3) It saves time if the same scenario is used frequently (develop it once, use it forever).

(4) It provides a consistent simulation experience (this is especially important if simulation is used for certification or in a longitudinal curriculum).

(5) A well-scripted scenario makes the simulation experience less dependent on the level of the instructor's expertise, because all simulators' responses are carefully preprogrammed.

(6) It requires a full-time simulator instructor to create scenarios.

Running a simulator on the fly

(1) There is no upfront time investment.

(2) It can be exhausting if the same scenario is used frequently.

(3) It is more flexible if the trainees take an action that was not anticipated during scenario development.

(4) It does not require a full-time simulation instructor.

(5) The way the scenario plays depends on the level of clinical knowledge of the instructor.

(6) It is less dependent on the instructor's computer programming skills.

Taking into account the pros and cons of these two methods, the logical conclusion is that if the same scenarios are going to be used on a regular basis, it would make sense to spend time to preprogram the scenarios, because it will save time in the long run. If simulation is used only occasionally, running a simulator on the fly is the best choice.

A variety of commercially available simulators with different levels of fidelity and realism raises a question as to which one should be used for a particular course. After many debates at the Society for Simulation in Healthcare, a consensus has been reached that the learning objectives dictate how much realism is sufficient [2]. For example, if the major goal of the training course is to teach procedural sedation and/or analgesia, using expensive surgical lights in the simulation theater will not significantly add to the course's educational value. Equally, if the purpose of the training course is to teach surgical residents appropriate chest tube placement, the presence of a real anesthesia machine will not help to reach this specific teaching point.

Summary

Simulators are very effective in healthcare education, and they can be used for teaching the safe administration of sedation and/or analgesia. There are a variety of commercially available simulators on the market today, from very affordable part task trainers and vital signs generators to highly sophisticated mannequin-based computer-driven high-fidelity simulators. Selection of an appropriate simulator or combination of simulators in most cases can be determined by the teaching and learning objectives of a particular training course, as well as by reference to the strategic plans of a given institution. Any simulator is capable of delivering an exciting and valuable educational experience to both the trainees and instructors.

References

1. Kozmenko V, Kaye AD, Hilton C. Theory and practice of developing an effective simulation-based curriculum. In Kyle RR, Murray WB, eds., *Clinical Simulation: Operations, Engineering and Management*. Burlington, MA: Academic Press, 2007; 135–52.

2. Society for Simulation in Healthcare discussion forum, 2009. www.ssih.org (accessed June 2011).

Further reading

Guyot P, Drogoul A, Honiden S. Power and negotiation: lessons from agent-based participatory simulations. Proceedings of the Fifth International Joint Conference on Autonomous Agents and Multiagent Systems (AAMAS-06); 27–33.

Idaho Bioterrorism Awareness and Preparedness Program. Training methodologies. www.isu.edu/irh/IBAPP/methodologies.shtml (accessed June 2011).

Knowles MS, Holton EF, Swanson RA. *The Adult Learner*, 6th edn. Burlington, MA: Elsevier, 2005.

Radcliff BJ. Why soft-skills simulation makes a hard case for sales training. Atlanta, GA: CompeteNet, 2005. www.competenet.com/downloads/SimulationWP-F1.pdf (accessed June 2011).

Serious games improving training and performance metrics. *Serious Games Market*. seriousgamesmarket.blogspot.com/2010/07/serious-games-improving-training-and.html (accessed June 2011).

Chapter 14

Sedation in the radiology suite

Brenda Schmitz

Introduction

The number of minimally invasive procedures and diagnostic imaging examinations requiring moderate sedation has increased greatly in the radiology department. While the interventional radiology suite has long been the location for many fluoroscopic and ultrasound-guided procedures, computed tomography (CT) and magnetic resonance imaging (MRI) are also modalities used for procedure guidance. Invasive procedures in radiology may be painful, anxiety-producing, and require the patient to remain still for an extended period of time. The American College of Radiology (ACR) and the Society of Interventional Radiology (SIR) have published practice guidelines for sedation and analgesia [1]. These guidelines can assist practitioners in providing appropriate and safe care for patients requiring sedation during diagnostic and therapeutic radiologic exams.

Contrast media in radiology

Many procedures in radiology are performed with the use of iodinated contrast media, and safe use of contrast media is important to everyday radiology practice. Although there are many types of iodinated contrast media available, with varied degrees of osmolarity, the one most commonly used in radiology procedures today is low-osmolar contrast medium (LOCM) of both ionic and nonionic types. Reports of adverse reactions from LOCM in the literature range from 0.2% to 0.7% [2–5]. High-osmolar contrast medium (HOCM) has an increased incidence of adverse reactions and is not used in most imaging centers today. Iso-osmolar contrast is also available, but the indication for use is not clear at this time. Contrast agents used in MRI are gadolinium-based and have lower risk of adverse reactions compared to LOCM. Adverse reactions to contrast media are referred to as anaphylactoid, as there is no evidence of an allergen–antibody relationship. However, the presentation and

Moderate and Deep Sedation in Clinical Practice, ed. Richard D. Urman and Alan D. Kaye.
Published by Cambridge University Press. © Cambridge University Press 2012.

treatment for these reactions is similar to an allergic-type reaction. A pre-procedure assessment of the following conditions is helpful to identify patients at an increased risk for adverse reactions:

- history of allergies, especially with a history of a significant reaction, such as anaphylaxis
- asthma
- renal insufficiency
- cardiac disease (angina, congestive heart failure, primary pulmonary hypertension, aortic stenosis)
- paraproteinemias such as multiple myeloma
- diabetes mellitus
- sickle cell anemia

Clinical signs of a contrast reaction, and suitable treatment methods, include the following:

- Mild reactions such as rash, uticaria, and pruritus often require no treatment, but the patient should be observed for 30–60 minutes to ensure that the symptoms resolve and do not progress to a more severe reaction. Diphenhydramine 25–50 mg PO/IV/IM may be given for patient comfort and relief of symptoms.
- Moderate to severe reactions such as wheezing, cough, and throat tightness require urgent attention with administration of oxygen, a beta-agonist such as albuterol via a metered-dose inhaler or nebulized delivery system, and, in cases of hemodynamic instability or airway compromise, subcutaneous or intramuscular epinephrine. Auto-injector delivery systems, such as an EpiPen, are quite useful to have available, as they are appropriately dosed and ready for immediate use.

Current guidelines do not support screening patients for seafood and shellfish allergies, as this has not been shown to increase the risk for an adverse reaction. Patients with a history of a prior reaction to contrast media are at risk for a recurrent reaction and should receive premedication prior to any future intravascular contrast study. There are several premedication protocols available [2], and they should be confirmed with the patient prior to the procedure. For emergency procedures, intravenous steroids have not been shown to be helpful when given less than 4–6 hours prior to contrast administration [2] (Table 14.1).

Procedures in interventional radiology requiring moderate sedation

Diagnostic venography/arteriography

A percutaneous catheter is inserted, often through a sheath placed in a peripheral artery (femoral, brachial) or vein. Contrast media is injected and the image is captured using fluoroscopy. Angiography is often performed to diagnose vessel stenosis and blockages, vascular malformations, aneurysms, and bleeding vessels, all within the viscera or in the extremities. When an abnormality is found, additional interventional procedures to treat the vessel are often performed immediately following angiography.

The most common site for arterial puncture is the left or right femoral artery, but other sites such as the brachial artery may be used as well. Once the skin puncture is made, a

Table 14.1. Prevention strategies for contrast media reactions

	Elective procedures	Emergency procedures
Option 1	Methylprednisolone 50 mg PO at 13 hours, 7 hours, and 1 hour before contrast injection, and diphenhydramine 50 mg IV, IM, PO 1 hour before contrast	Methylprednisolone sodium succinate 40 mg IV or hydrocortisone sodium succinate 200 mg IV every 4 hours until contrast given, and diphenhydramine 50 mg IV 1 hour prior to contrast injection
Option 2	Methylprednisolone 32 mg PO at 12 hours and 2 hours before contrast injection, and antihistamine (diphenhydramine) 50 mg IV, IM, PO 1 hour before contrast.	If allergic to methylprednisolone and other medications such as aspirin, NSAIDs, or asthmatic, may use dexamethasone sodium sulfate 7.5 mg or betamethasone 6.0 mg IV every 4 hours until contrast injection, and diphenhydramine 50 mg IV 1 hour prior to contrast administration
Option 3	Hydrocortisone 200 mg IV may be used for patients unable to take oral medications	Diphenhydramine 50 mg IV, IM, PO without steroid administration

vascular sheath is inserted. The vascular sheath contains a hemostatic valve that allows the passage of guidewires and various catheters to the intended location. Contrast is then injected by hand or power injector, and radiographic images are acquired.

Procedural and recovery considerations

- Pain assessment and management of anxiety are essential throughout the procedure and must be provided while at the same time allowing for the patient to cooperate with breath holds and/or to answer basic neurological assessment questions.
- Moderate sedation should be administered prior to local anesthetic injection and skin puncture and maintained throughout the procedure.
- Patients may experience nausea, warmth, and heat sensation during contrast injection.
- While contrast injection into the large vessels does not cause pain, special attention should be given during contrast injections to peripheral vasculature of the legs, arms, and head, as these can be quite painful, and analgesia should be administered prior to injection.
- The patient must remain still during image acquisition, because movement will negatively affect image quality.
- Contrast media volume varies depending on the number of vessels imaged or interventions deployed. It is important to maintain intravenous hydration with 0.9% saline at 100 mL/h to decrease the risk of contrast induced nephropathy (CIN) [2].
- A urinary catheter may be needed if the planned procedure and recovery period are long and require activity restrictions. Most arteriography exams last 1–2 hours, but additional time can be expected if interventional procedures follow the diagnostic exam.
- Post-procedure activity restrictions include bed rest with immobilization of the arterial-puncture-site limb for 4–6 hours unless a closure device is deployed in the puncture site

at the end of the procedure. When these devices are placed, bed rest is usually limited to 2 hours or per specific manufacturer guidelines.

- Complications of arteriography include bleeding from the puncture site, thrombosis at the insertion site or other accessed vessel, contrast reaction, embolus, and dissection.

Arterial interventions

When an artery becomes occluded or is abnormal, the treatment options are determined by the occlusion or abnormality type, location, and desired technical and clinical end point. There are several types of interventions, including:

- percutaneous transluminal angioplasty (PTA) with or without stent placement
- thrombolysis
- embolization

Percutaneous transluminal angioplasty

PTA is used to treat narrowed or occluded arteries and veins in the periphery or viscera. A catheter with a balloon attached is inserted through a sheath into a large peripheral artery or vein and directed to the occluded site under fluoroscopic guidance. The balloon is inflated and blood flow is restored. If appropriate, a stent is placed to maintain vessel patency.

Procedural and recovery considerations include the following:

- Arteriography or venography will precede interventional therapy. Monitor for contrast reaction.
- Patients need to maintain position and remain still, especially during imaging, balloon inflation, and stent deployment.
- Patients will most likely experience increased pain during angioplasty of peripheral vessels and may require additional analgesia prior to balloon inflation and stent deployment.
- Arterial spasm and ureteral, biliary, and gastrointestinal colic may occur during artery manipulation, requiring administration of nitroglycerine, verapamil, or papaverine directly to the affected vessel.
- Post-procedure, the puncture site should be assessed for bleeding, hematoma, and pain.
- Mild analgesia, such as with acetaminophen, is usually adequate; however, severe pain at the puncture site or intervention site should be evaluated immediately for complications such as bleeding, dissection, or thrombus.

Thrombolysis

A patient with acute or chronic peripheral arterial or bypass graft vessel occlusion with thrombus may present with acute pain and decreased or absent pulses in the affected limb. A thrombolytic drug such as tissue plasminogen activator (TPA) or urokinase is infused at a specific rate over several hours through a catheter positioned at the site of the occlusion. Repeat angiography is performed to assess vessel patency. The catheter may be left in place for an additional 24–48 hours to deliver a low dose of a thrombolytic agent. A thrombectomy catheter may be placed to mechanically remove the thrombus as well.

Percutaneous transcatheter embolization

Embolization of an artery or vein, often called bland embolization, is performed to occlude a vessel by administering an embolic agent made of liquid particulates, sclerosants, absolute ethanol, metal, coils, or glue to the site of the vessel abnormality. Choice of embolizing agent is based on the clinical application, target lesion, and specific technical and clinical considerations. Examples of indications for embolization therapy include treatment of bleeding, arteriovenous malformations, aneurysms, uterine fibroids, and varicoceles. In addition, bland embolization is used for preoperative devascularization of hypervascular organs and lesions to reduce intraoperative blood loss. All embolization procedures begin with selective angiography with contrast of the organ or lesion.

Procedural and recovery considerations for common arterial interventions are shown in Table 14.2.

Interventional oncology procedures

Percutaneous ablation techniques such as radiofrequency ablation (RFA) and cryotherapy are used to treat cancerous lesions of the liver, kidney, lung, and prostate. Ultrasound, MRI, or CT imaging is used to guide specialized catheters to the tumor site, where therapy is then delivered.

Radiofrequency ablation

During RFA, a needle probe with single or umbrella-type electrodes is placed through the skin directly to the tumor, connected to an electrical generator. Grounding pads are placed on the patient's thigh. A target temperature is set, and radiofrequency energy is delivered to the tumor through the electrodes, creating friction of ions and thus generating heat. Once the temperature reaches 60 °C, cell death occurs. Each ablation can take 10–30 minutes, depending on the number and size of lesions.

Although most RFA procedures can be performed with moderate sedation, deep sedation or general anesthesia may be needed to manage pain, discomfort due to positioning, and patient movement. RFA procedures are characterized by brief periods of intense stimulation and pain, often requiring an additional dose of sedative and/or analgesic. The sedation plan is often determined by operator preference and patient choice. Patients can experience moderate pain immediately after RFA and are managed with opioid analgesics. Patients are often discharged home the same day if pain can be controlled with oral medication. Procedure time can range from 1 to 3 hours.

Immediate post-procedure complications include:

- Lung RFA – pneumothorax is reported in 30–40% of patients [6], and serial chest x-rays are needed during the recovery phase for those that are small or asymptomatic. Most pneumothoraces are self-limiting and do not require a chest tube. Other complications include intercostal nerve injury and bleeding.
- Liver RFA – bleeding, especially in patients with abnormal coagulation, and nontarget embolization of the bowel or gallbladder. Brief or long-lasting shoulder pain is also reported.
- Renal RFA – retroperitoneal bleeding is reported in 15–20% of cases [6], but it is not significant enough to require transfusion or intervention in most cases. Intercostal nerve injury can occur during the procedure and is noted when the patient complains of pain, but if the patient is deeply sedated this will often go undetected.

Cryoablation

Most commonly used for renal cell carcinoma and in liver metastases, this procedure involves the placement of several cryoablation needles under CT or MRI guidance into

Table 14.2. Procedural and recovery care considerations for some common arterial interventions

Procedure	Procedural considerations	Recovery considerations
Uterine artery embolization	Epidural catheter placement may be considered prior to procedure for management of post-procedure pain. Moderate sedation is adequate for procedural management of pain and anxiety. Contrast media is utilized during arteriography for catheter placement. Abdominal pain and cramping generally occurs 30 minutes after the uterine artery is embolized and fibroid tumor necrosis begins.	Pain and cramping may be severe for 8–12 hours following the procedure. Systemic or epidural patient-controlled analgesia delivery systems are good options for patients. Assess respiratory status closely while patient-controlled pain medications are being titrated to avoid oversedation.
Chemoembolization	Selective angiography is performed to locate the lesion. A chemotherapeutic agent(s) is delivered directly to the tumor site. Next, an embolic agent, is injected at the site to reduce blood flow, thereby inducing direct ischemia to the tumor and trapping the chemotherapeutic agent, resulting in greater local drug concentration. Because the chemotherapeutic agents are not delivered systemically, side effects are minimal. Patients are given antiemetic agents and prophylactic antibiotics prior to the procedure. The procedure length is 1–2 hours.	Patients can develop post-embolization syndrome characterized by abdominal pain, nausea, vomiting, fever, and fatigue. Antiemetics, pain medications, and intravenous fluids should be continued during recovery. Patients will be admitted to the hospital for 24–48 hours for symptom management and observation.
Radioembolization (also called brachytherapy or selective internal radiation therapy, SIRT) for nonsurgical treatment of liver tumors	A selective hepatic angiogram is performed and a catheter is guided to a branch of the hepatic artery and placed near the liver tumor. Tiny microsphere beads containing yttrium-90, a radioisotope that emits beta-radiation, are infused into the blood supply of the tumor. The procedure can take 60–90 minutes. A pre-planning hepatic angiogram is performed several days prior to radioembolization to identify blood supply to the lesion. Coils may be inserted into vessels supplying the intestine or stomach to prevent migration of radioactive microspheres.	Abdominal pain, nausea, and fatigue are common after treatment. Patients are discharged home after they have recovered from sedation and the groin puncture site is stable.

Table 14.3. Central venous catheters: types and indications

Catheter type	Indications	Duration
Non-tunneled catheters: peripherally inserted central catheters (PICC), standard triple-lumen central catheters (CVAC), temporary dialysis catheters	IV antibiotic therapy and IV medications requiring central venous access Poor peripheral venous access Parenteral nutrition Hemodialysis access in acutely ill patient	Short to intermediate use
Tunneled catheters	Chemotherapy Hemodialysis Apheresis	Long term use
Implanted ports	Chemotherapy Intermittent IV therapy	Long term intermittent use

the tumor. Argon gas is delivered to the tip, where it expands and cools to temperatures below −100 °C, creating an "iceball" and destroying cancerous cells and a small amount of surrounding tissue. Two freeze–thaw processes are recommended to increase the efficacy of tumor ablation. Cryoablation may be performed under moderate sedation, but is often performed under deep sedation or general anesthesia because of prone positioning requirements and to limit any patient movement during needle probe placement.

Vascular access

Placement of central venous catheters in the interventional radiology department is accomplished with the use of both ultrasound and fluoroscopic guidance. The most common sites for tunneled central catheter insertion are the axillosubclavian, internal jugular, and external jugular veins. Catheters are placed for a variety of indications such as hemodialysis, chemotherapy, long-term intravenous antibiotic therapy, parenteral nutrition, or poor vascular access in an acutely ill patient. Several types of central venous catheters are available from various manufacturers (Table 14.3).

Procedural considerations

- Non-tunneled catheters are often placed with local anesthetic only; however, patients must maintain a turned neck position during catheter insertion and may require analgesia.
- Procedure length is minimal, and light to moderate sedation is all that is required.
- Attention must be paid to coordinating the patient's breathing during cannulation of the vein, to prevent air embolism.
- Regardless of the use of sedation or local anesthetic, patients should be placed on ECG monitoring during the procedure to assess for arrhythmias, which can occur during placement due to mechanical irritation from the catheter or guidewires near the right atrium.

Table 14.4. Biopsies: imaging techniques and sedation-related procedural considerations

Organ/site	Imaging modality	Procedural considerations
Superficial (including thyroid)	Ultrasound	Local anesthetic. Moderate sedation not needed in cooperative patients.
Liver	Ultrasound, CT, MRI, fluoroscopy	Analgesia is usually minimal, but patient may require sedation to limit movement and promote comfort. Major complications include hemorrhage, especially in the setting of cirrhosis and portal hypertension, and it may be life-threatening. Bed rest required post-procedure for 2–4 hours.
Abdominal (kidney, pancreas, spleen)	Ultrasound, CT, MRI	Based on location of lesion, sedation may be required to maintain patient position and provide analgesia.
Chest (lung)	Fluoroscopy, CT	Assess respiratory status closely, as patient is at risk for pneumothorax and bleeding when inadvertent puncture of a nontarget vessel occurs. May note a small amount hemoptysis after tissue sample obtained. Post-procedure chest x-ray needed to evaluate for pneumothorax.
Bone	CT, fluoroscopy	May be positioned supine or prone and require increased analgesia during procedure.

Percutaneous needle biopsy/core needle biopsy

Although fluoroscopy may be used, most needle biopsies are performed using ultrasound, CT, or MRI guidance. The type of image modality used depends upon the location, size, and accessibility of the lesion. While most superficial and abdominal lesions are amenable to ultrasound guidance, biopsies of the lung, bone, and spine are often performed using CT guidance. A new technique in liver imaging, MRI elastography [7], can identify fibrotic areas within the liver so that a more directed and precise core tissue sample can be obtained under MRI guidance. Special equipment and needles must be used that are MR-compatible, to avoid injuries to patient and staff from the magnetic field. A transjugular approach to liver biopsy may be required for patients with coagulopathy, whereby a core tissue sample is obtained by a catheter inserted in the jugular vein and guided to the primary vein.

Various biopsies, imaging techniques usually employed, and potential complications are listed in Table 14.4.

Dialysis and fistula/graft maintenance procedures

Patients receiving dialysis will often develop thrombosis and stenosis of the fistula or graft. Several treatment options are available, including angioplasty, stenting, thrombolysis, and thrombectomy with balloon techniques and mechanical devices. No one treatment has been shown to be more effective than the others [8], but the most important issues for prolonged graft patency are removal of the arterial clot, successful treatment of stenosis, and restoration of adequate graft blood flow. Stenosis and occlusions can also occur at the outflow tract of the fistula, and venous angioplasty has been shown to be effective; however, fistulas are known to have recurrent re-stenosis and must be followed every 3–6 months to maintain patency.

Procedural considerations

- Prior to any hemodialysis access intervention, the patient's potassium level and fluid volume status must be assessed if hemodialysis has not been performed recently due to fistula/graft dysfunction.
- The procedure begins with a venogram of the native venous system from the fistula/graft to the superior vena cava.
- Once all areas of stenosis and thrombosis are identified, moderate sedation should be administered and maintained prior to any balloon inflation or catheter manipulation, to minimize unwanted movement and provide analgesia.
- The procedure can take 1–2 hours if multiple occlusions are noted.
- Once the procedure has been successfully completed, patients may receive dialysis immediately. If the procedure is not successful, or if continuous thrombolytic therapy is required, a temporary central catheter may be placed to perform hemodialysis until the fistula is fully functional.

Drainage catheter placement

There are many types of drainage catheters placed under radiologic guidance to remove fluid accumulations from the body, such as chest tubes, nephrostomy tubes, and biliary tubes. In addition, a drainage catheter may be placed to remove fluid from an abscess located in the abdominal or pelvic cavity. Moderate sedation is used in most cases, because of the location and depth of the fluid collection, and discomfort related to catheter insertion. Specific procedural considerations are noted in Table 14.5.

Moderate sedation in MRI

Providing moderate sedation in the MRI suite presents both patient and environmental challenges. The most common need for moderate sedation in MRI arises from severe anxiety from claustrophobia while in the scanner. Reports in the literature indicate that 4–30% of patients undergoing an MRI exam experience anxiety that results in a nondiagnostic exam due to frequent movement [9]. Even when they are given oral anxiolytic agents, it is still difficult for patients to complete the study [10]. Other indications for moderate sedation include:

- interventional procedures performed under MRI guidance
- severe pain that limits the ability to maintain body position during the exam
- neurologic or behavior disorders that prevent the patient from tolerating the exam

It is important to limit patient movement in order to acquire clear diagnostic images, and in some instances patients require deep sedation or general anesthesia administered by an anesthesiologist.

MRI safety is paramount for patient and staff. An important point to remember is that the magnet is always "on" despite the presence of an exam in progress. The MRI area is divided into four zones:

- Zone I – general public areas outside the MRI environment.
- Zone II – interface area between public area and zone III. Typical activities include registration, safety screening, patient history, and insurance questions. Area is supervised by MR personnel.

Table 14.5. Drainage catheters: procedural and sedation considerations

Catheter type	Description	Procedural considerations	Sedation considerations
Biliary	A catheter is placed through the skin and liver into the bile ducts to drain bile, either externally into a drainage bag or internally into the small bowel.	Prophylactic antibiotics are often given, especially if known infection. Contrast is given through the catheter to confirm placement. Patients with underlying liver disease often have coagulopathy and are at risk for bleeding. If appropriate, a stent may be placed for areas of stricture.	Acute bacteremia may develop during procedure or in the recovery phase, leading to acute hemodynamic instability. Patients who are critically ill with known sepsis may require anesthesiology or intensivist-managed sedation. Patients may have altered mental status due to acute liver dysfunction.
Nephrostomy	A catheter is placed through the skin and kidney to the renal pelvis or calyx.	Prone position. Prophylactic antibiotics recommended. Contrast is injected into catheter to guide and confirm placement. Patients must be cooperative and follow directions.	Respiratory status must be monitored closely because of positioning. Obese and elderly patients are at risk for hypoventilation. Transient bacteremia may occur, causing altered hemodynamics during the procedure or immediately post-procedure. May require anesthesiology consultation for deep sedation in patients unable to follow direction and maintain position.
Gastrostomy/ jejunostomy	Catheter is placed through the abdominal wall directly to the stomach with fluoroscopic guidance.	Two techniques for catheter placement, one directly through the skin and the other through the patient's mouth and pulled out the abdominal wall using a snare catheter.	May be performed with local anesthetic, but often given moderate sedation as patients are often unable to cooperate due to underlying acute medical issues.
Abscess	Catheter is placed through the skin directly to the area of fluid collection.	Altered positioning due to fluid location, most likely will be supine.	Monitor respiratory status closely. Transient bacteremia may develop during catheter placement or

Table 14.5. (cont.)

Catheter type	Description	Procedural considerations	Sedation considerations
			immediately post-procedure, producing rigors, chills, and hypotension.
Chest	Catheter is placed in pleural space to drain blood, fluid, or air.	Supine or lateral (side-lying) position. Complications include pneumothorax and bleeding. Chest x-ray needed post-procedure.	Monitor respiratory status closely. Patient often dyspneic. Titrate sedation slowly to avoid oversedation once tube is placed and fluid removed and dyspnea resolved.
PleurX®	A catheter with a one-way valve that prevents inadvertent leakage of fluid or air is placed into the pleural or peritoneal space. Indicated for intermittent drainage of chronic effusions.	Supine position for placement, but patient with increased pleural fluid may have dyspnea and require slight head elevation.	Monitor respiratory status closely for patients with pleural effusions. Monitor for signs of pneumothorax when placing catheter in pleural space. Patient may require albumin with large fluid volume removal.

- Zone III – area is physically restricted to MR personnel by key locks or or other locking systems. This zone has free access to zone IV.
- Zone IV – scanner magnet room.

Ferromagnetic objects and equipment at the interface of zone III and IV and within zone IV produce a "missile effect" injury as they are pulled in to the bore of the scanner at a rapid speed. Commonly reported objects include infusion pumps and poles, wheelchairs, and scissors, and there is a report of an oxygen tank that led to a pediatric patient death [11]. Other injuries include skin burns from objects that produce heat while in the scanner, such as coiled monitor leads and certain medical implants, wires and staples, and objects such as bullets and shrapnel. Implanted objects such as certain aneurysm clips and surgical staples are also at risk of becoming dislodged. Acoustic injury can occur from the loud knocking sound made by the scanner, and patients should wear appropriately fitting earplugs and head-phones. For MRI-guided percutaneous procedures such as biopsies of the breast, prostate, and liver, all equipment, catheters, needles, and supplies must be nonferromagnetic and compatible for use in the scanner. The US Food and Drug Administration (FDA) labeling system for portable objects taken into the scanning room, as developed by the American Society for Testing and Materials (ASTM) International, is as follows:

- MRI safe (green square label): nonmetallic objects
- MRI conditional (yellow triangular label): no or negligible attractive forces
- MRI unsafe (red round label): not safe

While some equipment and medical devices may be deemed safe or conditional at lower magnet strength, such as 1.5 tesla, they may be found to be unsafe at higher strength, such as in the newer 3.0 tesla scanners. A listing of medical devices and implants tested for safety is available from the Institute for Magnetic Resonance Safety, Education, and Research [12]. Any item not listed as MRI safe or conditional must not be allowed in zone IV until testing is completed.

The American College of Radiology and the Joint Commission have published safety guidelines and alerts [13,14], and all personnel working in the MRI environment must review these guidelines and receive facility-specific safety training and screening prior to caring for patients in the environment. It is important to review the most current listing of approved medical devices, as this is updated frequently. For example, a recent review of the literature on patients with cardiac pacemakers [15] and guidelines from professional groups [16] clearly outline procedures that must be followed in order to safely perform imaging on these patients, and the benefits and risks must be clearly understood and discussed with the patient.

Prior to sedation, the patient must complete an MRI safety questionnaire and medical history. If the patient is not competent, a family member, guardian, or primary physician with knowledge of the patient's medical history must complete and sign the form. Direct visualization of the patient's respiratory status is not possible while the patient is in the scanner, and therefore the following MRI-safe monitoring equipment must be available: ECG, pulse oximetry, blood pressure, and capnography. The magnetic field will produce intermittent ECG tracing distortions despite filter settings, but heart rate and oxygenation are available by pulse oximetry. For patients with heart rhythm concerns, assessments may be made between imaging sequences. The capnograph provides a respiratory waveform and can be used as a respiratory rate monitor. Certain percutaneous procedures, such as cyroablation of a liver lesion, require the patient to perform breath holds and maintain a supine position for several hours, and are often performed under monitored anesthesia care. Breast biopsies, on the other hand, are many times performed with local anesthesia and minimal anxiolysis. Emergency equipment should be stored in zone II or III in the event of an emergency, the patient should be removed from zone IV immediately before resuscitative effort begins. Most emergency equipment, such as defibrillators, are ferromagnetic and could lead to a dangerous and possibly lethal situation for patient and staff. Emergency responders should not be allowed in zone IV unless they have been previously screened and trained in MRI safety.

References

1. ACR-SIR Practice Guideline for Sedation and Analgesia (res 45). American College of Radiology Guidelines and Standards Committee of the Commission on Interventional and Cardiovascular Radiology and the Society of Interventional Radiology, 2010. www.acr.org/guidelines (accessed February 2011).

2. American College of Radiology Committee on Drugs and Contrast Media. *ACR Manual on Contrast Media*, Version 7, 2010. www.acr.org/ SecondaryMainMenuCategories/ quality_safety/contrast_manual.aspx (accessed February 2011).

3. Davenport MS, Cohan RH, Caoili EM, Ellis JH. Repeat contrast medium reactions in premedicated patients: frequency and severity. *Radiology* 2009; **253**: 372–9.

4. Cochran ST, Bomyea K, Sayre JW. Trends in adverse events after IV administration of contrast media. *AJR Am J Roentgenol* 2001; **176**: 1385–8.

5. Wang CL, Cohan RH, Ellis JH, *et al.* Frequency, outcome, and appropriateness of treatment of nonionic iodinated contrast media reactions. *AJR Am J Roentgenol* 2008; **191**: 409–15.

6. Georgiades CS, Hong K, Geschwind JF. Pre- and postoperative clinical care of patients undergoing interventional oncology procedures: a comprehensive approach to preventing and mitigating complications. *Tech Vasc Interventional Rad* 2006; **9**: 113–24.

7. Yin M, Talwalkar JA, Glaser KJ, *et al.* Assessment of hepatic fibrosis with magnetic resonance elastography. *Clin Gastroenterol Hepatol* 2007; **5**(10): 1207–13.e2.

8. Bent CL, Sahni VA, Matson MB. The radiological management of the thrombosed arteriovenous dialysis fistula. *Clin Radiol* 2011; **66**(1): 1–12.

9. Meléndez JC, McCrank E. Anxiety-related reactions associated with magnetic resonance imaging examinations. *JAMA* 1993; **270**: 745–7.

10. Middelkamp JE, Forster BB, Keogh C, Lennox P, Mayson K. Evaluation of adult outpatient magnetic resonance imaging sedation practices: are patients being sedated optimally? *Can Assoc Radiol J* 2009; **60**: 190–5.

11. Kanal E, Barkovich AJ, Bell C, *et al.* ACR guidance document for safe MR practices: 2007. *AJR Am J Roentgenol* 2007; **188**: 1447–74.

12. Institute for Magnetic Resonance Safety, Education, and Research. www.imrser.org (accessed February 2011).

13. Shellock F. MRI safety website. www.mrisafety.com (accessed March 2011).

14. The Joint Commission. Preventing accidents and injuries in the MRI suite. *Sentinel Event Alert* 2008; **38**. www.jointcommission.org/sentinel_event_alert_issue_38_preventing_accidents_and_injuries_in_the_mri_suite (accessed March 2011).

15. Zikria JF, Machnicki S, Rhim E, Bhatti T, Graham RE. MRI of patients with cardiac pacemakers: a review of the medical literature. *AJR Am J Roentgenol* 2011; **196**: 390–401.

16. Levine GN, Gomes AS, Arai AE, *et al.* Safety of magnetic resonance imaging in patients with cardiovascular devices: an American Heart Association scientific statement from the Committee on Diagnostic and Interventional Cardiac Catheterization, Council on Clinical Cardiology, and the Council on Cardiovascular Radiology and Intervention: endorsed by the American College of Cardiology Foundation, the North American Society for Cardiac Imaging, and the Society for Cardiovascular Magnetic Resonance. *Circulation* 2007; **116**: 2878–91.

Chapter

15

Sedation in the endoscopy suite

Laura Kress, Donna Beitler, and Kai Matthes

Introduction

Approximately 2.8 million sigmoidoscopies and 14.2 million colonoscopies were performed in the USA in 2002 [1,2], and the majority of these procedures are performed in the office setting. An integral part of the practice of gastrointestinal endoscopy is adequate sedation and analgesia. The American Society of Anesthesiologists (ASA) has developed guidelines for sedation and analgesia by non-anesthesiologists [3]. These practice guidelines are systematically developed recommendations that assist the practitioner and patient in making decisions about health care. The guidelines provide basic recommendations that are supported by analysis of the current literature and by a synthesis of expert opinion, open forum commentary, and clinical feasibility data.

The level of sedation required depends upon the type of endoscopic procedure being performed. The American Society of Anesthesiologists (ASA) has classified four "levels" of sedation, often referred to as a continuum, from minimal sedation to general anesthesia (see Table 1.2). Most endoscopies are performed with the patient under *moderate sedation*, formerly known as *conscious sedation*. At this level of consciousness, the patient is able to make a purposeful response to verbal or tactile stimulation, and both ventilatory and cardiovascular function are maintained. There are instances that require a greater depth of sedation, which may become a general anesthetic [2]. Patient responsiveness during *deep sedation* involves purposeful responses to painful stimuli only. Airway support is sometimes required to maintain sufficient oxygenation [4]. At the level of *general anesthesia*, the patient is not arousable, even to painful stimuli. Airway support is frequently required, and cardiovascular function may be impaired [4–6].

Moderate and Deep Sedation in Clinical Practice, ed. Richard D. Urman and Alan D. Kaye.
Published by Cambridge University Press. © Cambridge University Press 2012.

The appropriate choice of agents and techniques for sedation/analgesia is dependent on the experience and preference of the individual practitioner, requirements or constraints imposed by the patient or procedure, and the likelihood of producing a deeper level of sedation than anticipated. Because it is not always possible to predict how a specific patient will respond to sedative and analgesic medications, practitioners intending to produce a given level of sedation should be able to rescue patients whose level of sedation becomes deeper than initially intended. For moderate sedation, this implies the ability to manage a compromised airway or hypoventilation in a patient who responds purposefully after repeated or painful stimulation. For deep sedation it implies the ability to manage respiratory or cardiovascular instability in a patient who does not respond purposefully to painful or repeated stimulation. Levels of sedation referred to in the recommendations relate to the level of sedation intended by the practitioner.

Sedation for upper gastrointestinal endoscopy is considered as safe, with only minimal risk for the patient. However, cardiopulmonary complications may account for over 50% of all reported complications. The majority of these incidents are based on aspiration, oversedation, hypoventilation, vasovagal episodes, and airway obstruction [7,8]. A prospective survey of 14,149 upper endoscopies indicated that the rate of immediate cardiopulmonary incidents was 2 per 1000 cases, with a 30-day mortality rate of 1 per 2000 cases [9]. A retrospective review of 21,011 procedures found the rate of cardiovascular complications was 5.4 per 1000 procedures [10]. The reported complications varied from mild transient hypoxemia to severe cardiorespiratory compromise and death.

The choice of the appropriate sedation modality is always a balance between optimizing the benefits of sedation and minimizing the potential risks. A survey by the American College of Gastroenterology physician members revealed that three-quarters of practitioners use an opioid combined with a benzodiazepine for sedation [11].

Pre-sedation patient assessment

The ASA agrees that appropriate pre-procedure evaluation increases the likelihood of satisfactory sedation and decreases the likelihood of adverse outcomes. The ASA recommends a classification of patients according to their individual risk factors, the ASA physical status classification system (see Table 3.2). This classification has been shown to correlate well with the risk of adverse events.

Clinicians administering sedation/analgesia should be familiar with sedation-oriented aspects of the patient's medical history and how these might alter the patient's response to sedation/analgesia. These include abnormalities of the major organ systems; previous adverse experience with sedation/analgesia as well as regional and general anesthesia; drug allergies, current medications, and potential drug interactions; time and nature of last oral intake; and history of tobacco, alcohol, or substance use or abuse. Patients presenting for sedation/analgesia should undergo a focused physical examination, including vital signs, auscultation of the heart and lungs, and evaluation of the airway. Pre-procedure laboratory testing should be guided by the patient's underlying medical condition and the likelihood that the results will affect the management of sedation/analgesia. These evaluations should be confirmed immediately before sedation is initiated.

The presence of underlying cardiopulmonary disease must be assessed, as these patients may not tolerate shifts in heart rate, blood pressure, and oxygen saturation that can occur with sedation. A history of obstructive sleep apnea and snoring should be assessed for presence of active or undiagnosed obstructive disease. A complete medication history must be obtained and documented. Patients who use opioid analgesics for chronic pain syndromes or who use illicit drugs may require larger doses of sedative medication to achieve an appropriate level of sedation for the procedure.

Patients undergoing sedation/analgesia for elective procedures should not drink fluids or eat solid foods for a sufficient period of time to allow for gastric emptying before their procedure, as recommended by the ASA guidelines for preoperative fasting (see Table 8.2). In urgent, emergent, or other situations in which gastric emptying is impaired, the potential for pulmonary aspiration of gastric contents must be considered in determining (1) the target level of sedation, (2) whether the procedure should be delayed, or (3) whether the trachea should be protected by endotracheal intubation. For additional pre-procedure assessment considerations, see Chapter 4.

Airway assessment

Positive-pressure ventilation, with or without tracheal intubation, may be necessary if respiratory compromise develops during sedation/analgesia. This may be more difficult in patients with atypical airway anatomy. In addition, some airway abnormalities may increase the likelihood of airway obstruction during spontaneous ventilation (Table 15.1).

Personnel and equipment

The careful monitoring of patients during and immediately after the administration of sedation is paramount in minimizing the potential risks. Rooms need to be large enough to accommodate the endoscopic and monitoring equipment, while still allowing for staff to move around the patient. In addition, the required emergency and resuscitation equipment should be located within the unit.

Emergency equipment required to be immediately available to the patient
- bag-valve mask and source of 100% oxygen
- suction equipment and portal suction machine
- airway and intubation equipment
- reversal medications

Emergency equipment required to be available on the unit
- defibrillator
- additional resuscitation medications required for advanced cardiac life support (ACLS)

Patients should be under constant surveillance by trained medical or nursing personnel from the start of sedation until the patient's consciousness returns to pre-sedation baseline. In addition to the endoscopist, during the procedure there should be a specially trained registered nurse exclusively assigned to the administration and monitoring of the sedation. A technician can be assigned to assist the endoscopist with equipment needs during the procedure. It is within the scope of practice of registered nurses (RNs) across the United States to administer and monitor patients receiving moderate sedation through the administration of opioids and benzodiazepines. Most states require the nurse to demonstrate competency in this skill through annual training. This education usually includes a didactic

Table 15.1. Factors that may be associated with difficulty in airway management

History	
Previous problems with anesthesia or sedation	
Stridor, snoring, or sleep apnea	
Advanced rheumatoid arthritis (limited neck extension)	
Chromosomal abnormality, e.g. trisomy 21 (atlantoaxial instability)	
Physical examination	
Habitus	Significant obesity (especially involving the neck and facial structures)
Head and neck	Short neck, limited neck extension Decreased hyoid–mental distance (less than 3 cm in an adult) Neck mass Cervical spine disease or trauma Tracheal deviation Dysmorphic facial features (e.g., Pierre-Robin syndrome)
Mouth	Small opening (less than 3 cm in an adult) Edentulous Protruding incisors Loose or capped teeth Dental appliances High arched palate Macroglossia Tonsillar hypertrophy Nonvisible uvula
Jaw	Micrognathia Retrognathia Trismus Significant malocclusion

course followed by a preceptorship with an experienced healthcare provider, where competency can be assessed and documented. Both the endoscopist and the RN should be knowledgeable in advanced cardiac life support techniques. Freestanding units are required to have access to an advanced cardiac life support team that can transfer the patient to a higher level of care should the need arise.

Patient monitoring for gastrointestinal endoscopy

According to the American Society for Gastrointestinal Endoscopy (ASGE) *Guidelines for Conscious Sedation and Monitoring During Gastrointestinal Endoscopy*, patients undergoing endoscopic procedures with moderate or deep sedation must have continuous monitoring before, during, and after the administration of sedatives [6]. Standard monitoring, airway and emergency equipment recommendations are listed below.

Standard noninvasive monitoring

- blood pressure*
- electrocardiogram (ECG)*
- oxygen and gas analyzer
- pulse oximetry (SaO$_2$)*
- capnography* (only if indicated)
- body temperature

*Minimal monitoring requirement for gastrointestinal endoscopy [6]

Standard airway and emergency equipment

- anesthesia machine
- oral suction
- emergency drugs (atropine, phenylephrine, succinylcholine)
- airway equipment (laryngoscope, endotracheal tubes, bag-valve mask [Ambu-bag])

Supplemental oxygen

Supplemental oxygen administration has been shown conclusively in controlled trials to reduce the incidence of desaturation, which can occur in up to 47% of patients undergoing endoscopic retrograde cholangiopancreatography (ERCP) without oxygen [12,13]. However, supplemental oxygen may mask hypoventilation [14,15]. Pulse oximetry is a "late sign" of airway obstruction, as hypercarbia occurs before hypoxia becomes evident in a decrease of SaO$_2$ values. During hypoventilation, a significant amount of CO$_2$ can accumulate in the patient, which may lead to CO$_2$ narcosis, before hypoxia becomes evident in desaturation. Capnography detects hypoventilation earlier and may be a more reliable monitor of ventilation.

Capnography

Particularly in prolonged therapeutic procedures such as ERCP, in which deeper levels of sedation are reached, capnography (end-tidal CO$_2$ monitoring) may be superior for evaluation of ventilation compared with pulse oximetry alone [16,17]. However, routine measurement of CO$_2$ has not yet been associated with any objective clinical outcome benefits. Oxygen insufflation via nasal prongs combined with an extranasal capnography line are currently available. Alternatively one can attach a plastic syringe needle to a standard capnography line. This can then be fixed into the side holes of the oxygen facemask near the mouth in close proximity to the exhaled air stream. Percutaneous capnography devices are becoming increasingly available and may provide more reliable data than end-tidal CO$_2$ detection techniques during spontaneous ventilation.

Assessment of sedation

An assessment of the patient's sedation level can be undertaken using an Observer's Assessment and Alertness/Sedation scale (Table 15.2).

Common procedures in gastrointestinal endoscopy

A vast majority of endoscopic procedures are diagnostic in nature and performed on relatively healthy patients with an ASA status of 1 or 2. However, some patients with significant

Table 15.2. Observer's Assessment and Alertness/Sedation (OAA/S) scale [18]

OAA/S score	Patient response	Speech	Facial expression	Eyes
5	Responds readily to name spoken in normal tone	Normal	Normal	Clear, no ptosis
4	Lethargic response to name spoken in normal tone	Mild slowing or thickening	Mild relaxation	Glazed or mild ptosis (less than half the eye)
3	Responds only after name is called loudly and/or repeatedly	Slurring or prominent slowing	Marked relaxation	Glazed and marked ptosis (more than half the eye)
2	Responds only after mild prodding or shaking	Few recognizable words		
1	Responds only after squeezing the trapezius			
0	Does not respond after squeezing the trapezius			

comorbidities may require elective or urgent endoscopic intervention with often inadquate preparation. Most endoscopic procedures are relatively short in duration and performed on an outpatient basis. Stimulation is in the form of varying abdominal comfort, or gag reflex during upper endoscopy. Rapid-onset and short-acting pharmacologic agents are preferred in order to improve practice efficiency by short induction and short recovery times. Anesthesia professionals are commonly involved in the care of high-risk patients with significant comorbidities [2].

Diagnostic and therapeutic endoscopic interventions include the following:

(1) esophagogastroduodenoscopy (EGD)

(2) proctoscopy/sigmoidoscopy/colonoscopy

(3) endoscopic retrograde cholangiopancreatography (ERCP)

Esophagogastroduodenoscopy (EGD)

EGD is the diagnostic and/or therapeutic examination of the upper gastrointestinal tract using a flexible endoscope. This procedure provides the possibility to obtain tissue specimens by performing a mucosal biopsy or staining of mucosal surface. Diagnostic EGD can be performed with little or no sedation, but potentially painful procedures such as esophageal dilatation require deeper levels of sedation or general anesthesia.

Stimulating events during EGD

(1) intubation of the esophagus

(2) passing the endoscope through the pylorus

(3) endoscopic intervention:

  (a) esophageal/gastric/duodenal biopsy

  (b) endoscopic mucosal resection (EMR)

  (c) endoscopic submucosal dissection (ESD)

(d) argon plasma coagulation (APC)

(e) endoscopic hemostasis

(f) variceal band ligation

(g) dilatation of esophageal strictures

(h) esophageal stenting

(i) photodynamic therapy

Proctoscopy/sigmoidoscopy/colonoscopy

Proctoscopy is the exam of the rectum using a rigid endoscope, which usually does not require intravenous anesthesia. Sigmoidoscopy and colonoscopy are the diagnostic and/or interventional examination of the sigmoid or the entire lower gastrointestinal tract up to the distal ileum using a flexible endoscope. Endoscopy of the lower gastrointestinal tract is considered less stimulating than that of the upper gastrointestinal tract, as there is no gag reflex involved.

Stimulating events during proctoscopy/sigmoidoscopy/colonoscopy

(1) introduction of the endoscope

(2) advancement of the endoscope against the bowel wall (diverticula, flexures, etc.)

(3) looping of the colonoscope with consecutive distention of the bowel

(4) endoscopic intervention:

(a) mucosal biopsy

(b) endoscopic mucosal resection (EMR)

(c) endoscopic submucosal dissection (ESD)

(d) argon plasma coagulation (APC)

(e) endoscopic hemostasis

(f) polypectomy

(g) dilatation and stenting of malignant strictures

Endoscopic retrograde cholangiopancreatography (ERCP)

ERCP is the radiographic examination of the biliary and/or pancreatic ducts using contrast injected endoscopically through the major or minor duodenal papilla. This procedure requires the skillful delivery of sedation and analgesia. If patients are too lightly sedated, they move, retch, or gag. If they are too deeply sedated, they may develop airway obstruction, hypoventilation, hemodynamic instability, and delayed emergence and recovery.

Stimulating events during ERCP

(1) intubation of the esophagus

(2) passing the scope through the pylorus

(3) shortening the scope

(4) cannulating the common bile duct or pancreatic duct

(5) sphincterotomy

(6) endoscopic intervention:

(a) stent placement

(b) balloon or basket extraction of biliary stones

(c) laser lithotripsy

Choice of sedation regimens

Sedation for gastrointestinal endoscopy is particularly challenging because of variability during most procedures, characterized by long nonstimulating periods interspersed with significantly stimulating events. Some endoscopic procedures are undertaken without sedation, while others may require general anesthesia. The administration of sedatives requires the placement of a peripheral intravenous line, which should be maintained until the patient is appropriately recovered, awake and alert, and hemodynamically stable.

Below are general patient characteristics associated with tolerance of upper endoscopy or colonoscopy with little or no sedation in a number of clinical trials.

Standard sedation anesthetic requirement:

- elderly
- nonanxious patients
- male gender
- absence of abdominal pain history

Less well studied are the factors that predict which patients are prone to experience great difficulty with sedation. The characteristics of difficult-to-sedate patients are recognized by most experienced endoscopists, and are listed below.

Increased sedation anesthetic requirement:

- a history of prior difficulty with conscious sedation
- prescribed or illicit benzodiazepine or opioid use
- heavy alcohol use

Sedation for gastrointestinal endoscopic procedures requires adequate patient management by trained individuals with theoretical and practical knowledge of the pharmacological properties of all medications used, and airway management skills which should include rescue interventions such as proper jaw-thrust maneuvers and positive-pressure ventilation using a bag-valve mask. Related risk factors, the depth of sedation, and the urgency of the endoscopic procedure play important roles in determining whether or not an anesthesiologist is consulted.

The choice of medication for deep sedation is largely operator-dependent, but it generally consists of a sedative such as a benzodiazepine used either alone or in combination with an opioid. The most commonly used benzodiazepines are midazolam and diazepam, with midazolam favored because of its fast onset, short duration, and high amnesic properties. Doses are titrated to patient tolerance depending upon age, other illnesses, use of additional medications, and the sedation requirements of the particular procedure. For prolonged therapeutic procedures such as ERCP, propofol has been demonstrated to be advantageous when compared to standard benzodiazepine/opioid sedation in terms of faster onset, deeper sedation, and faster recovery [4,19–30]. The ASGE recently published a position statement on gastroenterologist-directed administration of propofol, supporting its use by non-anesthesiologists [31]. However, according to current recommendations of the ASA and the propofol labeling, it can only be administered by practitioners trained in the administration of general anesthesia. Deep sedation requires intensive monitoring by individuals trained in emergency resuscitation and airway management [32].

Sedatives/anxiolytics

Patients undergoing sedation for gastrointestinal endoscopy may be premedicated with a benzodiazepine, preferably midazolam, because of its rapid onset and short-acting properties. Analgesia is usually accomplished with fentanyl, a short-acting potent opioid. Propofol is preferred over other anesthetics because of its rapid onset and short duration of action. However, multiple frequently repeated dosing of any of the aforementioned drugs can lead to drug accumulation and oversedation.

Benzodiazepines

Benzodiazepines (Table 15.3) act within the central nervous system at specific benzodiazepine receptor sites. Occupation of these receptors results in augmentation of gamma-aminobutyric acid (GABA), which is an inhibitory neurotransmitter resulting in depression of cortical function. Thus, benzodiazepines result in a dose-dependent continuum of effect from mild sedation through drowsiness and sleep to deep sedation. In addition to sedation, benzodiazepines have anxiolytic and amnesic effects.

Opioids

The analgesic effect of opioids (Table 15.4) is exerted mostly from binding to the mu-opioid receptor, which results in an analgesic effect as well as euphoria. Opioids also cause respiratory depression in a dose-dependent manner that may be reversed by opioid antagonists. Respiratory depression can occur with doses smaller than the dose needed to achieve altered consciousness. Opioids depress both the hypoxic and hypercarbic respiratory drive.

Most endoscopic procedures do not require strong analgesics, as there are usually only limited periods of modest stimulation. Fentanyl may be given in small boluses as an adjunct to the anesthetic regimen. The ventilatory-depressant effects of opioids should be noted, especially when they are used in combination with other sedatives. Patients undergoing sedation for endoscopy have an unprotected airway, may become apneic, and have the potential for aspiration.

Reversal agents

Because of the potential for cardiorespiratory complications associated with sedation, the practitioner should have knowledge of the pharmacology of and indications for reversal agents (Table 15.5).

Adjunct medications

Adjunct medications enhance the effects of opioids and sedatives, especially in the opioid-tolerant patient, and in patients with a history of alcohol and substance abuse. Some adjunct medications also have antiemetic qualities. Examples of adjunct medications include promethazine, droperidol, and diphenhydramine (Benadryl). Due to their superior antiemetic properties in comparison to older agents, serotonin-receptor antagonists (e.g., ondansetron and granisetron) are increasingly being used. Use of adjunct medications for long procedures will decrease the need for larger amounts of opioid analgesics, thereby reducing risks associated with these doses. Therefore, identification of high-risk patients and potential for longer therapeutic procedures is useful for optimal sedation practices.

Table 15.3. Benzodiazepines used for sedation

Drug (brand name)/action	Mode of administration	Pharmacokinetics	Comments
Midazolam hydrochloride (Versed) Short-acting benzodiazepine which produces sedation, anxiolysis, and amnesia	0.5–2.5 mg initial bolus IV Additional midazolam may be given in 0.25–1 mg IV doses to maintain desired level of sedation. For an otherwise healthy patient initial dose is 0.03 mg/kg, not to exceed 2.5 mg IV. Administer slowly with adequate time interval (2–3 min) between doses to assess for the effect of the previously administered dose. Decrease subsequent doses	*Onset*: 1–2.5 min *Peak*: 3–5 min *Duration*: 1–5 h *Elimination*: 1.8–6.4 h	Duration double in elderly and obese patients. *Respiratory*: central respiratory depressant and may produce apnea with rapid administration. Effects are pronounced with concomitant opioid administration. *Cardiovascular*: hypotension in hypovolemic patients, incidence increased with concomitant opioid administration. *Caution*: Do not use midazolam when the patient is taking a protease inhibitor.
Lorazepam (Ativan) Longer-acting benzodiazepine with amnesic and anticonvulsant properties	0.5–1 mg initial bolus IV. Additional lorazepam may be given in 0.25–0.5 mg doses IV to maintain desired level of sedation. **Not an FDA-approved indication**	*Onset*: 15–20 min *Peak*: 60–90 min *Amnesic effects*: 6–8 h after a single dose *Elimination*: 12 h	Must be diluted prior to administration in a peripheral vein. Give slowly to reduce side effects. *Caution*: Reduce dosage in the elderly or debilitated patient. The safety of lorazepam in pediatric patients has not been established.
Diazepam (Valium)	Up to 10 mg initial bolus IV (usually given in 1–2 mg doses). Up to 20 mg max IV dose.	*Onset*: 1–2 min *Peak*: 8 min *Elimination*: 0.83–2.25 days (18–54 h)	*Respiratory*: minimal respiratory depression *Cardiovascular*: minimal depressant effects *Caution*: May cause pain on injection, local irritation, and phlebitis.

Table 15.4. Opioids used for sedation

Drug (brand name)/ action	Mode of administration	Pharmacokinetics	Comments
Fentanyl citrate (Sublimaze) Short-acting narcotic analgesic	The initial dose is 25–100 µg IV administered over a 2 min period. Titrate 25–50 µg IV to patient response. Titration to desired level of sedation should be performed with adequate time interval (3–4 min) between doses.	*Onset*: 3–5 min *Duration*: 3 h	*Respiratory*: potent respiratory depressant alone and when combined with benzodiazepines. *Cardiovascular*: vagotonic producing bradycardia and hypotension in the hypovolemic patient. *Caution*: rapid administration may cause chest wall rigidity, leading to difficult ventilation.
Meperidine (Demerol)	Dilute and titrate 5–10 mg IV in increments	*Onset*: 3–5 min *Duration*: 1–3 h	In equal analgesic doses produces same sedation, respiratory depression, and incidence of nausea and vomiting as morphine. Use in caution with patients with renal insufficiency, liver failure, or CNS dysfunction. May exacerbate seizure disorder.
Morphine sulfate	1 mg IV increments; peak clinical effects not apparent for up to 20 min. Because of the late onset and long duration, morphine is not an ideal agent for sedation and therefore not commonly used.	*Onset*: 5–10 min, peak CNS effect delayed up to 20 min *Duration*: 2–4 h	*Respiratory*: potent respiratory depressant in presence of other sedatives. *Cardiovascular*: hypotension may follow administration to the hypovolemic patient. *Gastrointestinal*: nausea and vomiting. *Genitourinary*: urinary retention. Use with caution on patients with sphincter of Oddi dysfunction as it may increase pancreatic spasms.

Table 15.5. Reversal agents

Drug (brand name)/action	Mode of administration	Pharmacokinetics	Comments
Flumazenil (Romazicon)	IV administration over 15–30 s into a large vein. Initial dose is 0.2 mg IV over 15 s. If desired consciousness level is not achieved after 45 seconds, additional 0.2 mg IV doses administered at 60 s intervals until an adequate response is achieved or a maximum of four additional doses is administered. Maximum cumulative dose is 1 mg IV.	Has not been established as an effective treatment for hypoventilation due to benzodiazepine or combination benzodiazepine–opioid administration. May cause seizures in patients physically dependent on benzodiazepines.	*Caution*: the duration of action of this antagonist may be shorter than that of the drug.
Naloxone hydrochloride (Narcan) Opioid antagonists compete with opioids for the receptor site without causing an opioid effect	For the partial reversal of opioid-related respiratory depression following the use of opioids during procedures. A smaller dose of naloxone is usually sufficient. Naloxone should be titrated according to the patient's response. For the initial reversal of respiratory depression, naloxone should be injected in increments of 0.08–0.2 mg intravenously at 2–3 min intervals to the desired degree of reversal.	*Onset*: within 2 min of IV administration. *Peak*: 5–15 min *Duration*: 45 min	The elimination of naloxone is more rapid than that of opioids and therefore may result in the reappearance of narcosis. Patients should be monitored for a minimum of 2 h following administration of naloxone. It should be used with caution in patients with narcotic dependency as it can cause acute opioids withdrawal. Naloxone should be diluted for sedation reversal, as the doses are much smaller than for opioids overdose.

It should be noted that in December 2001 the Food and Drug Administration (FDA) issued a black-box warning for droperidol. This warning is intended to increase the physician's awareness of the potential for cardiac arrhythmias during drug administration, and to prompt the consideration of alternative medications for patients at high risk for cardiac arrhythmias. The warning states that cases of QT prolongation and/or torsades de pointes have been reported in patients receiving droperidol at amounts at or below recommended doses. Some of these cases have occurred in patients with no known risk factors for QT prolongation and have been fatal [7].

Pharyngeal anesthesia

Commonly used topical anesthetics include benzocaine, tetracaine, and lidocaine, which are administered by aerosol spray or gargling. Topical benzocaine is effective to prevent the gag reflex during insertion of the endoscope. The application should be limited to a single spray of 1 second duration in order to avoid methemoglobulinemia, a systemic side effect that may result if multiple doses are administered topically. Methemoglobinemia is a condition in which hemoglobin becomes methemoglobin by being oxidized and converted from Fe^{2+} to the ferric state (Fe^{3+}), or methemoglobin. Methemoglobin lacks the electron that is needed to form a bond with oxygen, and thus is incapable of oxygen transport, resulting in clinical hypoxia.

Complications

Complications during gastrointestinal endoscopy result mostly from interventional procedures. Hemorrhage following polypectomy is frequently seen and is managed endoscopically, but may require surgical intervention. Perforation during colonoscopy can lead to a distended abdomen with venous compromise and hemodynamic responses due to decreased preload. Variceal bleeding can lead to significant blood loss, which may lead to circulatory compromise and death. This emphasizes the need for healthcare personnel skilled in airway management and emergency resuscitative techniques to be present or immediately available in case any problem should arise.

Recovery

Patients may continue to be at significant risk for developing complications even following completion of the procedure. The critical period is usually the initial 15 minutes after removal of the endoscope. Patients should be continuously observed in an appropriately staffed and equipped area until they are near their baseline level of consciousness and no longer at risk for hypoxemia and cardiorespiratory depression. Discharge criteria should follow the institutional guidelines.

Medication reconciliation

Medication reconciliation was named as a 2005 National Patient Safety Goal by the Joint Commission [33]. With this announcement came the need to accurately and completely reconcile medications across the continuum of care, which includes reviewing and documenting the patient's medication history upon admission to the endoscopy suite. Use of a medication reconciliation tool is associated with significant improvements in patient safety. It helps ensure that pre-procedure medications are continued as needed and a copy of the revised medication list is given to the patient upon discharge from the unit.

Special considerations

Certain types of patients are at increased risk for developing complications related to sedation/analgesia unless special precautions are taken. In patients with significant underlying medical conditions (e.g., extremes of age; severe cardiac, pulmonary, hepatic, or renal disease; pregnancy; drug or alcohol abuse) pre-procedure consultation with an appropriate medical specialist (e.g., cardiologist, pulmonologist) may decrease the risks associated with moderate and deep sedation. In patients with significant sedation-related risk factors (e.g., uncooperative patients, morbid obesity, potentially difficult airway, sleep apnea), consultation with an anesthesiologist should be considered to help minimize adverse outcomes. When administering moderate or deep sedation to these challenging patients, the provider may request that an anesthesiologist be immediately available should problems arise.

Whenever possible, appropriate medical specialists should be consulted before administration of sedation to patients with significant underlying conditions. The choice of specialists depends on the nature of the underlying condition and the urgency of the situation. For severely compromised or medically unstable patients (e.g., anticipated difficult airway, severe obstructive pulmonary disease, coronary artery disease, or congestive heart failure), or if it is likely that sedation to the point of unresponsiveness will be necessary to obtain adequate conditions, practitioners who are not trained in the administration of general anesthesia should consult an anesthesiologist.

Summary

Millions of endoscopies are performed each year in the United States, most in the office-based setting with sedation provided by both anesthesia and non-anesthesia professionals. Most endoscopic procedures are relatively short in duration and performed on an outpatient basis. With appropriate patient selection, pre-procedure assessment, and intra- and post-procedure monitoring the provider can optimize the benefits of sedation while minimizing the potential risks to the patient.

References

1. Seeff LC, Richards TB, Shapiro JA, et al. How many endoscopies are performed for colorectal cancer screening? Results from CDC's survey of endoscopic capacity. Gastroenterology 2004; 127: 1670–7.

2. Matthes K. Gastrointestinal endoscopy in the office-based setting. In Shapiro F, ed., Manual of Office-Based Anesthesia Procedures. Philadelphia, PA: Lippincott Williams & Wilkins, 2007; 120–32.

3. American Society of Anesthesiologists Task Force on Sedation and Analgesia by Non-Anesthesiologists. Practice guidelines for sedation and analgesia by non-anesthesiologists. Anesthesiology 2002; 96: 1004–17.

4. Faigel DO, Baron TH, Goldstein JL, et al. Guidelines for the use of deep sedation and anesthesia for GI endoscopy. Gastrointest Endosc 2002; 56: 613–17.

5. American Society for Gastrointestinal Endoscopy. Training guideline for use of propofol in gastrointestinal endoscopy. Gastrointest Endosc 2004; 60: 167–72.

6. Waring JP, Baron TH, Hirota WK, et al. American Society for Gastrointestinal Endoscopy, Standards of Practice Committee. Guidelines for conscious sedation and monitoring during

gastrointestinal endoscopy. *Gastrointest Endosc* 2003; **58**: 317–22.

7. Benjamin SB. Complications of conscious sedation. *Gastrointest Endosc Clin N Am* 1996; **6**: 277–86.

8. Freeman ML. Sedation and monitoring for gastrointestinal endoscopy. *Gastrointest Endosc Clin N Am* 1994; **4**: 475–99.

9. Quine MA, Bell GD, McCloy RF, *et al.* Prospective audit of upper gastrointestinal endoscopy in two regions of England: safety, staffing, and sedation methods. *Gut* 1995; **36**: 462–7.

10. Arrowsmith JB, Gerstman BB, Fleischer DE, Benjamin SB. Results from the American Society for Gastrointestinal Endoscopy/U.S. Food and Drug Administration collaborative study on complication rates and drug use during gastrointestinal endoscopy. *Gastrointest Endosc* 1991; **37**: 421–7.

11. Cohen LB, Wecsler JS, Gaetano JN, *et al.* Endoscopic sedation in the United States: results from a nationwide survey. *Am J Gastroenterol* 2006; **101**: 967–74.

12. Crantock L, Cowen AE, Ward M, Roberts RK. Supplemental low flow oxygen prevents hypoxia during endoscopic cholangiopancreatography. *Gastrointest Endosc* 1992; **38**: 418–20.

13. Reshef R, Shiller M, Kinberg R, *et al.* A prospective study evaluating the usefulness of continuous supplemental oxygen in various endoscopic procedures. *Isr J Med Sci* 1996; **32**: 736–40.

14. Nelson DB, Freeman ML, Silvis SE, *et al.* A randomized, controlled trial of transcutaneous carbon dioxide monitoring during ERCP. *Gastrointest Endosc* 2000; **51**: 288–95.

15. Fu ES, Downs JB, Schweiger JW, Miguel RV, Smith RA. Supplemental oxygen impairs detection of hypoventilation by pulse oximetry. *Chest* 2004; **126**: 1552–8.

16. Soto RG, Fu ES, Vila H, Miguel RV. Capnography accurately detects apnea during monitored anesthesia care. *Anesth Analg* 2004; **99**: 379–82.

17. Vargo JJ, Zuccaro G, Dumot JA, *et al.* Automated graphic assessment of

respiratory activity is superior to pulse oximetry and visual assessment for the detection of early respiratory depression during therapeutic upper endoscopy. *Gastrointest Endosc* 2002; **55**: 826–31.

18. Chernik DA, Gillings D, Laine H, *et al.* Validity and reliability of the Observer's Assessment of Alertness/Sedation scale: study with intravenous midazolam. *J Clin Psychopharmacol* 1990; **10**: 244–51.

19. Heuss LT, Schnieper P, Drewe J, Pflimlin E, Beglinger C. Safety of propofol for conscious sedation during endoscopic procedures in high-risk patients: a prospective, controlled study. *Am J Gastroenterol* 2003; **98**: 1751–7.

20. Heuss LT, Schnieper P, Drewe J, Pflimlin E, Beglinger C. Conscious sedation with propofol in elderly patients: a prospective evaluation. *Aliment Pharmacol Ther* 2003; **17**: 1493–501.

21. Goff JS. Effect of propofol on human sphincter of Oddi. *Dig Dis Sci* 1995; **40**: 2364–7.

22. Walker JA, McIntyre RD, Schleinitz PF, *et al.* Nurse-administered propofol sedation without anesthesia specialists in 9152 endoscopic cases in an ambulatory surgery center. *Am J Gastroenterol* 2003; **98**: 1744–50.

23. Koshy G, Nair S, Norkus EP, Hertan HI, Pitchumoni CS. Propofol versus midazolam and meperidine for conscious sedation in GI endoscopy. *Am J Gastroenterol* 2000; **95**: 1476–9.

24. Jung M, Hofmann C, Kiesslich R, Brackertz A. Improved sedation in diagnostic and therapeutic ERCP: propofol is an alternative to midazolam. *Endoscopy* 2000; **32**: 233–8.

25. Rex DK, Overley C, Kinser K, *et al.* Safety of propofol administered by registered nurses with gastroenterologist supervision in 2000 endoscopic cases. *Am J Gastroenterol* 2002; **97**: 1159–63.

26. Seifert H, Schmitt TH, Gultekin T, Caspary WF, Wehrmann T. Sedation with propofol plus midazolam versus propofol alone for interventional endoscopic procedures: a prospective, randomized

study. *Aliment Pharmacol Ther* 2000; **14**: 1207–14.

27. Sipe BW, Rex DK, Latinovich D, *et al.* Propofol versus midazolam/meperidine for outpatient colonoscopy: administration by nurses supervised by endoscopists. *Gastrointest Endosc* 2002; **55**: 815–25.

28. Vargo JJ, Zuccaro G, Dumot JA, *et al.* Gastroenterologist-administered propofol for therapeutic upper endoscopy with graphic assessment of respiratory activity: a case series. *Gastrointest Endosc* 2000; **52**: 250–5.

29. Vargo JJ, Zuccaro G, Dumot JA, Shermock KM, Morrow JB, Conwell DL, Trolli PA, Maurer WG. Gastroenterologist-administered propofol versus meperidine and midazolam for advanced upper endoscopy: a prospective, randomized trial. *Gastroenterology* 2002; **123**: 8–16.

30. Wehrmann T, Kokabpick S, Lembcke B, Caspary WF, Seifert H. Efficacy and safety of intravenous propofol sedation during routine ERCP: a prospective, controlled study. *Gastrointest Endosc* 1999; **49**: 677–83.

31. Vargo JJ, Cohen LB, Rex DK, Kwo PY. Position statement: nonanesthesiologist administration of propofol for GI endoscopy. *Gastrointest Endosc* 2009; **70**: 1053–9.

32. American Society of Anesthesiologists (ASA). Guidelines for office-based anesthesia. Park Ridge, IL: ASA, 1999 (last affirmed 2009). www.asahq.org/For-Healthcare-Professionals/Standards-Guidelines-and-Statements.aspx (accessed June 2011).

33. The Joint Commission. Using medication reconciliation to prevent errors. *Sentinel Event Alert* 2006; **35**. www.jointcommission.org/sentinel_event_alert_issue_35_using_medication_reconciliation_to_prevent_errors (accessed June 2011).

Chapter 16

Sedation in the interventional cardiology suite

Erika G. Puente, Alberto Uribe, and Sergio D. Bergese

Introduction

Almost a century after the introduction of cardiac catheterization, and with the development of further interventional cardiology techniques, the cardiology suite has progressed from a solely diagnostic facility. Now it is a more elaborate suite that currently allows the application of multiple techniques for the diagnosis and treatment of a large number of cardiac diseases.

In this context, the complexities of some procedures have increasingly demanded that the management of patients undergoing them also evolves. Additionally, availability of and demand for these procedures has also grown, and they are now frequently performed on a routine or daily basis in most healthcare facilities. Today these increasingly complex procedures are being performed on more acutely ill patients, presenting a challenge to provide adequate patient safety and achieve procedural success. The ultimate goal of the cardiovascular specialist is to be able to perform a successful procedure while ensuring that the patient remains comfortable and has adequate pain control (Table 16.1).

In order to achieve these goals, the patient should be managed with sedative medications sufficient to decrease excessive movement, while at the same time avoiding sedative-induced hemodynamic changes and hypoventilation.

Guidelines for sedation and/or analgesia by non-anesthesiologists provide some direction on sedation techniques for medical diagnostic and therapeutic procedures, but specific guidelines for the anesthetic management of patients in the cardiac catheterization and electrophysiology laboratories by non-anesthesia specialists have not yet been developed [1,2].

Moderate and Deep Sedation in Clinical Practice, ed. Richard D. Urman and Alan D. Kaye.
Published by Cambridge University Press. © Cambridge University Press 2012.

Table 16.1. Goals of sedation and/or analgesia during interventional cardiology procedures

Minimize physical discomfort
Minimize pain
Minimize negative psychological response to treatment
Provide some degree of amnesia
Gain the patient's cooperation
Adequate ventilation (patent airway) and oxygenation (normal breathing)
Minimal variation in hemodynamic parameters
Enable safe discharge from the outpatient unit

Table 16.2. Equipment in the procedure room

Fluoroscopy machine
Procedure table
Screens
Sterile table
Blood analysis machine
Infusion pumps

The cardiology suite

The cardiology suite is designed to meet certain safety parameters. It is typically divided into two main areas, the procedure room and the control room. The control room, which is a nonsterile area, is divided from the procedure room with permanent visual access through special radiation-shielded windows. The person inside the control room has visual access to the procedure room and is able to record and monitor the procedure, as well as to communicate at all times with the personnel on the other side. The control room contains a fully functional workstation that allows the technician to control the fluoroscopy machine, record digital data, and monitor the patient's vital signs and ECG readings (Figure 16.1).

The procedure room is where the intervention is carried out and, therefore, where the equipment used to perform the procedure is located. The cardiologist, nurses, and technicians in the room will work together to provide adequate patient care and monitoring. All personnel who have access to the procedure room during an active procedure must wear protective garments or lead aprons for protection against radiation exposure. These aprons should be of the correct size and should cover reproductive and endocrine organs such as the thyroid gland.

The equipment inside the procedure room consists of the fluoroscopy machine, a procedure table, screens for viewing the procedure, a sterile table for the catheters and supplies, a blood analysis machine, and infusion pumps (Table 16.2 and Figure 16.2).

Monitoring equipment includes blood pressure, vital signs, and ECG monitors, a pulse oximeter, a cardioverter/defibrillator, emergency medications, and airway equipment. It is recommended that there should always be a ventilator, an anesthesia cart, and perhaps a

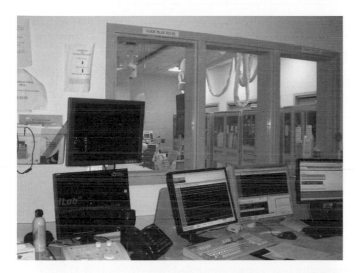

Figure 16.1. Control room with fully functional workstation and radiation-shielded windows.

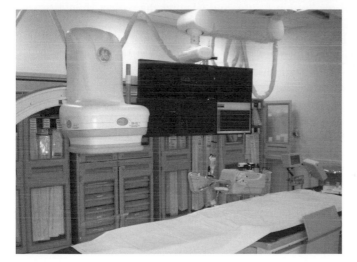

Figure 16.2. Set up in the procedure room, with fluoroscopy machine, procedure table, screens, and infusion pumps.

fiberoptic cart available nearby, or at least a plan in place to access these pieces of equipment, if necessary.

In the procedure room, the physician who carries out the procedure is responsible not only for performing the procedure but also for supervising sedation/analgesia and monitoring of the patient, with the assistance of supporting personnel. Gaitan *et al.* surveyed 95 cardiac electrophysiology programs and found that nurses provided most of the sedation services, including 38% of cases in which patients underwent deeper sedation levels and could not be aroused [3]. This indicates the importance of providing adequate training and guidance for the personnel involved in administering sedation to patients undergoing interventional procedures in the cardiology suite.

Nevertheless, the fact that the physician performing the procedure has to also supervise the sedation and monitor the patient at the same time represents a challenge and, therefore requires the assistance of supporting personnel. Thus, the person in charge of administering the sedation and monitoring the patient should be a well-trained professional dedicated to this task only. These professionals should receive additional and specialized training in basic life support and airway management, pharmacology and interactions of sedatives and analgesics. They should also be trained in the theory and practice of sedation, patient monitoring requirements and interpretation, complications of sedation and analgesia, and recovery and discharge criteria [2].

Patient evaluation

All patients to be scheduled for an interventional cardiac procedure should undergo a rigorous screening and detailed pre-procedure evaluation for medical risk factors that might predispose the patient to complications during the procedure. Most complications are likely to be associated with hemodynamic stability and airway maintenance. Patients considered at higher risk are those who are morbidly obese, have chronic obstructive pulmonary disease (COPD), obstructive sleep apnea, congestive heart failure, are ASA Class 3, have a known or potentially difficult airway, those taking medications that may interfere with the sedation requirements, and those with hemodynamic instability (e.g., poorly controlled hypertension) [1,2].

When deciding the type of medication to use, and whether the patient should receive sedation and/or general anesthesia, the proceduralist must take into consideration the patient's specific needs, and this may involve consulting an anesthesia professional. Table 16.3 lists some of the criteria to consider when deciding if the patient is an appropriate candidate for sedation. For more in-depth discussion, see Chapter 4.

When evaluating patients who will be undergoing interventional cardiac procedures, it is important to remember that these patients usually have a history of prior cardiac disease. Some patients may have a history of previous cardiac diagnostic catheterizations, stent placements, surgeries, arrhythmia interventions (conversion with medication or ablation), echocardiograms, intracardic device placement (pacemaker/defibrillator), and a medication regimen that may need to be reviewed. It is not uncommon that patients scheduled for interventional cardiac procedures may also have a history of prior failed interventions. In such cases, a thorough pre-procedure evaluation should be performed to rule out any possible complications associated with the sedation and/or analgesic technique or medications. If a previous procedure failed because of airway management problems or hemodynamic instability, or if deeper sedation was required, then performing the procedure under general anesthesia should be considered.

In some cases, a pre-procedure evaluation may allow the physician to intervene and prepare the patient beforehand to enable the patient to undergo the procedure without

Table 16.3. Suggested criteria for patients undergoing sedation

Inclusion criteria	Possible exclusion criteria
*ASA class 1 and 2	*Uncooperative patient or significant language barrier
*ASA class 3 in stable condition	*Significant comorbidities
*Meet criteria for outpatient diagnostic or surgical procedure	*History of sedation/anesthesia complications
*Able to provide informed consent	*Drug allergies to intended medications
	*Concern for a difficult airway
	*No companion or caregiver for 24 h available at home after the procedure
	*Opioid – dependent patient

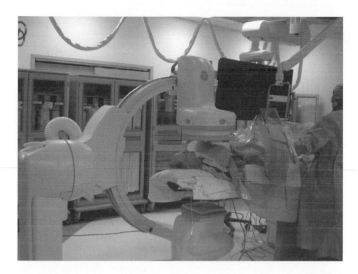

Figure 16.3. Set-up and location of the fluoroscopy machine. Note the proximity to the patient's head.

general anesthesia. Among the interventions that might help in such cases are those designed to improve diuresis and/or respiratory function.

Because of the set-up of catheterization and electrophysiology laboratories, respiratory function and airway assessment are particularly important and require special attention. Airway access may become difficult because the fluoroscopy machine generally surrounds the patient's head and is placed very close, impeding visualization and providing inadequate space to maneuver equipment for respiratory assistance. In addition, the fluoroscopy table does not have the ability to elevate the head as operating room tables do (Figure 16.3).

If the patient meets any of the criteria for difficult mask ventilation or endotracheal intubation, additional efforts should be made to inform the personnel of the possible dangers of oversedation. The importance of proper sedation and airway monitoring should be reinforced, and special attention should be paid to the location of airway supplies [1].

Interventional procedures in the cardiology suite

Table 16.4 lists the interventional procedures commonly performed in the cardiac catheterization and electrophysiology laboratory, along with their sedation requirements and complications.

Sedation and pharmacology

Sedation provides comfort and makes the procedure less unpleasant for the patient; at the same time, it facilitates the performance of the procedure by reducing patient movement. Sedation is achieved by utilizing drugs that induce a state of decreased consciousness to some degree. Several scales have been developed to measure the patient's level of consciousness, including the Modified Observer's Assessment of Alertness/Sedation (MOAA/S) scale. This widely used scale is derived from the original Observer's Assessment of Alertness/Sedation (OAA/S), and utilizes only the responsiveness component of that scale (Tables 16.5 and 16.6) [8,9].

Most of the procedures performed in the cardiac catheterization and electrophysiology laboratories require mild to moderate levels of sedation, and this is determined by an OAA/S

Table 16.4. Interventional procedures, sedation, and complications in the cardiology suite

Lab	Procedure	Sedation	Common complications
Cardiac catherization lab	Percutaneous coronary interventions	Moderate or deep sedation or general anesthesia	Significant blood loss Arrhythmia Perforation of calcified conduits
	Percutaneous ventricular assist devices	Moderate or deep sedation or general anesthesia	Significant blood loss Arrhythmia
	Percutaneous closure of septal defects	Moderate or deep sedation or general anesthesia	Hypotension Thrombosis Significant blood loss Intraprocedure air embolism Device embolization, thrombosis Embolization during or following the procedure Device-related arrhythmias Cardiac perforation with or without cardiac tamponade [1,4]
	Percutaneous peripheral arterial revascularization	Epidural anesthesia or moderate/deep sedation or mixed	Hypercoagulation Transient painful extremity ischemia Epidural or spinal hematoma if regional anesthesia is used in the setting of anticoagulation
	Percutaneous valve repair and replacement (currently under investigation and in clinical trials)	General anesthesia [1,4]. Invasive monitoring (arterial line and TEE) [4]	Unstable hemodynamics Myocardial ischemia Significant arrhythmias
Electrophysiology lab	Electrophysiology studies	Moderate or deep sedation or general anesthesia	Minor bleeding Temporary hemodynamic instability Arrhythmias Significant blood loss
	Catheter ablation	Moderate or deep sedation or general anesthesia during electrical cardioversion [5]	Arrhythmia Cardiac decompensation [6] Cardiac perforation Embolism

Table 16.4. *(cont.)*

Lab	Procedure	Sedation	Common complications
Electrophysiology lab	Electrical cardioversion	Brief period of deep sedation and amnesia to avoid recall of discomfort caused by the electrical shock [7] Consider post-procedure continuous ECG monitoring	Mild sternal pain Arrhythmias Embolism
	Implantable cardioverter defibrillators	Local anesthesia combined with moderate/deep sedation or general anesthesia during defibrillation threshold (testing of the device)	Transient ischemic attack Myocardial infarction Stroke Cardiac tamponade Hypercapnea Pneumothorax Cardiopulmonary arrest due to refractory ventricular fibrillation Pulseless electrical activity Cardiogenic shock Embolic events [5]
	Biventricular pacemakers and defibrillation lead placement	Local anesthesia combined with moderate/deep sedation or general anesthesia during defibrillation threshold (testing of the device)	Pneumothorax Hypercapnea Coronary sinus perforation Cardiac perforation Cardiac tamponade Myocardial infarction Stroke Embolic events
TEE	Transesophageal echocardiography (TEE)	Moderate or deep sedation or general anesthesia [5]	Aspiration Sore throat
ICE	Intracardiac echocardiography (ICE)	Moderate sedation [5]	Aspiration Sore throat

Procedural sedation: to achieve adequate relaxation, analgesia, and amnesia, and to maintain patients arousable to respond to verbal commands, with adequate spontaneous ventilation [1]. Dexmedetomidine is recommended in patients with respiratory compromise. Dexmedetomidine is not recommended in the electrophysiology lab because its sympatholytic action could interfere with the induction of arrhythmias [4].

and/or a MOAA/S score of ≥ 3, where the patient is still awake and responds to his or her name called out loudly and repeatedly. This level of sedation is not expected to compromise the patient's vital signs and protective reflexes, and the patient is expected to maintain normal spontaneous breathing. Efforts should be made to provide pain relief by means of local

Table 16.5. Observer's Assessment of Alertness/Sedation (OAA/S) scale

Score	Sedation level	Responsiveness	Speech	Facial expression	Eyes
5	Alert	Responds readily to name	Normal	Normal	Clear, no ptosis
4	Light	Lethargic response to name	Mild slowing	Mild relaxation	Glazed or mild ptosis
3	Moderate	Response only after name is called loudly	Slurring or prominent slowing	Marked relaxation	Glazed and marked ptosis
2	Deep	Response only after mild prodding or shaking	Few recognizable words	None	None
1	Deep sleep	Response only after painful stimulus	None	None	None

Table 16.6. Modified Observer's Assessment of Alertness/Sedation (MOAA/S) scale

6	Appears alert and awake, responds readily to name spoken in normal tone
5	Appears asleep, but responds readily to name spoken in normal tone
4	Lethargic response to name spoken in a normal tone
3	Responds only after name is called out loudly or repeatedly
2	Does not respond to mild prodding or shaking
1	Does not respond to noxious stimulus

anesthetic infiltration at the site of the catheter placement, or by regional anesthesia. In addition, longer procedures (>2 hours) are not uncommon and can make the patient restless and uncomfortable even after administration of significant amounts of intravenous sedatives and analgesics. A unique characteristic of many of the procedures performed in the cardiology suite is that they involve brief periods of intense stimulation followed by long periods of minimal stimulation. It is important to anticipate a patient's response to painful stimulation and titrate sedative drugs appropriately in order to avoid over- or undersedation.

Maintaining the desired level of sedation can be challenging, and there is always a risk of "overshooting" to the next level. Patients may undergo short periods of deeper sedation levels (OAA/S and/or MOAA/S score $\leq$ 2), and sometimes this cannot be avoided. Therefore, supporting personnel should be trained to manage the next level of sedation safely and to be able to rescue the patient by keeping the airway patent and supporting normal breathing.

Furthermore, to avoid overdosing and the resultant complications, fast-onset and short-acting drugs are preferred (Tables 2.3, 2.4, 2.6, and 16.7). Long-acting drugs should be used

Table 16.7. Sedative/analgesic drugs and reversal agents recommended for procedural sedation and/or analgesia in the cardiac suite

Drug	Dosing	Observations
Midazolam	*Healthy adults < 60 y/o:* 1–2.5 mg / 2 min slow IV; with CNS depressant ↓ dose 30%. *Adults > 60 y/o or chronically ill:* 1–1.5 mg/2 min slow IV; with CNS depressant ↓ dose 50%. *Maintenance:* titrate to increments of 25% of initial dose required to achieve adequate sedation.	*Half-life:* 1–4 h *Onset:* 1–2 min *Duration:* 30–60 min *Mechanism:* Short-acting benzodiazepine with sedative, amnesic, and anxiolytic effects. *Advantages:* Availability, good safety profile, reversible (flumazenil). *Disadvantages:* Requires another agent for analgesia, poor reliability, repeat dosing usually required, respiratory depression and hypotension [10]. *Interactions:* CNS depressants may enhance effects (antihistamines, antiemetics, hypnotics, barbiturates, alcohol).
Fentanyl	*Adults:* 25–50 µg slow IV push Maximum of 200 µg for pain control/sedation/intubation	*Half-life:* 3–4 h *Onset:* 1–2 min *Duration:* 30–60 min *Mechanism:* Synthetic opioid with narcotic analgesic effects. Fast- and short-acting as a mu-opioid receptor agonist. *Advantages:* Availability, good safety profile, minimal cardiovascular depression, reversible (naloxone). *Disadvantages:* Cough, itching, nausea, vomiting, respiratory depression, requires another agent for sedation, poor reliability, repeat dosing usually required [10]. *Interactions:* CNS depressants may enhance effects (antihistamines, antiemetics, sedatives, hypnotics, barbiturates, and alcohol) [11].
Flumazenil	*Adults:* 200 µg every 1–2 min until desired effect (max 3 mg/h)	*Half-life:* 3–4 h *Onset:* 1–2 min *Peak effect:* 6–10 min *Duration:* 45 min *Mechanism:* Reverses the effect of benzodiazepine overdoses by competitive inhibition at the benzodiazepine binding site on the $GABA_A$ receptor. *Advantages:* Rapid onset of action and reverses the effect of benzodiazepines.

Table 16.7. (cont.)

Drug	Dosing	Observations
		Disadvantages: Use not recommended in patients with benzodiazepine withdrawal or in status epilepticus.
Naloxone	*Adults:* 0.2–2.0 mg IV Additional dose as needed	*Half-life:* 1–1.5 h *Onset:* 1 min *Duration:* 15–45 min *Mechanism:* Reverses the effect of opioid overdose. It acts as a mu-opioid receptor competitive antagonist and counteracts the life-threatening depression of the central nervous system and respiratory system. *Advantages:* Fast opioid reversal, good safety profile. *Disadvantages:* Not recommended for routine use; resedation may occur when naloxone effects wear off.

with caution, because their effects can be unpredictable and they may predispose to unwanted interactions, which may be beyond the ability of supporting personnel to manage. Although the ideal characteristics for sedative drugs have not yet been validated in the medical literature, it is widely accepted that they should have a rapid onset of action, allow for a quick recovery of cognitive and physical faculties following the procedure, and have a predictable pharmacokinetic and pharmacodynamic profile. It is also important to realize that repeated administration of sedative drugs such as benzodiazepines, opioids, and propofol can result in significant accumulation of these drugs, leading to exaggerated sedative side effects. The reader is encouraged to review principles of drug pharmacokinetics and pharmacodynamics such as each individual drug's half-life and context-sensitive half-time (Chapter 2).

Usually a combination of fentanyl and midazolam has been the standard practice for many years. Both medications have a similar onset and duration of action and have relatively good safety profiles. Another advantage is that both medications are reversible and have antidotes to counteract their effects in cases of overdose. Midazolam is a benzodiazepine that provides a fast onset of action and short-term sedative, amnesic, and anxiolytic effects. Since midazolam does not have analgesic properties; it is often combined with an analgesic such as fentanyl. Fentanyl is a synthetic opioid that also has a fast onset and short-term analgesic effects. When combined, midazolam and fentanyl can be titrated to desired effect. The only downside to this combination is that these medications can enhance each others' effects, and the provider must be careful when administering supplemental doses. The potential for cardiac and respiratory depression is not to be underestimated, and these medications should be administered slowly and in incremental doses [10].

Ultimately, the goal is to provide an optimal level of sedation for each individual patient, appropriate for the specific scheduled procedure. Nevertheless, the ability to achieve the desired level of sedation will depend on the characteristics and dosing of the different drugs selected as well as on the individual patient's dose-related response to the drugs.

This goal of optimal sedation is usually achieved with a combination of sedative drugs and opioid analgesics. Besides the drugs recommended in Tables 2.3, 2.4, 2.6, and 16.7, there are other drugs that can be used to achieve adequate sedation levels in patients undergoing interventional procedures (Chapter 2). These drugs should be used by experienced and appropriately trained personnel because of the significant risk of overdose.

Propofol is a widely used and popular sedative-hypnotic drug with a rapid onset, distribution, and clearance, and therefore a short duration of action. It also has antiemetic effects and allows for a more rapid recovery of cognitive function. This intravenous drug is used to provide moderate to deep sedation. However, it is associated with a higher risk of hypotension, respiratory depression, and airway obstruction. It does not provide analgesic effects and requires additional opioid analgesics for pain relief, thus potentiating its sedative effects and further increasing the risk of cardiorespiratory depression. Propofol does not have a reversal agent to counteract its effect.

Dexmedetomidine is an alpha-2-agonist that acts centrally and provides both sedative and analgesic effects. It is becoming more popular for procedural sedation because of its dual properties and relatively safe profile. It causes minimal respiratory depression, but may cause bradycardia and hypotension. Other limitations of dexmedetomidine include a slow onset and longer duration of action, and the fact that the duration of action depends on the duration of infusion as well as the infusion rate.

When providing procedural (minimal, moderate, or deep) sedation to patients in the cardiac suite, every patient should be monitored closely by properly trained personnel. Usually, the set-up of the cardiac catheterization and electrophysiology laboratory favors patient monitoring by the cardiologist. Nevertheless, supporting personnel should also be trained to monitor vital signs through continuous blood pressure monitors or arterial lines, electrocardiography, and pulse oximetry. Monitoring of respiration should also be performed (see Chapter 5).

Summary

With the evolution of modern interventional cardiology techniques, the cardiology suite has become a frequent place where the diagnosis and treatment of patients requires the use of procedural sedation. Complex and lengthy procedures often performed on patients with significant co-morbidities require the sedation provider to have adequate knowledge of pharmacology principles, training in airway management, and a thorough understanding of cardiovascular physiology.

References

1. Faillace RT, Kaddaha R, Bikkina M, et al. The role of the out-of-operating room anesthesiologist in the care of the cardiac patient. *Anesthesiol Clin* 2009; 27: 29–46.

2. Knape JTA, Adriaensen H, van Aken H, et al. Guidelines for sedation and/or analgesia by non-anaesthesiology doctors. *Eur J Anaesthesiol* 2007; 24: 563–7.

3. Gaitan BD, Trentman TL, Fassett SL, Mueller JT, Altemose GT. Sedation and analgesia in the cardiac electrophysiology laboratory: a national survey of electrophysiologists investigating who, how, and why? *J Cardiothorac Vasc Anesth* 2011 Jan 18 [Epub ahead of print].

4. Shook DC, Savage RM. Anesthesia in the cardiac catheterization laboratory and electrophysiology laboratory. *Anesthesiol Clin* 2009; 27: 47–56.

5. Gross WL, Faillace RT, Shook DC, Daves SM, Savage RM. New challenges for anesthesiologists outside of the operating room: the cardiac catheterization and electrophysiology laboratories. In Urman R, Gross W, Philip BK, eds., *Anesthesia Outside of the Operating Room.* Oxford: Oxford University Press, 2011; 179–97.

6. Hall SC. Anesthesia outside the operating room. In Twersky R, Philip B, eds., *Handbook of Ambulatory Anesthesia,* 2nd edn. New York, NY: Springer, 2008; 253–79.

7. Litt L, Young WL. Procedures performed outside the operating room. In Stoelting RK, Miller RD, eds., *Basics of Anesthesia,* 5th edn. Philadelphia, PA: Churchill Livingstone, 2007; 550–60.

8. Yeganeh N, Roshani B, Almasi A, Jamshidi N. Correlation between Bispectral Index and predicted effect-site concentration of propofol in different levels of target-controlled, propofol induced sedation in healthy volunteers. *Arch Iran Med* 2010; **13**: 126–34.

9. Yuen VM, Irwin MG, Hui TW, Yuen MK, Lee LH. A double-blind, crossover assessment of the sedative and analgesic of intranasal dexmedetomidine. *Anesth Analg* 2007; **105**: 374–80.

10. Brown TB, Lovato LM, Parker D. Procedural sedation in the acute care setting. *Am Fam Physician* 2005; **71**: 85–90.

11. Fentanyl citrate. [Drug data sheet.] www.adaweb.net/Portals/0/Paramedics/documents/fentanylcitrate.pdf (accessed June 2011).

Further reading

Galvagno SM, Kodali B. Patient monitoring. In Urman R, Gross W, Philip BK, eds., *Anesthesia Outside of the Operating Room.* Oxford: Oxford University Press, 2011; 20–7.

Hession PM, Joshi GP. Sedation: not quite that simple. *Anesthesiol Clin* 2010; **28**: 281–94.

Joe RR, Chen LQ. Anesthesia in the cardiac catheterization lab. *Anesthesiol Clin North America* 2003; **21**: 639–51.

Chapter

17

Sedation in the emergency department

Heikki E. Nikkanen

Introduction

The demands made on a modern emergency department (ED) are such that having an internal capacity to provide a range of procedural sedation is essential to its functioning. Patients arrive at every hour of the day, with pathology that may require sedation for diagnosis or treatment. The requirement for urgent action is greater than in an outpatient office or clinic, where cases are typically planned. Patients in the ED may be critically ill, or have a threat to an organ or limb which must be dealt with rapidly. Imposing on colleagues from the department of anesthesia to provide sedation for these patients is logistically difficult, given the after-hours and unplanned nature of these cases. Emergency physicians (EPs) with training and board certification in emergency medicine have the skills to recognize these situations, and to assess the risks and benefits of procedural sedation in caring for these patients. In addition, the EP has advanced airway management and resuscitation training to manage complications arising from sedation [1,2].

Cases requiring sedation in the ED include, but are certainly not limited to, reduction of a dislocation or fracture, especially those involving a proximal joint or requiring significant manipulation; abscess drainage, notably those which are large, complex, or in sensitive areas; cardioversion; placement of tube thoracostomy; debridement or suturing of a wound; lumbar puncture; foreign body removal; or painful examination. In some EDs, sedation of a patient in order to tolerate CT or MRI may also be within the scope of the emergency physician.

Development of a procedural sedation program

In the United States, the provision of anesthesia in hospitals is governed by regulation 482.52 set forth by the Centers for Medicare and Medicaid Services (CMS) within the Department of Health and Human Services (HHS). In 2010, CMS released a clarifying

Moderate and Deep Sedation in Clinical Practice, ed. Richard D. Urman and Alan D. Kaye.
Published by Cambridge University Press. © Cambridge University Press 2012.

memo, in which deep sedation was classified as anesthesia, along with general and regional types. This requires the provider to be an anesthesiologist; certified registered nurse anesthetist (CRNA); anesthesia assistant; non-anesthesiologist MD or DO; or oral surgeon, dentist, or podiatrist qualified to administer anesthesia under state law. The hospital's anesthesia services policies, which are typically overseen by the department of anesthesia, govern the circumstances under which a non-anesthesiologist physician, such as an EP, can provide "anesthesia services," which includes deep sedation. There is debate about whether this clarification and the underlying rule violate the Joint Commission guidelines on specialty self-determination. Moderate sedation remains within the scope of practice of the "appropriately trained medical practitioner," but nevertheless the hospital anesthesia service is responsible for developing policies and procedures to govern its use.

A good working relationship between the department of anesthesia and the ED is thus of great importance in creating and maintaining a procedural sedation program. Initial development of the training, program logistics, and ongoing quality assurance should be done jointly with the department of anesthesia. Having a track record of providing successful and safe moderate sedation is a strong prelude to developing a deep sedation program. Actively opening the discussion with the hospital leadership and anesthesiology department may not immediately result in success, but is more likely to do so than the passive approach.

ED representation on a hospital sedation and anesthesia committee will also ensure that issues unique to emergency medicine are raised regularly. Other specialties using procedural sedation have very different needs. Endoscopy, cardiac catheterization, transesophageal echocardiography, or dental procedures typically require a longer, but less profound, sedation than is required in an ED. Gaining approval for providing deep and dissociative sedation and using short-acting sedative agents, such as propofol and etomidate, can be of significant benefit for care of the ED patient. Both moderate and deep sedation have been shown to be safe tools in the hands of emergency physicians [3–7]. These data can be used to reinforce the position of the ED regarding this issue.

Personnel requirements for moderate and deep sedation, as well as for the "dissociative" sedation obtained via ketamine, vary depending on the practice setting. A reasonable standard for most EDs in the United States, and one advocated in clinical practice guidelines, is to have a dedicated medical professional, usually a nurse, administer medications and monitor the patient for moderate or dissociative sedation [8]. On the basis of the CMS regulation, however, a nurse cannot provide deep sedation. CMS guidelines have also been interpreted in the past to mean that one provider cannot perform both deep sedation and the procedure. Many institutions therefore require a dedicated physician to provide deep sedation, who does not perform or supervise the procedure simultaneously. For single-coverage EDs, this may present a significant problem.

Special considerations for ED patients

Two issues exist which set patients presenting to the ED apart from others requiring sedation. They are the variables of the last oral intake and the urgency of the required procedure. Striking a balance between safety and prompt treatment is a prime consideration for the emergency physician [9]. Unfortunately, there is little evidence on which to base the decision. It is worth noting that there is no established relationship between fasting and aspiration complication in ED procedural sedation [10].

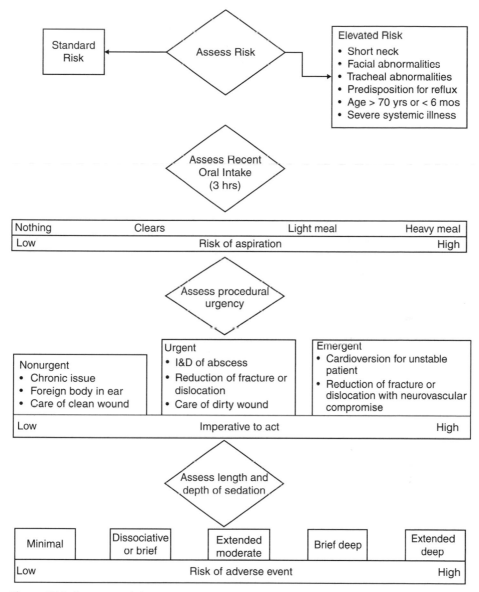

Figure 17.1. Four-step sedation assessment.

Risk factors predisposing a patient to aspiration include prolonged duration of sedation, greater depth of sedation, age over 70, greater degree of underlying illness, history of a difficult airway, and presence of pathology conducive to reflux. Regarding the type of oral intake, solid food and acidic particulates are more likely to cause aspiration pneumonitis [11,12].

A consensus clinical practice advisory published by the American College of Emergency Physicians (ACEP) evaluated the existing literature applicable to the emergency patient and augmented this with an expert panel's opinion. They developed a four-step process to evaluate the risks and benefits of providing sedation (Figure 17.1) [8]. Based on this assessment, a maximum level of sedation is suggested (Figure 17.2).

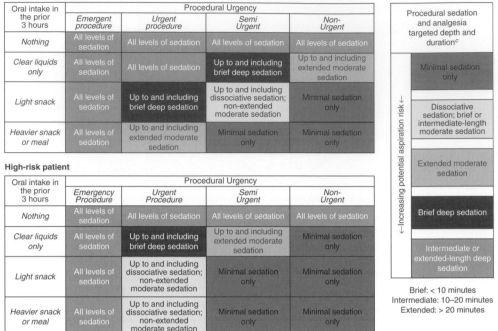

Figure 17.2. Suggested limits of length and depth of sedation. Reprinted with permission from Green *et al.* [9].

Selection of sedation agents

Although many agents can be used to achieve either moderate or deep sedation in the ED, only a small number are in common use, either singly or in combination. The drug and dose should be primarily chosen as a function of the sedation assessment. Given a choice between otherwise equivalent drugs, the recovery time is also an important factor. For many ED sedations, propofol is chosen for its effects and short duration of action.

Midazolam/fentanyl

Most common is the pairing of an opioid and a benzodiazepine, to provide relief of pain and to cause sedation. Midazolam has a rapid onset of action, and a superior amnesic effect compared with other benzodiazepines [13]. Benefits of the use of midazolam include amnesia to the procedure and the ability to reverse its effects. However, longer procedural and recovery times are seen. A study comparing midazolam and etomidate at doses of 0.035 mg/kg and 0.10 mg/kg respectively showed a significantly longer time from initiation to recovery (16 vs. 32 minutes, $p < 0.001$) and a higher number of doses needed [14]. Regarding opioids, fentanyl is preferred for procedural sedation in the ED due to its rapid onset of action and short duration, as well as the relative lack of cardiovascular effect [15].

Propofol

Propofol has generated significant debate in the emergency medicine literature regarding its use in procedural sedation. Its ability to rapidly generate deep sedation was cause for concern that its use would result in inadvertent general anesthesia. Experience with its use by emergency physicians in thousands of cases shows that its safety profile in the hands of the EP is as good as or better than that of other available agents. It produces sedation reliably, with a very rapid onset and very short duration. In one study, it was found to be as effective as midazolam without adverse effects. In the same study, the recovery time was 15 minutes for propofol, compared to 76 minutes for midazolam [16]. For a practice environment with limited time and resources, this represents a significant advantage. An evaluation of the cost-effectiveness of propofol relative to midazolam shows savings of time and cost [17]. A prospective study of 116 patients using propofol in the ED for procedural sedation showed it to be safe and well received by patients and physicians [18]. Compared to etomidate in a randomized controlled trial (RCT) of 214 patients, it was similar in adverse events and recovery time, but etomidate caused myoclonus in 20% of patients. Successful sedation was achieved in 97% of patients who received propofol, compared to 90% with etomidate [19].

Etomidate

Etomidate has been used for years as an induction agent for endotracheal intubation. Its properties of rapid action, short duration, and cardiovascular stability also make it attractive for procedural sedation. In one study of 150 ED procedures performed with etomidate, five patients developed hypoxemia and required assisted ventilation. In 95% of cases, recovery to pre-procedure level of consciousness occurred within 30 minutes. Patient satisfaction was very high [20]. A double-blind RCT with 44 patients comparing etomidate against midazolam in fracture reduction showed a recovery time of 15 minutes and 32 minutes, respectively. Success of the procedure was 100% for the etomidate group, and 86% for the midazolam group. Side effects and adverse events were rare, but equal in the two groups.

Ketamine

Ketamine's effects do not easily fit into the previously discussed sedation scale. A significant benefit is the preservation of airway reflexes and respiratory drive, which makes it a better agent in cases where aspiration or hypoxemia are more significant risks. Respiratory depression has been described at the time of injection, which can be mitigated by infusing it over 1–2 minutes. Increases in blood pressure and heart rate are ubiquitous but mild, and easily controlled with sympatholytic agents. No reports have been made of cardiac ischemia resulting from ketamine administration. In a review of trials of ketamine, only one cardiorespiratory event with a poor outcome was identified in over 70,000 uses [21]. Ketamine alone has predictable and rapid effects when administered intramuscularly. It is used commonly in children. A phenomenon known as "emergence" in adults given ketamine causes discomfort in patients and physicians alike. There are a number of strategies which may be employed to counter this effect. A simple strategy some authors recommend is to coach patients that they can control or choose the dream they will have. A soothing atmosphere has been anecdotally seen to have beneficial effects, but may not be feasible in a busy ED. One study suggests that addition of midazolam 0.07 mg/kg IV at the time of ketamine administration decreases the incidence of this side effect from 50% to 7% [22]. This relatively high dose resulted in a few incidences of respiratory depression requiring transient ventilatory support. A smaller dose of benzodiazepine may be given either just before emergence, or on an as-needed basis. A large meta-analysis suggests that emergence dysphoria is present in only 1.4% of cases, although there is a wide variation in studies including adults [23]. Hypersalivation may also occur, which can be controlled by pretreatment with atropine 0.01 mg/kg IM or IV. The most feared complication, laryngospasm, occurs in 1.4% of cases [24]. Despite a number of studies, no clear risk factors have been identified in the ED sedation population. This complication can usually be managed with bag-valve mask ventilation, although rarely intubation is required.

Combining ketamine and propofol in a 1 : 1 mixture has been tested in a prospective trial which enrolled 114 patients, with the hypothesis that the cardiovascular effects would be balanced and emergence reaction minimized [25]. A median dose of 0.75 mg/kg of each agent was used, with an interquartile range (IQR) of 0.6–1.0 mg/kg. Three patients required bag-valve mask ventilation, four required airway repositioning, and three had mild emergence dysphoria. Median time to recovery was 15 minutes (IQR 12–19 minutes), and satisfaction scores were high for physicians, nurses, and patients. This combination, "ketofol," offers another pharmacologic option which appears safe and effective, although not clearly of any benefit over other options. Below are a few representative cases describing procedural sedation management of patients in the ED setting.

Example cases

Case 1

A 5-year-old girl arrives to the ED after a fall from a bicycle. Her physical examination and radiographic evaluation show a fracture of the left radius and ulna. There is no tenting of the skin, and her neurovascular examination is normal distal to the injury. She has no other significant injury, and her medical history is unremarkable. The reduction and splinting of the fracture will require sedation. She weighs 20 kg. Her last meal was milk and cookies, ingested 2 hours before arrival.

In this circumstance, ketamine is a reasonable choice. It is well tolerated in children, with a lower incidence of the emergence phenomenon than in adults. A dose of 20–40 mg (1–2 mg/kg) IV over 2–3 minutes would be a reasonable dose. If IV access cannot be obtained, ketamine is the only sedative agent that is reliable via the IM route, at a dose of 4–5 mg. Many patients do not require glycopyrrolate or atropine, unless the procedure is in the oropharynx. An analgesic for pain or a benzodiazepine for emergence reaction can be considered as needed. This case would be classified as semi-urgent, and based on the ACEP guideline, dissociative sedation could be performed without further delay.

Case 2

A 72-year-old woman comes to the ED with lightheadedness and palpitations. Her blood pressure is 64/36 and an electrocardiogram shows atrial fibrillation with a rapid ventricular rate of 140. ST segment depressions are seen inferiorly. The blood pressure does not respond to a bolus of normal saline. Given the patient's shock state and evidence of end-organ dysfunction, the decision is made to perform a synchronized cardioversion. She weighs 65 kg. Her last meal was beef stroganoff, consumed immediately before arrival.

In this instance, there are a few choices. Propofol could be used, given its short action, at a reduced dose, given the patient's age and comorbidity. A typical initial sedation dose for a healthy adult is 1 mg/kg; this patient might only need 80% of this dose, or about 50 mg. Alternatively, etomidate has good cardiovascular stability, although a longer duration of action. If this agent were selected, a dose on the lower side of the range 0.1–0.2 mg/kg should be selected. A reasonable amount would be 6 mg. Finally, given the significant concerns about worsening her hemodynamic status, ketamine could be used at a dose of 1–2 mg/kg. Assuming the cardioversion is successful, a dose of midazolam, ativan, or another benzodiazepine could be used to blunt the emergence reaction. Given the very short duration of the procedure, the risk–benefit equation of giving an adjunct opioid likely argues against its use. Although she is a higher-risk patient based on age and comorbid conditions, the procedure would be classified as emergent, based on her hemodynamic instability and ischemic ECG. The sedation could therefore be done without delay.

Case 3

A 40-year-old man with a history of hypertension, opioid abuse, and renal insufficiency is brought to the ED after he notes his arm has been swollen at the antecubital area for the past three days. Physical evaluation augmented with ultrasound shows a large subcutaneous abscess with septations which will require a complicated drainage. He has normal vital signs with the exception of a blood pressure of 164/90, and there is no evidence of lymphangitic spread or surrounding cellulitis. He is just finishing up a sandwich as he is brought in for evaluation. Although he has no drug allergies, he does have a severe allergic reaction to eggs. His weight is 90 kg.

This patient has somewhat limited options. Local anesthesia will likely not be sufficient to permit a proper drainage. His egg allergy precludes the use of propofol. Ketamine could be used, but it could worsen his hypertension, and there is a risk of an uncomfortable and long recovery from the sedation. Etomidate, at a dose of 14 mg IV (0.15 mg/kg, rounded up), remains a choice for this patient. Midazolam could also be used, but titration of the dose is often required and results in a longer recovery time than propofol or etomidate. An adjunctive dose of an opioid analgesic should be given, such as fentanyl in doses of 50–100 μg IV, repeated as needed. Given the semi-urgent nature of his procedure and his oral intake, his sedation should be delayed for at least 3 hours.

Summary

Emergency physicians have the skills needed to safely administer moderate and deep procedural sedation. Representation on the hospital sedation committee is important in developing an independent moderate and deep sedation practice. Brief deep sedation is more suited to the majority of ED cases. Decisions on appropriate fasting time must be taken on a case-by-case basis.

References

1. Hockberger RS, Binder LS, Graber MA, et al. American College of Emergency Physicians Core Content Task Force II. The model of the clinical practice of emergency medicine. Ann Emerg Med 2001; 37: 745–70.
2. Allison EJ, Aghababian RV, Barsan WG, et al. Core content for emergency medicine. Task Force on the Core Content for Emergency Medicine Revision. Ann Emerg Med 1997; 29: 792–811.
3. Mallory MD, Baxter AL, Yanosky DJ, et al. Emergency physician-administered propofol sedation: a report on 25,433 sedations from the Pediatric Sedation Research Consortium. Ann Emerg Med 2011; 57: 462–8.

4. Burton JH, Miner JR, Shipley ER, *et al.* Propofol for emergency department procedural sedation and analgesia: a tale of three centers. *Acad Emerg Med* 2006; **13**: 24–30.

5. Green SM, Roback MG, Krauss B, *et al.* Predictors of airway and respiratory adverse events with ketamine sedation in the emergency department: an individual-patient data meta-analysis of 8,282 children. *Ann Emerg Med* 2009; **54**: 158–68.

6. Peña BMG, Krauss B. Adverse events of procedural sedation and analgesia in a pediatric emergency department. *Ann Emerg Med* 1999; **34**: 483–91.

7. Couloures KG, Beach M, Cravero JP, Monroe KK, Hertzog JH. Impact of provider specialty on pediatric procedural sedation complication rate. *Pediatrics* 2011; **127**: e1154–60.

8. Godwin SA, Caro DA, Wolf SJ, *et al.* American College of Emergency Physicians. Clinical policy: procedural sedation and analgesia in the emergency department. *Ann Emerg Med* 2005; **45**: 177–96.

9. Green SM, Roback MG, Miner JR, Burton JH, Krauss B. Fasting and emergency department procedural sedation and analgesia: a consensus-based clinical practice advisory. *Ann Emerg Med* 2007; **49**: 454–61.

10. Roback MG, Bajaj L, Wathen JE, Bothner J. Preprocedural fasting and adverse events in procedural sedation and analgesia in a pediatric emergency department: are they related? *Ann Emerg Med* 2004; **44**: 454–9.

11. Olsson GL, Hallen B, Hambraeus-Jonzon K. Aspiration during anaesthesia: a computer-aided study in 185,358 anaesthetics. *Acta Anaesthesiol Scand* 1986; **30**: 84–92.

12. Green SM, Krauss B. Pulmonary aspiration risk during ED procedural sedation: an examination of the role of fasting and sedation depth. *Acad Emerg Med* 2002; **9**: 35–42.

13. Muse DA. Conscious and deep sedation. In Harwood-Nuss A, Wolfson AB, eds., *The Clinical Practice of Emergency Medicine*, 3rd edn. Philadelphia, PA: Lippincott Williams & Wilkins, 2001; 1761.

14. Hunt GS, Spencer MT, Hays DP. Etomidate and midazolam for procedural sedation: prospective, randomized trial. *Am J Emerg Med* 2005; **23**: 299–303.

15. Blackburn P, Vissers R. Pharmacology of emergency department pain management and conscious sedation. *Emerg Med Clin North Am* 2000; **18**: 803–27.

16. Havel CJ, Strait RT, Hennes H. A clinical trial of propofol vs. midazolam for procedural sedation in a pediatric emergency department. *Acad Emerg Med* 1999; **6**: 989–97.

17. Hohl CM, Nosyk B, Sadatsafavi M, Anis AH. A cost-effectiveness analysis of propofol versus midazolam for procedural sedation in the emergency department. *Acad Emerg Med* 2008; **15**: 32–9.

18. Zed PJ, Abu-Laban RB, Chan WW, Harrison DW. Efficacy, safety and patient satisfaction of propofol for procedural sedation and analgesia in the emergency department: a prospective study. *CJEM* 2007; **9**: 421–7.

19. Miner JR, Burton JH. Clinical practice advisory: emergency department procedural sedation with propofol. *Ann Emerg Med* 2007; **50**: 182–7.

20. Vinson DR, Bradbury DR. Etomidate for procedural sedation in emergency medicine. *Ann Emerg Med* 2002; **39**: 592–8.

21. Strayer RJ, Nelson LS. Adverse events associated with ketamine for procedural sedation in adults. *Am J Emerg Med* 2008; **26**: 985–1028.

22. Sener S, Eken C, Schultz CH, Serinken M, Ozsarac M. Ketamine with and without midazolam for emergency department sedation in adults: a randomized controlled trial. *Ann Emerg Med* 2011; **57**: 109–14.

23. Green SM, Roback MG, Krauss B, *et al.* Predictors of emesis and recovery agitation with emergency department ketamine sedation: an individual-patient data meta-analysis of 8,282 children. *Ann Emerg Med* 2009; **54**: 171–80.

24. Green SM, Roback MG, Krauss B, *et al.* Predictors of airway and respiratory adverse events with ketamine sedation in the emergency department: an individual-patient data meta-analysis of 8,282 children. *Ann Emerg Med* 2009; **54**: 158–68.

25. Willman EV, Andolfatto G. A prospective evaluation of "ketofol" (ketamine/propofol combination) for procedural sedation and analgesia in the emergency department. *Ann Emerg Med* 2007; **49**: 23–30.

Chapter

18

Sedation in the intensive care setting

Ghousia Wajida and Jeffrey S. Kelly

Introduction

The intensive care unit (ICU) represents a dynamic, complex milieu in which individual patient pathophysiology and multimodal therapeutic interventions interact unpredictably, mandating frequent patient reevaluation to potentially alter ongoing medical management based upon patient response (or lack thereof) and current clinical conditions. The patient's care team is constantly challenged under such circumstances to determine the risk–benefit ratio of any individual therapy as well as the interplay of various therapies and their effect upon patient homeostasis. Adjunctive administration of sedatives and analgesics to minimize the critically ill patient's physical discomfort and psychoemotional stress exemplifies this dynamic patient care environment, with under- and oversedation being a known risk for adverse patient outcomes. Thus, it is important for ICU caregivers to have a comprehensive understanding of ICU sedation and how to safely provide such care in appropriately selected patients. The goals of this chapter are: (1) to emphasize thorough patient evaluation to identify appropriate ICU sedation candidates, (2) to review common indications for ICU sedation administration, (3) to understand the risks inherent in under- and oversedation, (4) to review the basic pharmacology and administration techniques of commonly utilized ICU sedatives and analgesics, and (5) to encourage readers to utilize sedation scales to guide ongoing sedation administration and minimize the chance of under- or oversedation.

Patient selection, indications, and risks

Common sense dictates that sedation should usually not be a top priority in any ICU patient demonstrating significant instability in airway patency, oxygenation/ventilation, and/or

Moderate and Deep Sedation in Clinical Practice, ed. Richard D. Urman and Alan D. Kaye.
Published by Cambridge University Press. © Cambridge University Press 2012.

Table 18.1. Possible etiologic causes of ICU agitation and delirium

Metabolic	Hypoglycemia, nonketotic hyperosmolar states, acidosis, hyponatremia, hypernatremia, hypercalcemia, hyperammonemia, acute hepatic encephalopathy, uremia
Respiratory	Hypoxemia, hypercapnia, increased work of breathing, patient–ventilator dyssynchrony
Ischemia	Ischemia (myocardial, cerebral, intestinal), hypotension (absolute or relative), shock (cardiogenic, distributive, hemorrhagic)
Infections	Systemic infections, sepsis, encephalitis, meningitis, brain abscess
Medications	Withdrawal syndromes (opioids, benzodiazepines, alcohol), overdose (stimulants, SSRIs, salicylates, antipsychotics), serotonin syndrome (linezolid, opioids, valproate, tramadol, monoamine oxidase inhibitors), neuroleptic malignant syndrome, anticholinergics, antihistamines, corticosteroids
Miscellaneous	Hypertensive encephalopathy, posterior reversible leukoencephalopathy syndrome (PRES), seizure/nonconvulsive status epilepticus, stroke, hypothermia, hyperthermia, hypothyroidism, hyperthyroidism, autoimmune encephalopathy (thrombotic thrombocytopenic purpura, lupus)
Modifiable	Pain, sleep deprivation, absence of day–night cycling, unfamiliar personnel/environment, extremes of environmental temperatures, physical restraints, visual, auditory, or language barriers, inability to communicate
Preexisting patient-specific factors	Posttraumatic stress disorder, substance abuse, dementia

hemodynamics. Initial interventions in such patients should appropriately focus on ensuring airway patency, initiating supplemental oxygen therapy, utilization of noninvasive or invasive mechanical ventilation, and/or resuscitation with intravenous (IV) fluids and vasoactive agents in parallel with diagnosis/definitive treatment of precipitating medical conditions.

As soon as vital functions have stabilized and definitive treatment has begun, each patient should be systematically evaluated to exclude other etiologies for motor agitation, disruptive behaviors, or ventilator dyssynchrony (Table 18.1). Any correctable factors so identified should receive appropriate diagnostic and therapeutic interventions, as misguided administration of sedation in this setting may mask ongoing signs/symptoms of the underlying condition(s), delay their diagnosis and treatment, and potentially result in adverse or paradoxical effects related to sedation administration.

The patient should then be assessed for hepatorenal function, intravascular volume status, cardiovascular reserve, and reliance of hemodynamics upon underlying sympathetic drive. Many critically ill patients demonstrate hemodynamic profiles that are in large part maintained by exaggerated levels of central sympathetic tone; sedation of any kind under these conditions poses a significant risk for hypotension (particularly in patients with preexisting volume depletion). Furthermore, specific sedatives and analgesics also have known pharmacologic effects on contractility, vascular tone, and sympathetic–parasympathetic balance. Certain sedative medications rely upon hepatic inactivation or have active metabolites that require renal elimination. These agent-specific properties should be integrated with the patient's hemodynamic evaluation and metabolic profile in order to choose the most appropriate sedation regimen in a given patient.

Given that large numbers of ICU nurses underestimate the pain experienced by the critically ill, each patient must receive frequent assessments for pain (utilizing the commonly available Visual Analog Scale in appropriately responsive patients) followed by administration of analgesia (most commonly opioids) as indicated. ICU survivors frequently recall significant pain associated with their ICU stay (even during routine nursing and respiratory care), and the stress response associated with unrelieved pain can result in undesirable effects such as tachycardia, hypertension, increased oxygen consumption, hypercoagulability, immunosuppression, persistent catabolism, diaphragmatic splinting, ineffective cough/secretion clearance, and impaired respiratory gas exchange. This emphasizes an "analgesia first" approach to avoid undertreating pain (often providing sedation as a side effect), followed by reevaluation for additional sedation requirements. Use of analgesics for sedation in the absence of pain is usually best avoided, given possible adverse effects (respiratory depression, dysphoria) and the widespread availability of more appropriate sedative agents.

Common indications for administration of ICU sedation (alone or in combination) include:

(1) patient comfort (pain, anxiolysis, amnesia, end-of-life care)
(2) decrease oxygen consumption (work of breathing, intracranial pressure, mixed venous desaturation)
(3) facilitate mechanical ventilation, oxygenation, and/or ventilation
(4) facilitate nursing/respiratory care and patient mobilization
(5) facilitate diagnostic and therapeutic procedures
(6) facilitate wake–sleep cycles
(7) adjunctive administration with neuromuscular blocking agents

Inadequate levels of sedation in ICU patients may place them at additional risk for adverse consequences, which may include any or all of the following:

(1) physical/psychological discomfort (pain, anxiety, awareness)
(2) autonomic stress response (hypertension, tachycardia)
(3) increased oxygen consumption
(4) ventilator dyssynchrony with increased work of breathing
(5) impairment with bedside nursing and respiratory care interventions
(6) bedside provider injury
(7) patient-initiated discontinuation of support (self-extubation, enteric tube/Foley catheter removal)
(8) subsequent sedation administration to oversedation levels

Similarly, excessive levels of ICU sedation are associated with a number of undesirable effects, including, but not limited to, the following:

(1) respiratory depression
(2) impairment of serial clinical assessments (particularly mentation/neurologic status)
(3) hypotension and bradycardia
(4) paradoxical effects (disinhibition, increased motor agitation)
(5) development of delirium
(6) prolonged "hangover" effects upon discontinuation

(7) withdrawal symptoms

(8) immunosuppression

(9) development of tolerance requiring escalating sedation dosing

(10) increased mechanical ventilation time

(11) increased ICU length of stay/costs

(12) complications from immobility (deep vein thrombosis, pressure ulcers, deconditioning)

Delirium, an acute fluctuation in mental status accompanied by an altered level of consciousness, inattention, and disorganized thinking, is a recently recognized and underdiagnosed complication of critical illness. It occurs in up to 80% of ICU patients and is an independent risk factor for increased ICU/hospital length of stay, prolonged neurocognitive impairment, discharge to long-term care facilities, and mortality. Variables associated with ICU development of delirium include advanced age, sensory (i.e., hearing and/or visual) impairment, loss of day–night circadian cycling, use of physical restraints, preexisting cognitive dysfunction (i.e., dementia), and sedation utilization (particularly benzodiazepine administration).

Specific agents and modes of administration

Clinical practice guidelines for the prolonged administration of sedative and analgesic agents in critically ill patients have been developed by the Society of Critical Care Medicine and represent the most current, evidence-based, expert panel approach to ICU sedation. Readers are encouraged to apply these guidelines to their ICU sedation management practice, and we have included this document in our reading list to promote its utilization.

While the occasional ICU patient (such as high spinal cord injuries or patients requiring mechanical ventilation for neuromuscular weakness) may be adequately managed with scheduled enteral administration of sedative or analgesic agents, IV administration is appropriately indicated in the vast majority of the critically ill. Intermittent IV techniques minimize IV fluid intake, limit pharmacy costs, and obligatorily mandate frequent, serial patient evaluations to guide and modify ongoing sedation care. Conversely, intermittent IV administration promotes potential "peaks and valleys" of over- and undersedation, increases personnel time expenditure/costs, increases cumulative agent doses over time, is more difficult to order, and is impractical with certain sedative and analgesic agents. In contrast to an intermittent IV approach, administration by continuous IV infusion minimizes the risks of such "peaks and valleys," decreases bedside personnel time/costs, and minimizes cumulative drug doses. Continuous infusion techniques alternatively require more IV access sites, present drug compatibility issues, lead to larger daily IV fluid intake, may increase duration of mechanical ventilation and ICU/hospital length of stay, increase pharmacy costs, and predispose patients to more diagnostic imaging procedures as well as withdrawal syndromes. Sedatives and analgesics that are commonly administered in the ICU are further detailed below, with agent-specific dosing guidelines summarized in Table 18.2.

Opioids

Opioids represent the "gold standard" for analgesics and are mentioned first among specific drug classes to reemphasize the need for an "analgesia first" approach to ICU sedation.

Table 18.2. Common ICU sedatives, analgesics, and dosing

Drug class	Agent	Intermittent IV administration	Continuous IV infusion rate
Opioid	Morphine	0.025–0.15 mg/kg q 1–2 h	0.05–0.35 mg/kg/h
	Hydromorphone	0.01–0.03 mg/kg q 1–2 h	0.007–0.015 mg/kg/h
	Fentanyl	0.5–1.5 μg/kg q 30–60 min	1–10 μg/kg/h
	Meperidine	12.5–25 mg q 10 min × 2 (shivering)	Not applicable
Benzodiazepine	Midazolam	0.02–0.1 mg/kg q 30 min – 2 h	0.03–0.2 mg/kg/h
	Lorazepam	0.015–0.06 mg/kg q 2–6 h	0.015–0.1 mg/kg/h
Intravenous anesthetic	Propofol	Not applicable	10–75 μg/kg/min
Alpha-2-agonist	Dexmedetomidine	Not applicable	0.2–0.7 μg/kg/h (± 1 μg/kg load over 10 min)
Butyrophenone antipsychotic	Haloperidol	0.03–0.15 mg/kg q 30 min – 6 h	0.04–0.15 mg/kg/h

These agents work systemically via central mu receptors to modify the perception of painful sensory input. They can also be administered neuraxially (epidural or subarachnoid) to treat pain in appropriately selected ICU patients, but such use is beyond the scope of this chapter. Benefits of opioids include analgesia, sedation (at higher doses), relative hemodynamic stability, cough suppression, and reversibility (naloxone). Potential undesirable side effects of opioids may include respiratory depression, impaired mentation, unreliable amnesia, nausea and vomiting (via central chemoreceptor trigger zone stimulation), ileus, urinary retention, dysphoria (when administered in the absence of pain), vagal effects, and pharmacologically active metabolites (the latter two with specific opioid agonists).

Morphine, a naturally occurring opioid derived from the poppy seed, represents the gold standard against which other analgesics are compared. With IV administration, its central nervous system (CNS) effects peak in 15–30 minutes and peak respiratory depression occurs at approximately 60 minutes, with an expected analgesic duration of up to 4 hours. Morphine may predispose patients to an increased risk of hypotension from multiple mechanisms, including vagal-mediated bradycardia, arteriolar dilatation from histamine release, and/or venodilation. Histamine release may also result in urticaria and bronchospasm. Morphine-6-glucuronide, a hepatic metabolite with potency approaching that of the parent drug, may accumulate in patients with impaired renal function; other opioid analgesics may be more appropriate in such patients.

Hydromorphone is a semisynthetic opioid with 5–6 times the potency of morphine and a similar duration of analgesic action. Its advantages over morphine include less histamine release and metabolism to inactive metabolites.

Fentanyl is a synthetic opioid with approximately 100 times the potency of morphine. While fentanyl's high lipid solubility gives it a very rapid onset of action (30–60 seconds) and analgesic peak (3–5 minutes), this physicochemical property also explains fentanyl's short duration of analgesia (30–60 minutes), due to its redistribution into more poorly perfused peripheral tissues. Similar to hydromorphone, fentanyl is metabolized by the liver to inactive metabolites. It can also cause bradycardia (particularly in large doses), but does not stimulate histamine release. One very rare complication of fentanyl administration is skeletal muscle rigidity (most commonly at high doses), which can potentially impair oxygenation and ventilation. Prolonged administration by infusion may lead to fentanyl accumulation at the mu receptor (so-called increased context-sensitive half-time), with resultant delay in dissipation of its clinical effects (particularly respiratory depression) upon infusion discontinuation.

Meperidine, a synthetic opioid 7–10 times less potent than morphine, has an onset and duration of action intermediate between those of morphine and fentanyl. Meperidine administration is likely to result in hypotension due to decreased sympathetic tone, histamine release, and negative inotropic properties, and its antimuscarinic effects may result in tachycardia, mydriasis, and drying of secretions. Meperidine's active metabolite normeperidine has a long elimination half-time and can accumulate in patients with renal dysfunction, causing myoclonus and seizure activity. Meperidine use in patients on antidepressants (either selective serotonin reuptake inhibitors or monoamine oxidase inhibitors) has resulted in fatal drug interactions, and it has also been associated with the development of delirium when utilized for perioperative analgesia. Meperidine is thus a poor choice for analgesic therapy in the critically ill, given the more favorable pharmacology of other opioids. One possible meperidine indication in the ICU would be intermittent, low-dose (12.5–25 mg) IV administration for shivering associated with either the immediate perianesthetic period or post-resuscitation application of therapeutic hypothermia.

After the patient's analgesic needs have received proper treatment, he or she should be reevaluated for adequacy of sedation in conjunction with the ongoing clinical condition and medical care plan. Those identified as requiring additional sedation should then undergo a secondary assessment as to (1) the probable duration of sedation going forward and (2) the anticipated need to rapidly wean sedation to periodically evaluate neurologic function and/or facilitate expedient tracheal extubation. These factors dictate whether a short- or long-duration sedative is most appropriate in a given patient.

Benzodiazepines

Benzodiazepines are the cornerstone for sedation management in critically ill patients via their positive modulation on gamma-aminobutyric acid (GABA), the main CNS inhibitory neurotransmitter. They work by attaching to the $GABA_A$ receptor to increase chloride conductance into neurons, resulting in hyperpolarization and higher stimulation requirements for the neuron to reach firing threshold. Benefits of benzodiazepines include sedation, anxiolysis, anterograde amnesia, anticonvulsant effects, hemodynamic stability (at usual sedative doses), muscle relaxation (at higher doses), lowered intracranial pressure, and reversibility (flumazenil). Potential undesirable effects of this drug class include dose-dependent respiratory depression (although less so than with opioids), absence of analgesia, venoirritation (with lorazepam), paradoxical agitation (perhaps due to their amnesic properties), and association with the development of delirium.

Midazolam is a water-soluble benzodiazepine that does not generally cause pain on bolus injection. It is converted into a lipid-soluble form at physiologic pH, resulting in a rapid (2–5 minutes) onset and relatively short (approximately 45–60 minutes) duration of action after single-dose IV administration. Midazolam is converted by the liver to the active metabolite alpha-hydroxymidazolam, which can accumulate in patients with renal dysfunction. It is the preferred sedative agent for short-term ICU sedation (particularly in patients not requiring serial neurologic evaluations), as well as for treatment of acutely agitated ICU patients.

In contrast to midazolam, lorazepam is a relatively insoluble agent that must be commercially suspended with polyethylene glycol and propylene glycol for IV administration. This hyperosmolar preparation is venoirritating and causes pain on IV bolus administration. Lorazepam is less lipid-soluble than midazolam, resulting in a slower onset (5–15 minutes) and making it less useful for acute ICU sedation indications. Alternatively, it has a longer duration of clinical sedation (4–8 hours) because of its low dissociation rate from the benzodiazepine receptor, and it is converted by the liver to inactive glucuronide metabolites. These properties explain both lorazepam's preferred suitability for longer-term ICU sedation and its association with patient transitioning to a state of delirium at relatively modest daily doses (perhaps related to persistent amnesic effects). Long-term lorazepam administration by infusion (particularly at high rates for prolonged periods) has been associated with reversible acute tubular necrosis, lactic acidosis, and hyperosmolar states.

Intravenous anesthetics

Propofol is an IV general anesthetic agent that demonstrates sedative and hypnotic properties at lower doses. Similar to benzodiazepines, it works via the $GABA_A$ receptor by decreasing the rate of GABA dissociation. Propofol is metabolized by the liver to inactive metabolites, and its kinetic behavior is unaltered by significant hepatic or renal disease. Because propofol is an insoluble isopropyl phenol, it must be emulsified in a soybean oil/glycerol/egg phosphatide vehicle for IV administration. This vehicle provides 1.1 kcal/mL of energy (which must be accounted for in the patient's daily nutritional evaluation), and serves as a rich medium for bacterial overgrowth when contaminated. Sodium metabisulfite (which may produce allergic reactions in sulfite-sensitive patients) is therefore added as a preservative to commonly used generic propofol formulations, and strict aseptic handling, with changes of propofol infusion bottles/tubing at least every 12 hours is mandatory. Propofol's high lipid solubility results in a rapid (approximately 30–60 seconds) onset of action and a short (5–10 minutes) duration of clinical action after IV bolus administration, due to its redistribution into more poorly perfused tissues. While such characteristics are ideal for induction of anesthesia in the operating room, they make propofol bolus administration in the ICU unfeasible except for specific, short-term, procedure-based situations (such as endotracheal intubation). Propofol sedation in the ICU is thus almost exclusively administered using a titrated continuous IV infusion.

Propofol's main advantage in the ICU is its rapid onset and short, predictable recovery profile (even after long-term administration), which makes it useful in patients requiring serial neurologic assessments or those undergoing rapid weaning from mechanical ventilation. Other potential benefits in selected ICU patients may include anticonvulsant effects, antiemetic activity, decreased cerebral metabolic rate/intracranial pressure, depression of airway reflexes, and possible bronchodilatory properties. The most common side effect of ICU propofol administration is dose-dependent hypotension, which precludes its consistent use in many hemodynamically unstable ICU patient populations. Additional undesirable propofol traits in selected ICU patients may include absence of analgesia, unreliable amnesia, myoclonus, hypertriglyceridemia, elevation of pancreatic enzymes, and pain with peripheral administration. High-dose (80–100 µg/kg/min) propofol infusion administered for more than 48 hours places the patient at risk for propofol infusion syndrome (PRIS), a potentially fatal complication manifested by hypotension, bradycardia/asystole, heart failure, rhabdomyolysis, severe metabolic acidosis, hyperlipidemia, renal failure, and fatty liver infiltration. Pediatric patients appear to be at particular risk for PRIS, and the Food and Drug Administration (FDA) has specifically recommended against prolonged propofol sedation in this patient population.

Alpha-2-agonists

Dexmedetomidine is a centrally acting, presynaptic alpha-2-agonist recently approved for short-term (< 24 hours) ICU sedation. Compared to clonidine, dexmedetomidine is 7–10 times more selective for central alpha-2-receptors, with a shorter duration of action. It causes sedation via potassium and calcium channels located in the locus ceruleus of the brainstem to cause neuronal hyperpolarization, resulting in a decreased rate of central neuronal firing. Dexmedetomidine's main advantages are its preservation of central respiratory drive as well as its ability to reliably allow patient arousal from the sedated state to assess neurologic function. It also has analgesic-sparing, anxiolytic, and antisialogogue properties (which may be desirable in certain ICU patient groups), and is associated with a lower incidence of delirium than the benzodiazepines. Dexmedetomidine's lowering of the thermoregulatory (i.e., shivering) threshold may be of potential benefit during utilization of therapeutic hypothermia after successful resuscitation from ventricular fibrillation or ventricular tachycardia. The main side effect of dexmedetomidine is hypotension and bradycardia (particularly when a loading dose is administered), with volume-depleted patients and/or those with high levels of underlying sympathetic tone being at higher risk for this complication. Additional dexmedetomidine concerns include incomplete analgesia, incomplete amnesia, suppression of adrenal steroidogenesis, and higher cost compared to other IV sedation alternatives. A typical ICU infusion rate of dexmedetomidine has expected onset of clinical effect within 10 minutes, and an IV loading dose can be utilized in addition for situations requiring more rapid sedation therapy.

Antipsychotics

Haloperidol is a minimally sedating butyrophenone antipsychotic agent primarily administered in the ICU to treat delirium (as detailed above). It reliably maintains hemodynamic stability, has no respiratory depressant properties, demonstrates antiemetic activity, and also has anxiolytic effects. Undesirable characteristics of haloperidol include lack of both analgesia and amnesia, lowering of the seizure threshold, and ventricular arrhythmias (including torsades de pointes) from QT prolongation. Similar to other antipsychotics, haloperidol can cause akathisia (restless leg syndrome) and dystonic extrapyramidal symptoms, and it is also associated with the development of neuroleptic malignant syndrome in non-ICU patients.

Patient monitoring and sedation scales

Frequent reassessment of the patient's sedation level facilitates titration of the chosen agent(s) to a predetermined end point (minimizing the risk of under- or oversedation) as the dynamic course of critical illness changes over time. Such an approach lowers cumulative sedative doses, limits duration of sedation therapy, and minimizes the development of agent-specific side effects, tolerance, and/or withdrawal. This concept has led to the development of multiple, relatively straightforward sedation monitoring scales that accurately describe degrees of sedation into well-defined categories to guide sedation titration to a predefined goal, minimize interobserver variability between bedside caregivers, and facilitate communication among the patient's medical care team. An example of one common sedation scale (the Riker Sedation–Agitation Scale) is shown in Table 18.3. Once a stable level of sedation is achieved with the chosen sedation scale, it is recommended that sedation be discontinued once daily to allow spontaneous arousal in those ICU patients whose clinical condition is unlikely to deteriorate with scheduled sedation interruption. This so-called "daily awakening" has been shown to decrease both duration of mechanical ventilation and ICU length of stay.

Because spontaneous movement, hypertension, and tachycardia are neither sensitive nor specific objective markers of inadequate sedation and analgesia in the critically ill, a number of cerebral function monitors (CFM) have been developed over the last decade that process raw cortical EEG signals and mathematically convert them to an analog numerical scale using proprietary software. CFM's underlying assumption is that consciousness results from cortical electrical activity, and that suppression of such activity can indicate progressive decrements in consciousness. One CFM commonly utilized is the Bispectral Index (BIS), with readings of 100 being completely awake, 40–60 considered low probability for consciousness under general anesthesia, and 0 being compatible with an isoelectric EEG. CFMs are primarily utilized in the operating room to monitor for anesthesia levels and

Table 18.3. Sedation scale example: Riker Sedation–Agitation Scale

Score	Sedation–agitation description	Description of patient behavior/response
7	Dangerous agitation	Pulling at endotracheal tube, thrashing, climbing over bed rails, trying to remove support devices (Foley, etc.)
6	Very agitated	Does not calm with frequent verbal reminders, requires physical restraints, bites endotracheal tube
5	Agitated	Mildly agitated, attempts to sit up, calms with verbal instructions
4	Calm and cooperative	Awakens easily, follows commands
3	Sedated	Difficult to arouse, awakens to verbal/gentle tactile stimulation but drifts off again, obeys simple commands
2	Very sedated	Arousable to physical stimulation, does not follow commands, may move spontaneously
1	Unarousable	Minimal or no response to noxious stimulation, does not follow commands

Features and descriptions (absent or present)

---

1. Acute onset or fluctuating course

  A. Is there evidence of an acute change in mental status from baseline?

  B. Did the (abnormal) behavior fluctuate during the past 24 hours, i.e., tend to come and go or increase and decrease in severity as evidenced by fluctuations in sedation scale or the Glasgow Coma Scale measurements?

---

2. Inattention

Did the patient have difficulty focusing attention as evidenced by a score of less than 8 correct answers on either the visual (10 simple pictures) or auditory (squeeze hand or nod when the letter A is spoken in a random letter sequence) components of the Attention Screening Examination (ASE)?

---

3. Disorganized thinking

For patients not on mechanical ventilation, determination whether the patient's thinking is disorganized or incoherent, such as rambling or irrelevant conversation, unclear or illogical flow of ideas, or unpredictable switching from subject to subject. For patients being maintained on mechanical ventilation, is there evidence of disorganized or incoherent thinking as evidenced by incorrect answers to 3 or more of the 4 following questions and inability to follow the commands below?

Questions

(1) Will a stone float on water?   (2) Are there fish in the sea?

(3) Does 1 pound weigh more than 2 pounds?   (4) Can you use a hammer to pound a nail?

Commands:

(1) Are you having unclear thinking?

(2) Hold up this many fingers [examiner holds 2 fingers in front of the patient].

(3) Now do the same thing with the other hand [without holding the 2 fingers in front of the patient].

---

4. Altered level of consciousness (any level other than alert, such as being vigilant, lethargic, stupor, or coma)

Alert: spontaneously fully aware of environment and interacts appropriately

Vigilant: hyperalert

Lethargic: drowsy but easily aroused, unaware of some elements in the environment or not spontaneously interacting with the interviewer; becomes fully aware and appropriately interactive when prodded minimally

Stupor: difficult to arouse, unaware of some or all elements in the environment or not spontaneously interacting with the interviewer; becomes incompletely aware and inappropriately interactive when prodded strongly; can be aroused only by vigorous and repeated stimuli and as soon as the stimulus ceases, stuporous subject lapses back into an unresponsive state

Coma: unarousable, unaware of all elements in the environment with no spontaneous interaction or awareness of the interviewer so that the interview is impossible even with maximal prodding

---

Overall CAM-ICU assessment (Features 1 and 2 and either Feature 3 or 4): YES/NO

Figure 18.1. The CAM-ICU Delirium Assessment Tool.

minimize patient recall of unpleasant intraoperative events. They have yet to be widely accepted for ICU sedation monitoring, and little correlation exists between sedation scale and BIS readings. While ICU CFM utilization cannot be routinely recommended, its application to patients receiving adjunctive neuromuscular blockade administration can provide some assurance that such patients are sufficiently sedated and unlikely to recall their pharmacologically weakened state.

The Society of Critical Care Medicine recommends that ICU patients be routinely assessed for the presence of delirium, which is most commonly diagnosed and monitored utilizing the Confusion Assessment Method for the ICU (CAM-ICU) (Figure 18.1). Delirium exists when the patient exhibits both features 1 and 2 along with *either* feature 3 or feature 4. CAM-ICU assessments should be coordinated with daily interruptions in sedation when at all possible, and can be completed by trained bedside providers within 2 minutes.

Summary

ICU sedation should be guided by the current/anticipated course of the individual patient's critical illness, their degree of underlying organ system dysfunction, the known pharmacologic properties of available sedating agents, and the projected duration of sedation required. Treatment of pain with opioids as clinically indicated usually represents the most appropriate initial intervention, followed by adjunctive sedation administration utilizing additional agent(s) with the best risk–benefit profile for a given patient. Titration to a defined sedation end point via application of commonly used sedation scales should occur whether an intermittent IV or continuous infusion technique is chosen. Delirium has recently been identified as a significant problem contributing to adverse ICU outcomes and should also be monitored for, using the CAM-ICU monitoring tool. Specific sedating agents may have an impact on the development of delirium, and this should be incorporated into the ICU sedation decision-making process.

Further reading

American Society of Anesthesiologists Task Force on Intraoperative Awareness. Practice advisory for intraoperative awareness and brain function monitoring: a report by the American Society of Anesthesiologists Task Force on Intraoperative Awareness. *Anesthesiology* 2006; **104**: 847–64.

Brush DR, Kress JP. Sedation and analgesia for the mechanically ventilated patient. *Clin Chest Med* 2009; **30**: 131–41.

Carson SS, Kress JP, Rodgers JE, *et al.* A randomized trial of intermittent lorazepam versus propofol with daily interruption in mechanically ventilated patients. *Crit Care Med* 2006; **34**: 1326–32.

Chanqu, G, Jaber S, Barbotte E, *et al.* Impact of systematic evaluation of pain and agitation in an intensive care unit. *Crit Care Med* 2006; **34**: 1691–9.

Dasta JF, Kane-Gill SL, Pencina M, *et al.* A cost-minimization analysis of dexmedetomidine compared with midazolam for long-term sedation in the intensive care unit. *Crit Care Med* 2010; **38**: 497–503.

Girard TD, Jackson JC, Pandharipande PP, *et al.* Delirium as a predictor of long-term cognitive impairment in survivors of critical illness. *Crit Care Med* 2010; **38**: 1513–20.

Jacobi J, Fraser GL, Coursin DB, *et al.* Task Force of the American College of Critical Care Medicine (ACCM) of the Society of Critical Care Medicine (SCCM), American Society of Health-System Pharmacists (ASHP), American College of Chest Physicians. Clinical practice guidelines for the sustained use of sedatives and analgesics in the critically ill adult. *Crit Care Med* 2002; **30**: 119–41.

Kam PC, Cardone D. Propofol infusion syndrome. *Anaesthesia* 2007; **62**: 690–701.

Olsen ML, Swetz KM, Mueller PS. Ethical decision making with end-of-life care: palliative sedation and withholding or withdrawing life-sustaining treatments. *Mayo Clin Proc* 2010; **85**: 949–54.

Pandharipande PP, Pun BT, Herr DL, *et al.* Effect of sedation with dexmedetomidine vs lorazepam on acute brain dysfunction in mechanically ventilated patients: the MENDS randomized controlled trial. *JAMA* 2007; **298**: 2644–53.

Rea RS, Battistone S, Fong JJ, Devlin JW. Atypical antipsychotics versus haloperidol for treatment of delirium in acutely ill patients. *Pharmacotherapy* 2007; **27**: 588–94.

Sessler CN, Varney K. Patient-focused sedation and analgesia in the ICU. *Chest* 2008; **133**: 552–65.

Shehabi Y, Riker RR, Bokesch PM, *et al.* Delirium duration and mortality in lightly sedated mechanically ventilated intensive care patients. *Crit Care Med* 2010; **38**: 2311–18.

Strøm T, Martinussen T, Toft P. A protocol of no sedation for critically ill patients receiving mechanical ventilation: a randomised trial. *Lancet* 2010; **375**: 475–80.

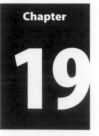

Chapter

19

Pediatric sedation

Corey E. Collins

Introduction

The delivery of sedation to children presents a significant challenge to many clinicians on a daily basis. While tremendous evidence exists to guide the clinician through the pharmacology, physiology, and medical issues involved, the final sedative regimen is most likely based on the specific training of the provider and the experience that individual brings to the procedure. Collectively, all providers tasked with providing sedation to children must acknowledge the inherent limitations of their experiences and training; only then can clinicians bring sober and intelligent judgment to this critical arena.

In this short chapter, a comprehensive review of pediatric sedation is not possible. The numerous resources available should be sought for in-depth guidance and specific data on particular procedures, coexisting diseases, and drugs. As always, clinicians have an obligation to understand the specific challenges of their environment and the patients in their care.

This chapter will present a general approach to pediatric sedation, focusing on the unique variables children bring to this clinical setting. In this practical discussion, the emphasis will be on (1) the specific settings for pediatric sedation and the interplay between setting and sedation plan, (2) clinical preparation, and (3) the potential limitations or complications that must be understood.

Pediatric sedation oversight

With the proliferation of indications for pediatric sedation, there has been a corresponding increase in the guidelines and patient safety measures intended to reduce the risk of

Moderate and Deep Sedation in Clinical Practice, ed. Richard D. Urman and Alan D. Kaye.
Published by Cambridge University Press. © Cambridge University Press 2012.

complications and error. Numerous agencies worldwide have developed, implemented, and validated specific guidelines for the training of sedation personnel, criteria necessary for sedation locations, the recovery and discharge of sedation patients, and the continuous quality improvement (CQI) applicable to sedation practices. In the United States, the American Academy of Pediatrics, the American Society of Anesthesiologists, the American Academy of Pediatric Dentistry, and the American Academy of Emergency Medicine have published such guidelines [1–4]. The American Academy of Pediatrics *Guidelines for monitoring and management of pediatric patients* are especially pertinent [4].

The development of a pediatric sedation program has historically occurred in response to clinical needs, and often without institutional oversight. Current recommendations, however, include a mandate for an institutional oversight body with responsibility for setting credentialing requirements, CQI process, and other safety and clinical concerns. Current Joint Commission policy requires this oversight to be led by the department of anesthesiology in each facility. This is particularly important for pediatric patients.

At a minimum, any personnel responsible for the provision of sedative drugs to children are expected to obtain credentialing through an institutional oversight committee. It is typically required that such clinicians have advanced training in pediatric care and maintain current certification in Pediatric Advanced Life Support (PALS) and perhaps Advanced Cardiac Life Support (ACLS) if care is provided to adolescents. Despite these credentials, it must be acknowledged that clinicians may have specific deficiencies in requisite skills such as bag-mask ventilation, direct laryngoscopy, or interpretation of clinical monitoring data. Such deficiencies, once recognized, should serve as an impetus for focused training and lead the individual clinician to seek specific training to improve these skills. Each institution should develop a process to assist with such training, and should seek resources within and outside the institution to meet these needs.

While it is fortunate that serious complications are quite rare in pediatric sedation, this does not absolve clinicians from maintaining all skills necessary to treat complications quickly and with confidence. Sedation providers must be able to rescue a child from a plane of sedation deeper than their credentials specify. In other words, if credentialed to provide deep sedation, the clinician must maintain the skills necessary to support a child whose sedation level has descended to deep sedation. Lack of competency in patient rescue techniques may lead to adverse outcomes.

Risks and adverse events in pediatric sedation

The determination of adverse-event rates in pediatric sedation has been elusive. Variation in event definition, nonuniform data collection, interinstitution variation in staffing, credentialing, or procedural technique make pooled, multivariate analysis of adverse outcomes problematic. Bhatt and a multidisciplinary consensus group produced a set of definitions related to pediatric sedation that seeks to recognize the requirement for clinical intervention as a critical element for an adverse event [5]. In other words, an "adverse event" is any clinical situation that prompts a specific intervention aimed at limiting a perceived threat to the patient's welfare. Other adverse event reports have focused on specific clinical parameters to define events such as measured pulse oximetry, blood pressures, or clinical signs such as stridor or retractions.

While many sedation regimens have been evaluated and compared for safety or outcomes, it is often not possible to answer the simple question, "What is the safest sedation protocol for procedure *x*?" Low complication rates overall, and confounding variables, make conclusive controlled trials practically impossible to conduct. Furthermore, many medications employed for pediatric sedation have not been fully evaluated and approved by the Food and Drug Administration (FDA), and "off-label" use is common. Therefore, the clinician must recognize these limitations and seek to define "safe sedation" appropriately.

Data on adverse-event rates for pediatric sedation are available from a number of sources. Once again, it is critical that the available data be scrutinized, as the absence of complications in these trials indicates the reality that rare events require enormous datasets to establish statistically significant trends. It can be too easy to erroneously declare that a sedation regimen is "safe" merely because the data were not sufficiently powered.

The latest report of the multicenter Pediatric Sedation Research Consortium calculates an overall adverse-event rate of 339.6 per 10,000 [6]. Oxygen desaturation was most frequently reported, with an incidence of 156.5 per 10,000. No deaths occurred and only one cardiac arrest, in a child with significant underlying disease. Overall, there were 1/400 respiratory-related events and 1/200 patients required some form of ventilator support (mask ventilation, oral airway placement). These data underscore the critical nature of competent airway management skills as a foundation for all safe pediatric sedation programs [6]. As in pediatric anesthesia, the highest priority must be careful and attentive airway care and vigilance for any deterioration in breathing.

Unique pediatric anatomy and physiology

Children present for sedation for many reasons and at all ages. Knowledge of specific developmental issues (anatomical, physiological, behavioral) is a prerequisite before provision of sedative drugs. Considering the preceding discussion on adverse airway events, a brief review of the pediatric airway is offered [7].

As a child ages, the airway matures into the adult configuration at adolescence. Infants and toddlers have relatively large tongues and their larynx resides relatively higher in the neck and is anteriorly tilted. Overall, children have more reactive airways; they are more likely to exhibit laryngospasm, or suffer more pronounced arterial desaturation should laryngospasm or bronchospasm occur. These facts make the sedated child more likely to experience an adverse airway event than an adult and may lead to more pronounced desaturation. The clinician should consider the increased risk of airway-related events as an inverse relationship to age.

The small child's cardiovascular system tends toward higher vagal tone, leading to a bradycardic response with autonomic stimulation. For small infants who rely on heart rate to increase cardiac output during times of stress, vagal discharge during airway manipulation, for example, can lead to decreased blood pressure or abnormal heart rhythms such as nodal bradycardia or junctional rhythms. During sedation, anticipation of this response and consideration of anticholinergic use (e.g., atropine or glycopyrrolate administration) is recommended.

Pulmonary function in the infant or small child is constrained by a reduced functional residual capacity, leading to more rapid oxygen depletion should apnea occur. Oxygen consumption is higher on a proportional basis compared with adults but tidal volumes are relatively similar. Small children increase their respiratory rates to meet their increased oxygen requirements, and therefore sedation-related decreases in respiratory rates combined with impaired pulmonary volumes of oxygen reserve can lead to an alarmingly rapid fall in oxygen saturation. Also, smaller children are much more prone than adults to apnea with sedation when drugs such as benzodiazepines, intravenous anesthetics such as propofol, and opioids are combined.

Behavioral concerns

As children develop, the ability to communicate, understand, conceptualize, or manage shifts from simply responding to environmental stimuli to complex reasoning and mature interaction with others. As children of all ages present for sedation, the provider must consider the child's developmental stage to form an appropriate plan. Small infants may be lulled by a cooperative and calm parent. However, children 2–5 years of age will exhibit a range of behaviors that must be considered. Refusal to take medications by mouth would prompt consideration of other routes (intramuscular, subcutaneous, rectal). Increased agitation may hinder the effect of sedatives, prompting additional doses that may cause an unexpected increase in sedation. Older children may accept intravenous lines, be more accepting of explanations, and transition more smoothly to the procedure area. They may, however, begin to associate the clinical setting with a threat and refuse to cooperate. Most clinicians will start to respect a child's refusal for a procedure around age 12 years [8]. By adolescence, most developmentally intact children will exhibit behavior similar to adults, although this is not a certainty; though intellectually capable of understanding the complex connections between the need for a procedure and reassurance that sedation will reduce discomfort, an adolescent may still lack the emotional control to cooperate fully.

Pharmacology

Many drugs used for pediatric sedation have been in clinical use for decades and were released for use with minimal pre-market safety trials in children. Current safety data are usually the result of retrospective analysis of rare events or comparative studies of specific regimens. The pharmacodynamics and pharmacokinetics of typical sedatives in children has slowly emerged for many agents over the years. It is important to note that sedative drugs are often used "off-label" for clinical sedation: propofol is only labeled for adult sedation; ketamine safety and effectiveness below the age 16 has not been established. Table 19.1 presents the most commonly used drugs for procedural sedation and analgesia [9].

The pharmacology of sedative drugs in children is a complex field that must consider the child's age, renal function as a means for elimination of many drugs, liver function as a means of transformation of certain drugs to active forms and other drugs to inactive forms, and the interplay of total body water, protein synthesis, or distribution characteristics. Needless to say, this complex array of considerations makes the accurate prediction of clinical effects of even a single sedative agent difficult, and of multiple agents nearly impossible. The clinician can, however, develop experience with sedative drugs and learn to titrate agents to a specific clinical end point. There must be patience with certain medications, as the delivery may require crossing the blood–brain lipid barrier (benzodiazepines) and others may distribute rapidly to the muscles and delay onset or require additional boluses for effect (pentobarbital). Combining agents can improve clinical effect through synergism, but such synergism is responsible for the increased adverse events with specific combinations (midazolam + fentanyl). Therefore, most sedation protocols use a single agent with careful criteria and limited options for additional agents of another drug

Table 19.1. Drugs for procedural sedation and analgesia

Drug	Pediatric dosing	Onset (min)	Duration (min)	Comments
Sedative-hypnotics				
Chloral hydrate	*Oral:* 25–100 mg/kg, after 30 min can repeat 25–50 mg/kg. *Maximum total dose:* 2 g or 100 mg/kg (whichever is less) Single use only in neonates	*Oral:* 15–30	*Oral:* 60–120	Effects unreliable if age > 3 years
Diazepam	*Intravenous:* initial 0.05–0.1 mg/kg, then titrate slowly to maximum 0.25 mg/kg	*Intravenous:* 4–5	*Intravenous:* 60–120	Reduce dose when used in combination with opioids
Etomidate	0.1 mg/kg intravenous; repeat if inadequate response	*Intravenous:* < 1	*Intravenous:* 5–15	Adverse effects include respiratory depression, myoclonus, nausea, and vomiting
Midazolam	*Intravenous (0.5–5 years):* initial 0.05–0.1 mg/kg, then titrated to maximum 0.6 mg/kg *Intravenous (6–12 years):* initial 0.025–0.05 mg/kg, then titrated to maximum 0.4 mg/kg	*Intravenous:* 2–3	*Intravenous:* 45–60	
	Intramuscular: 0.1–0.15 mg/kg *Oral:* 0.5–0.75 mg/kg *Intranasal:* 0.2–0.5 mg/kg *Rectal:* 0.25–0.5 mg/kg	*Intramuscular:* 10–20 Oral: 15–30 *Intranasal:* 10–15 *Rectal:* 10–30	*Intramuscular:* 60–120 Oral: 60–90 *Intranasal:* 60 *Rectal:* 60–90	Reduce dose when used in combination with opioids. May produce paradoxical excitement
Methohexital	*Rectal:* 25 mg/kg *Intravenous:* 0.5–1.0 mg/kg	*Rectal:* 10–15	*Rectal:* 60	Avoid if temporal lobe epilepsy or porphyria
Pentobarbital	*Intravenous:* 1–6 mg/kg, titrated in 1–2-mg/kg increments every 3–5 min to desired effect Intramuscular 2–6 mg/kg, maximum 100 mg	*Intravenous:* 3–5 *Intramuscular:* 10–15	*Intravenous:* 15–45 *Intramuscular:* 60–120	May produce paradoxical excitement. Avoid in patients with porphyria

Table 19.1. (cont.)

Drug	Pediatric dosing	Onset (min)	Duration (min)	Comments
	Oral or rectal (<4years): 3–6 mg/kg, maximum 100 mg *Oral/rectal (>4 years):* 1.5–3 mg/kg, maximum 100 mg	*Oral or rectal:* 15–60	*Oral or rectal:* 60–240	
Propofol	*Intravenous:* 1.0 mg/kg, followed by 0.5 mg/kg repeat doses as needed	*Intravenous:* < 1	*Intravenous:* 5–15	Frequent hypotension and respiratory depression.
Thiopental	*Rectal:* 25 mg/kg	*Rectal:* 10–15	*Rectal:* 60–120	Avoid in patients with porphyria
Analgesics				
Fentanyl	*Intravenous:* initial 1.0 μg/ kg up to 50 μg/dose, may repeat every 3 min, titrate to effect	*Intravenous:* 3–5	*Intravenous:* 30–60	Reduce dosing when combined with benzodiazepines
Morphine	*Intravenous:* initial 0.05–0.15 mg/kg up to 3 mg/dose, may repeat every 5 min, titrate to effect	*Intravenous:* 5–10	*Intravenous:* 120–180	Reduce dosing when combined with benzodiazepines
Dissociative drug				
Ketamine	*Intravenous:* 1–1.5 mg/kg slowly over 1 min; may repeat dose every 10 min as needed	*Intravenous:* 1	*Intravenous:* dissociation 15; recovery 60	Multiple contraindications.[a] Unpleasant dreams or hallucinations rare in children. Often given with concurrent atropine or glycopyrrolate to counter hypersalivation
	Intramuscular: 4–5 mg/kg, may repeat (2–4 mg/kg) after 10 min	*Intramuscular:* 3–5	*Intramuscular:* dissociation 15–30; recovery 90–150	
Inhalational drug				
Nitrous oxide	Preset mixture with minimum 30% oxygen self-administered by demand valve mask (requires cooperative child) Continuous flow nasal mask in	< 5	< 5 following discontinuation	Requires specialised apparatus and gas scavenger capability. Several contraindications

Table 19.1. (*cont.*)

Drug	Pediatric dosing	Onset (min)	Duration (min)	Comments
	uncooperative child with close monitoring			
Reversal drugs (antagonists)				
Naloxone	*Intravenous or intramuscular:* 0.1 mg/kg/ dose up to maximum of 2 mg/dose, may repeat every 2 min as needed	*Intravenous:* 2	*Intravenous:* 20–40 *Intramuscular:* 60–90	If shorter acting than the reversed drug, serial doses may be required
Flumazenil	*Intravenous:* 0.02 mg/kg/ dose, may repeat every 1 min up to I mg	*Intravenous:* 1–2	*Intravenous:* 30–60	If shorter acting than the reversed drug, serial doses may be required

Reproduced with permission from Krauss and Green [9].
Alterations in dosing may be indicated depending on the clinical situation and the practitioner's experience with these drugs. Individual dosages may vary when used in combination with other drugs, especially when benzodiazepines are combined with opioids.
a Ketamine is absolutely contraindicated in children younger than 3 months (higher risk of airway complications) and in setting of known or suspected psychosis (can exacerbate condition). Relative contraindications include age younger than 12 months; procedures involving stimulation of posterior pharynx; history of tracheal surgery or stenosis; active pulmonary infection or disease (including upper respiratory infection); known or suspected cardiovascular disease; head injury associated with loss of consciousness; altered mental status; emesis; central nervous system masses, abnormalities, or hydrocephalus; glaucoma or acute globe injury; porphyria; thyroid disorder or thyroid medication.

family; this is especially true for nursing sedation protocols, where an additional agent can cause a child to quickly descend from light sedation to deep sedation or even general anesthesia.

Synergism between medications used for sedation and outpatient management of pediatric conditions can lead to erratic effects. For example, many medications used for the treatment of attention-deficit disorder are stimulants and will lead to a relative tolerance to sedation. Conversely, some antidepressants increasingly prescribed to children can augment the depressant effects of sedatives.

Clinical sedation for procedures is a dynamic process with a variable level of stimulation and invasiveness. Thus the onset, depth, and duration of sedation must be titrated and controlled with a certain amount of sophistication and understanding of both the medications employed and the procedure itself. The ideal medication regimen optimizes the onset and potency of sedation in direct preparation and synchronization with the level of noxious stimulation. Clearly, this ideal is nearly impossible to realize, mostly because of the latency in delivery of drug to the site of action in the central nervous system and the resultant neurochemical effect, the variability of sensitivity of each patient to a given drug, inaccuracies in the drug dose delivered, or estimation of the true severity of noxious stimulation. The reality therefore becomes a process of "best-guess" drug dosing or algorithms that initiate drug dosing on weight-based criteria alone, with additional drug doses or options dictated by the subsequent response of the child. Many sedation protocols successfully employ this tactic, but a certain failure rate is guaranteed because of the impossibility that any protocol will include options necessary to address all scenarios. Nevertheless, it is important to emphasize that protocols help reduce the real human effect of trying to succeed by deviating from established rules and guidelines.

Overview of the sedation process and medication selection

Final planning of a safe and effective sedation regimen must account for many diverse factors. Figure 19.1 presents a schematic depiction of these factors. Pain management and sedation are most effective when the clinician is attentive to objective measures of patient distress. While a number of pain scales are routinely available and validated, use for sedation can be difficult. These scales are intended to grade pain and direct appropriate intervention, while sedation protocols must evaluate pain and distress in a dynamic setting. Therefore, knowledge of these pain scales improves accurate clinical judgment but cannot substitute for vigilance and training for sedation (Figure 19.2).

Common pediatric sedation scenarios
Radiology

Children are often negatively affected by radiological examinations, however brief. Often, a radiograph can be obtained with restraints alone, or a computed tomography (CT) can be completed with a parent's assistance. More lengthy studies such as magnetic resonance imaging (MRI) are poorly tolerated by most children and require sedation or general anesthesia. MRI has the additional requirement for an immobile child, not just a sedated child.

An undersupply of anesthesiology teams has resulted in the successful development of nurse-administered pediatric sedation protocols. Most often with a supervising physician, nurses assess and medicate children according to set criteria. The drug pentobarbital is frequently used, as it often results in a deeply sedated and motionless child for 60–90 minutes, sufficient for most MRI examinations. Infusions of drugs such as propofol or dexmedetomidine can result in adequate sedation with the added benefit of prompt offset. These protocols are less appropriate for invasive radiologic procedures with a painful component (e.g., arterial puncture or percutaneous biopsy). Dexmedetomidine provides modest analgesia, but pentobarbital and propofol do not.

Sedation for a CT scan can be accomplished using bolus sedatives such as propofol, remifentanil, or midazolam ($\pm$ fentanyl) to provide brief deep sedation that will last 8–10 minutes. Chloral hydrate has been used for decades for radiology sedation but the erratic pharmacology, long latency before onset of sedation, and long half-life has made it less desirable. Its safety profile and history, however, means that it is still used as a reasonable agent for nurse-administered sedation programs.

Lastly, sedation may be needed to obtain a radiograph (e.g., extremity film) in a traumatized child. This may be well managed with an oral or intravenous sedative, such as midazolam, lorazepam, or chloral hydrate, prior to arrival at the radiology suite.

Failure of sedation in the radiology suite may result in referral of the patient to the anesthesia service. Success may be improved by evaluation of the child's state before starting the sedation to assess his/her anxiety, parental anxiety, patient maturity, and the ability of the sedating clinician to assuage and pacify the child.

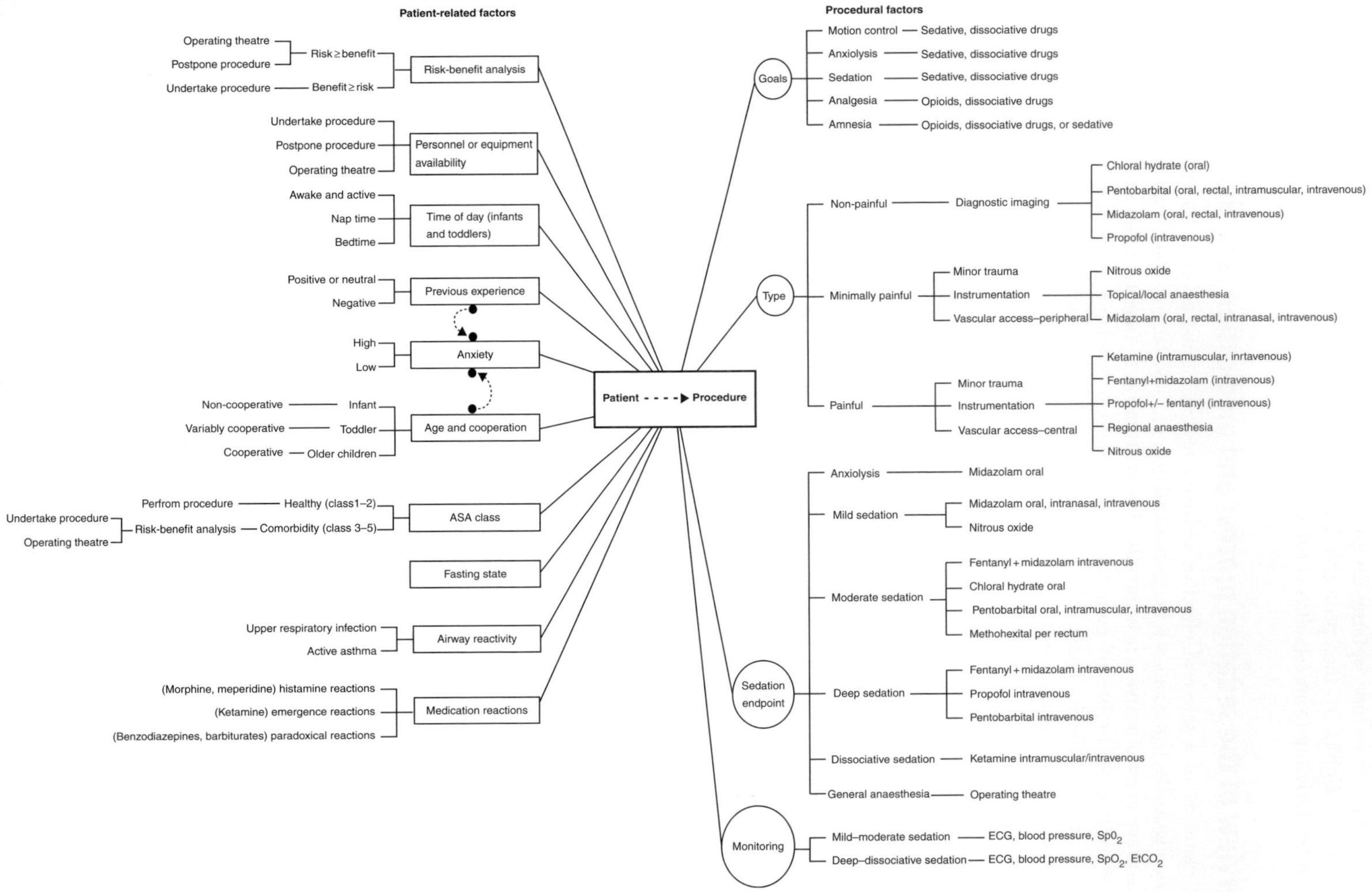

Figure 19.1. Factors determining medication choices and sedation end points. SpO$_2$, oxygen saturation; EtCO$_2$, end-tidal carbon dioxide. Reprinted with permission from Krauss and Green [9].

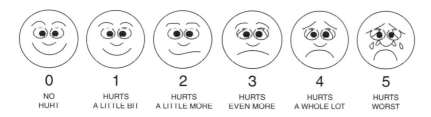

	DATE / TIME					
Face 0 - No particular expression or smile 1 - Occasional grimace or frown, withdrawn, disinterested 2 - Frequent to constant quivering chin,clenched jaw						
Legs 0 - Normal position or relaxed 1 - Uneasy, restless, tense 2 - Kicking, or legs drawn up						
Activity 0 - Lying quietly, normal position, moves easily 1 - Squirming, shifting back and forth, tense 2 - Arched, rigid or jerking						
Cry 0 - No cry (awake or asleep) 1 - Moans or whimpers; occasional complaint 2 - Crying steadily, screams or sobs, frequent complaints						
Consolabillity 0 - Content, relaxed 1 - Reassured by occasional touching, hugging or being talked to, distractible 2 - Difficult to console or comfort						
TOTAL SCORE						

Figure 19.2. Two examples of commonly used pediatric pain scales: the Wong–Baker Faces Pain Rating scale (above) and the FLACC scale (below).

Emergency department

Pediatric sedation in the midst of a critical event such as trauma, fractures, or acute illness requires a dedicated, team approach. It is unlikely that a single agent will permit procedural sedation, and residual sedative effects can complicate evaluation of the child's mental status. The ideal regimen will have prompt onset and offset, minimally effect the vital signs, provide potent analgesia for painful interventions, and not obtund the respiratory drive.

Ketamine is advantageous in many settings, as it exhibits many features of an ideal agent. It has prompt onset, potent analgesic and amnesic effects, and relatively short effective duration. It can be administered by mouth, rectum, blood, or intramuscular injection. Ketamine has the undesirable tendency to cause salivation, and the additional secretions are thought by some to increase the risk of coughing or laryngospasm. An anticholinergic agent such as glycopyrrolate or atropine can be coadministered. Lastly, there continues to be significant concern regarding the propensity for ketamine to cause an agitated dysphoric state, typically referred to as "dissociation," where the patient experiences negative psychic phenomenon. This is pharmacologically related to ketamine's similarity to phencyclidine (the street drug "acid"). In children such negative experiences are less significant than in adults, and ketamine therefore remains a reasonable and frequently deployed sedative agent in emergency departments in the United States.

Considerable debate continues over the use of propofol by non-anesthesiologists. Propofol infusions may provide hypnosis, amnesia, and anesthesia but no analgesia. Careful clinical monitoring is needed to detect apnea or airway obstruction. It can be difficult to maintain adequate sedation if stimulation occurs or a painful procedure is attempted. The addition of a potent analgesic can improve sedation for painful procedures but concomitantly increases the risk of apnea and airway compromise.

Endoscopy

Numerous clinical reports document the options for endoscopic procedures under sedation. The low complication rates for a variety of protocols support the overall safety of sedation in the endoscopy suite, though standards for sedative administration and patient monitoring are forthcoming [10].

Propofol as a sole agent provides excellent conditions in a timely manner. Typically, a sedation clinician is necessary to monitor for excess sedation or apnea. The concomitant administration of other sedatives will increase the risk of apnea and airway compromise, though with added benefit of improved amnesia and immobility (e.g., propofol + fentanyl). When deeper levels of sedation are desired, a sedation clinician dedicated to monitoring the child is necessary.

Pediatric intensive care unit

Critically ill children present an exceptionally significant set of challenges. Sedation must be considered in the context of the child's immediate clinical state, the level of sedation considered necessary, the potential risks of any administered sedative drugs, and the experience of the staff providing care. Many units adopt routines for specific clinical needs, perhaps to the exclusion of other available protocols. Yet the safety of a familiar protocol will likely offset any risks of attempting to maintain competence in a multitude of sedation techniques. Unfortunately, a lack of rigorous evidence regarding the safety and efficacy of the many possible regimens makes local practice highly variable and often dogmatic.

For example, a recent systematic review on the safety and efficacy of sedation for intubated children in a pediatric ICU reported only one high-quality study available and concluded that "high-quality evidence to guide clinical practice is still limited" [11]. The extreme range of clinical situations, from deep sedation for painful procedures and nonphysiological ventilation strategies such as high-frequency oscillation ventilation to mild sedation for a minor dressing change, places a high demand on excellent clinical judgment, maintenance of competence with numerous drugs, and a willingness to scrutinize local practice.

Of the available sedation strategies, most pediatric units employ a combination of opioid analgesics with benzodiazepines for sedation, with titration of infusions to meet clinical needs (morphine or fentanyl with midazolam). Dexmedetomidine has found increasing use in the pediatric ICU, as it provides excellent titratable sedation and analgesia with relatively few adverse events. Similar to clonidine, its selective alpha-agonism for receptors in the brain results in sedation that is very similar to physiological sleep. Its use in children has been described most commonly for ventilated children. The major adverse events include bradycardia, hypertension, and hypotension [12]. Propofol infusion was much more common before the recognition of the propofol infusion syndrome, a poorly understood constellation of cardiovascular instability, metabolic acidosis, hyperkalemia, and rhabdomyolysis associated with prolonged exposure to high-dose propofol infusions and linked to numerous pediatric deaths [13]. While propofol remains an excellent sedative drug for the pediatric ICU, its use now requires careful clinical monitoring and caution.

Neonatal units face even more rigorous challenges. Prolonged ventilation of premature infants with profound systemic morbidities is often required. While it is clear that sedation is required for neonates, drug choice, dosing, and safety issues are poorly described. Cochrane reviews for mechanically ventilated neonates failed to establish recommendations regarding the use of opioids or midazolam [14,15]. Other agents have been described, including dexmedetomidine and remifentanil. Certain agents may be avoided in this population because of the potential for neurological injury (e.g., ketamine) or because they contain potentially injurious chemical excipients such as benzyl alcohol or propylene glycol (midazolam, lorazepam) [16]. Table 19.2 lists a suggested schedule for neonatal ICU sedation and analgesia, based on practice at the Brigham and Women's Hospital in Boston, MA (personal correspondence, R. Patnode, 2011).

Specific drugs

The following are general comments regarding the most frequently used sedatives, with particular emphasis on the unique characteristics of each [7].

Propofol

Propofol is an intravenous anesthetic agent that when delivered at lower doses, or as an infusion, can be used to induce various levels of sedation. At lower dose ranges mild to moderate sedation can be obtained in children, though the lack of analgesia may cause erratic clinical effect during periods of stimulation. Propofol has the tendency to decrease respiratory effort in a dose-dependent way. The synergistic response with other sedatives can be profound with propofol. Irritation at the site of injection or infusion is common and sometimes results in unexpected patient movement that may dislodge an IV or surprise the clinician.

When used for sedation, small boluses may be given and the patient closely monitored for clinical effect. Over the course of a few minutes, if the desired effect is not achieved, additional small boluses may be given. With patience and close monitoring most children will respond successfully to the technique for all but the most stimulating procedures.

Midazolam

Midazolam is a fast-acting benzodiazepine that may be administered orally, intravenously, or nasally to achieve mild to moderate sedation. As with all benzodiazepines, excess dose can induce general anesthesia and profound respiratory depression. An atypical behavioral response may occur, resulting in agitation.

When given orally, a typical dose of 0.5 mg/kg will result in mild sedation after 15–20 minutes. The taste is bitter and is poorly tolerated unless masked in flavored syrup. Duration of effect can be erratic but usually lasts approximately 30–60 minutes. Intravenous delivery of 0.025–0.5 mg/kg will result in mild to moderate sedation in approximately 2 minutes, with a clinical effect lasting 30–60 minutes. Nasal administration has been used

Table 19.2. Drugs for procedural sedation and analgesia in the neonatal intensive care unit

Clinical scenario	Medication	Notes
Minimally invasive procedures: blood draws, IV start	24% sucrose PO PRN	Note that these painful experiences do require some intervention to prevent stress and future enhanced pain-related agitation
Lumbar puncture	Morphine or fentanyl; lidocaine	
Dressing change	Morphine or fentanyl; sucrose	
Elective intubation	Fentanyl or morphine bolus followed by infusion; consider midazolam	
Mechanical ventilation	Fentanyl infusion and/or midazolam infusion	Patient may require additional PRN boluses of morphine, fentanyl, or midazolam for episodic agitation or pain
Postoperative analgesia	Morphine or fentanyl; acetaminophen	Titrate analgesics to pain scores

Medication	Doses	Notes
Morphine	0.05–0.15 mg/kg IV or SQ q 2–4 h	Prolonged exposure will require weaning
Fentanyl	1–3 µg/kg IV q 2–4 h Infusion dose: 0.2–2 µg/kg/h titrated	Infuse slowly < 1µg/kg/min to avoid hypotension, rigid chest, bradycardia
Midazolam	0.05–0.1 mg/kg bolus	Full term only
Lidocaine infiltration	1 mL/kg max using 0.5% solution	Local injection may obviate need for systemic sedatives and analgesics. Generally avoided for infants <34 weeks gestational age
Oral sucrose solution	24% sucrose 0.5–1.5 mL PO PRN	Oral sucrose has been shown to be effective for procedural analgesia in young infants
Acetaminophen	10–15 mg/kg PO/PR/PGT q 6 h	Max 24 h dose = 90 mg/kg

Adapted from personal correspondence with Rita Patnode, RN, Brigham and Women's Hospital, Boston, MA, 2011.

for the uncooperative child, although mucosal irritation causes nearly universal distress, and therefore this route should be reserved for special circumstances only.

Chloral hydrate

Chloral hydrate 50–100 mg/kg oral delivery provides reliable moderate sedation or sleep in most children following 30–60 minutes of latency. Most often a quiet environment will facilitate the onset of sleep. Once asleep, most children will tolerate a calm transfer to another location or procedure suite without rousing. Sedation typically persists for approximately 1 hour, although a full return to baseline level of consciousness may require far longer. Because of the characteristics of chloral hydrate, it is generally not advised to add additional sedative drugs should adequate sedation not be achieved.

Ketamine

As a phencyclidine derivative, ketamine administration may induce concerning psychological responses in children, although experience suggests that children are less prone to this phenomenon than adults. Sialorrhea (excessive salivation) may occur and increase the risk of an adverse respiratory event; anticholinergic coadministration may be advisable. The relatively high risk for nausea and vomiting may warrant antiemetic therapy.

Intramuscular dosing of 3–5 mg/kg may be used for an uncooperative child, with onset of sedation typically within 5–15 minutes. Oral dosing of 3–6 mg/kg will typically sedate the child in approximately the same time. Intravenous doses of 1–2 mg/kg can provide a cooperative and well-sedated child. Ketamine is the only typical pediatric sedative drug with excellent analgesic properties and minimal respiratory depression.

Nitrous oxide

Recognized since the eighteenth century for its sedative and analgesic qualities, 50% nitrous oxide in oxygen provides excellent mild to moderate sedation for brief procedures or examinations. Additional sedatives should be avoided, as excessive sedation or anesthesia may occur. The onset of sedation may be delayed depending on the child's minute ventilation, anxiety level, or other factors that cause decreased delivery of the gas. Recovery from nitrous oxide is prompt and predictable; most patients will return to baseline level of consciousness within 5–10 minutes of discontinuation.

Pentobarbital

This barbiturate has been used to induce sleep of sufficient duration to permit longer radiologic studies such as MRI. A dose of 4–6 mg/kg can be given via the oral or intravenous route. Onset of sleep is typically within 10–15 minutes. Paradoxical emergence agitation can occur and can complicate recovery significantly. This "rage reaction" can threaten patient safety and may necessitate intervention such as supplemental sedation (midazolam), restraint, or hospitalization.

Clonidine and dexmedetomidine

Alpha-2-adrenergic receptor agonists such as clonidine and dexmedetomidine are well known to cause sedation, anxiolysis, and hypnosis. Clonidine 2–4 µg/kg orally can produce effective sedation and analgesia, though onset times can be greater than 60–90 minutes. While clonidine is less specific for receptors in the central nervous system, dexmedetomidine exhibits highly selective preference for the receptors located in the locus ceruleus, the region responsible for producing sleep in humans. For this reason, dexmedetomidine has emerged as a unique sedative drug capable of inducing a controlled state of moderate to deep sedation without depressing ventilation, blunting laryngeal reflexes, or significantly depressing cardiovascular parameters. When it is administered as a bolus dose of 0.5–1 µg/kg over 10 minutes and followed by an infusion of 0.5–1 µg/kg/h, most patients are moderately sedated with spontaneous ventilation and will tolerate endoscopy, examinations, minor surgical procedures, or mechanical ventilation. Due to interaction with cardiac alpha receptors, bradycardia and hypotension can occur and may limit its use in certain children. Limited pediatric safety data are available, and labeled use is for adults only at this time.

Summary

Practical pediatric sedation remains a considerable challenge for many clinicians. The many factors that inherently affect pediatric physiology, pharmacology, and behavior must be recognized by all clinicians attempting to sedate children. Institutional oversight must seek to balance the needs of patients with the risks of sedation. The individual clinician should seek continuous improvement of personal training and experience to further his or her ability to care for sedated children.

References

1. Woolley SM, Hingston EJ, Shah J, Chadwick BL. Paediatric conscious sedation: views and experience of specialists in paediatric dentistry. *Br Dent J* 2009; **207**: E11; discussion 280–1.

2. Cote CJ, Wilson S. Guidelines for monitoring and management of pediatric patients during and after sedation for diagnostic and therapeutic procedures: an update. *Paediatr Anaesth* 2008; **18**: 9–10.

3. Guideline for monitoring and management of pediatric patients during and after sedation for diagnostic and therapeutic procedures. *Pediatr Dent* 2008; **30**: 143–59.

4. American Academy of Pediatrics, American Academy of Pediatric Dentistry. Guidelines for monitoring and management of pediatric patients during and after sedation for diagnostic and therapeutic procedures: an update. *Pediatrics* 2006; **118**: 2587–602.

5. Bhatt M, Kennedy RM, Osmond MH, *et al.* Consensus-based recommendations for standardizing terminology and reporting adverse events for emergency department procedural sedation and analgesia in children. *Ann Emerg Med* 2009; **53**: 426–35 e4.

6. Cravero JP, Blike GT, Beach M, *et al.* Incidence and nature of adverse events during pediatric sedation/anesthesia for procedures outside the operating room: report from the Pediatric Sedation Research Consortium. *Pediatrics* 2006; **118**: 1087–96.

7. Miller RD, ed. *Anesthesia*, 6th edn. Philadelphia, PA: Churchill Livingstone, 2005.

8. Lewis I, Burke C, Voepel-Lewis T, Tait AR. Children who refuse anesthesia or sedation: a survey of anesthesiologists. *Paediatr Anaesth* 2007; **17**: 1134–42.

9. Krauss B, Green SM. Procedural sedation and analgesia in children. *Lancet* 2006; **367**: 766–80.

10. Dar AQ, Shah ZA. Anesthesia and sedation in pediatric gastrointestinal endoscopic procedures: a review. *World J Gastrointest Endosc* 2010; **2**: 257–62.

11. Hartman ME, McCrory DC, Schulman SR. Efficacy of sedation regimens to facilitate mechanical ventilation in the pediatric intensive care unit: a systematic review. *Pediatr Crit Care Med* 2009; **10**: 246–55.

12. Yuen VM. Dexmedetomidine: perioperative applications in children. *Paediatr Anaesth* 2010; **20**: 256–64.

13. Papaioannou V, Dragoumanis C, Theodorou V, Pneumatikos I. The propofol infusion "syndrome" in intensive care unit: from pathophysiology to prophylaxis and treatment. *Acta Anaesthesiol Belg* 2008; **59**: 79–86.

14. Bellu R, de Waal K, Zanini R. Opioids for neonates receiving mechanical ventilation: a systematic review and meta-analysis. *Arch Dis Child Fetal Neonatal Ed* 2010; **95**: F241–51.

15. Ng E, Taddio A, Ohlsson A. Intravenous midazolam infusion for sedation of infants in the neonatal intensive care unit. *Cochrane Database Syst Rev* 2003: CD002052.

16. Shehab N, Lewis CL, Streetman DD, Donn SM. Exposure to the pharmaceutical excipients benzyl alcohol and propylene glycol among critically ill neonates. *Pediatr Crit Care Med* 2009; **10**: 256–9.

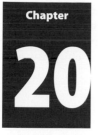

Chapter

20

Sedation in the office/outpatient setting

Debra E. Morrison and Kristi Dorn Hare

Introduction

The office/outpatient setting as a site for surgical procedures is, metaphorically, a small lifeboat (not a pirate ship!) on the high seas at a distance from the port or the mother ship, the hospital, far from immediate assistance. Whether the site is a detached procedural area on the campus of a large medical center, a freestanding outpatient surgical suite, or a single procedure room in a physician's office, the metaphor is appropriate. The lifeboat and her crew must be equipped, skilled, and disciplined adequately to handle emergencies without immediate help from the outside and, as a team, must act in concert with one another. On the campus of a medical center, even a detached outpatient area may have access to anesthesia providers, skilled staff, monitoring equipment, and rescue capability. There is usually an on-site rapid response and/or a code team, and specialty consultants when needed. However, those advanced teams will not be as close as they would be in the main hospital operating room, emergency department, or intensive care unit room. Help is even more remote in a freestanding outpatient surgical suite or a physician's office, when reliance is upon the municipal emergency response system (911). In any case the crew of the lifeboat must be prepared to perform primary resuscitation as the first responders.

There must be a shared culture of safety. A standard policy and procedure, a working document, should be developed, followed, examined, and revised when appropriate. Whether or not the setting/organization undergoes official accreditation, the policy and procedure should follow national patient safety guidelines. There should be adherence to the policy and a recommended standard of safety.

Moderate and Deep Sedation in Clinical Practice, ed. Richard D. Urman and Alan D. Kaye.
Published by Cambridge University Press. © Cambridge University Press 2012.

Patients and procedures should be selected for appropriateness in the specific setting, and the plan for sedation should be appropriate to the patient, the procedure, and the setting. A pre-procedure safety checklist (time-out) should be developed, and routine debriefing should occur after each procedure in order to improve process, efficiency, and safety.

The team

The procedural team functioning far from immediate assistance must of necessity be highly skilled and experienced. In his book *The Checklist Manifesto* [1], Dr. Atul Gawande discusses the team, rather than individual aspects of health care. The book is as much about teamwork as it is about checklists, and he explains, "In a world in which success now requires large enterprises, teams of clinicians, high-risk technologies, and knowledge that outstrips any one person's abilities, individual autonomy hardly seems the ideal we should aim for."

In many private offices, physicians routinely perform procedures with the help of medical assistants (MAs). This is fine for procedures requiring local anesthetic only. If sedation is being used, a registered nurse (RN) or team of RNs with education and experience in sedation is needed. The RN must be adequately equipped with medications for sedation (IV and PO), reversal agents, emergency medications, monitoring equipment, and equipment for immediate resuscitation. The RN(s) and the physician should have current BLS/ACLS certification. There is no substitute for preparedness and experience. Ideally, the RN doing sedation should have a critical care background of at least 2 years and the confidence to command the attention of the surgeon/practitioner/physician when necessary, in order to "stop the assembly line" and focus all care on the patient. This will ensure that the RN will recognize problems and be prepared to intervene.

The RN must be aware of the details of each procedure, in order to anticipate challenges and problems, and must be able to read cues from both the surgeon/practitioner/physician and the patient in order to administer sedation safely. She/he should be intimately involved with patient evaluation. She/he must be aware of and respectful of other members of the operative team. The RN should be an advocate for the surgeon/practitioner/physician as well as for the patient. The nurse who is administering sedation and monitoring the patient should not be responsible for assisting with the procedure to the degree that she/he is distracted from care of the patient.

The surgeon/practitioner/physician should form a partnership with the RN, who should be empowered to be the guardian of all. The concerns of the RN should never be dismissed, and the surgeon/practitioner/physician should lead the rest of the team in respect for the RN, especially if she/he expresses concerns. A nurse who fears derision or dismissal may not be quick to speak up with concerns for the patient and may worry silently, hoping that the procedure will soon be over, thus delaying successful intervention if there is a problem. A surgeon/practitioner/physician may enter "the zone" while performing a procedure, but should develop a "third ear" open to communication from the RN performing sedation and monitoring the patient. Even at a critical period during the procedure, the physician should be able to at least acknowledge any communication from the nurse. The surgeon/practitioner/physician should plan well and anticipate necessary equipment and contingencies in advance, so that the procedure proceeds as smoothly and quickly as possible.

Although MAs, schedulers, and surgical or other technologists will not be directly involved in sedation, they should be considered intregral members of the team. Their perceptions, impressions, patient interactions, and helping hands help smooth the process and add to patient safety and procedural success.

Each person on the team should be valued and respected for his/her contribution, and each should understand the concerns and responsibilities of the others. Everyone should be able to perform at greater than 100% of his/her job when necessary. This may be ultimately accomplished by working together and surviving crises, or accelerated by team training/practice/simulation/drills, formal or informal in nature. Individuals can also improve their skills and add to collective knowledge and skill by attending workshops and conferences. Well-trained team members who work in concert are ultimately happier. They are more efficient and cost-effective if they are able to perform consistently and predictably and respond effectively to problems before they develop into disasters.

Care in particular revolves around the patient, and not the procedure, the surgeon/practitioner/physician, the RN, or any other individual.

The setting

The setting for any sedation procedure needs to be safe, first of all. It must be fully equipped and staffed with everything needed for the planned procedure and for sedation, as well as for recognition of problems and immediate rescue and resuscitation.

There are vast resources available to procedure areas within medical centers. If the outpatient area is on a medical center site, many hospital support systems should be available: equipment, sterile equipment, supplies, specialty consultants, and rapid response teams.

If the outpatient setting is remote, or in a private office, much more care should be taken in sedation, and in planning and preparation for adverse events. If the office is busy and carries out many procedures, the staff will become adept at preparing for them. If the procedures are infrequent, there will be gaps in preparation and efficiency. Steps are much more likely to be omitted without constant practice. In all cases, it is best to have procedure plans in a book or on cards. These plans list the equipment needed, and the expectations of the MD regarding that case. These plans are invaluable to aid the staff in adequately preparing for procedures, as well as providing a checklist to discover well in advance of the procedure if a crucial item is missing. It is frustrating, inconvenient, and potentially dangerous to find when the procedure is under way that a needed piece of equipment or medication cannot be obtained. It causes delay, negatively influences the morale of all members of the team, and can potentially harm patients. Once again, the more remote the location, the more diligent the preparation must be, since there are no immediate resources to call on.

Policy and procedure

An appropriate policy and procedure should be developed, based on National Patient Safety Goals [2] and AORN recommendations [3–5]. This should cover all aspects of the practice.

Culture of safety

The Association of periOperative Registered Nurses (AORN) advocates a culture of safety. Their position statements attest that it is the right of every patient to receive the highest level of care in all settings, with all providers collaboratively striving to create an environment of safety. They insist that every patient scheduled for an invasive procedure deserves to have an RN throughout the continuum of care, including an RN circulator [3–5]. All members of the perioperative/procedural team should be able to work as a team, allowing open discussion of concerns, near-misses, and errors, identification of systems issues, and advocacy of process improvements without fear of reprisal. Learning and improvement are enhanced by a debriefing of adverse events, without blame, by the entire team. Patients and their families are necessarily part of the team. Each member of the team should be a patient advocate. AORN advocates reducing error, educating staff, and creating collaborative strategies to strengthen the culture of safety. Economic concerns must not supersede patient safety: lack of patient safety will ultimately be cause for economic concern.

Safety standards should be consistent with National Patient Safety Goals as outlined by the Joint Commission, American Society of Anesthesiologists, and University HealthSystem Consortium guidelines [2,6–8].

Procedure selection

The scope of practice of the surgeon/practitioner/physician(s) involved determines the range of procedures possible in a given procedural setting. The physician should pare the list to include only those procedures that are appropriate to the detached outpatient or office setting, and schedule other procedures in a setting equipped for the complexity of the procedure or anticipated length of recovery/time to discharge, such as the medical center campus or in the hospital itself.

Criteria for selection

- Consider the length of each procedure, and schedule only procedures that can be completed and fully recovered from in the period of a working day.
- If a procedure involves blood loss, schedule in a facility where transfusion is an option.
- Procedures should be amenable to local anesthesia with minimal or moderate sedation: schedule procedures that require deeper sedation or anesthesia, even if appropriate for the location, for a day when anesthesia care can be provided.
- If a procedure may be amenable to sedation in some patients, but not definitely amenable to sedation in all patients, it is reasonable to schedule patients on a day when both sedation and anesthesia are available. Evaluate patients and consent them for both contingencies. This allows a greater range of options without aborting the procedure and rescheduling.

Patient selection

Pre-evaluate patients to screen for criteria that contraindicate procedures under sedation, particularly in the office/outpatient setting. Screening can commence with the first patient encounter, when a patient is being evaluated for candidacy for the procedure. A scheduler or clerk can be given a list of simple screening questions to be directed to each patient who calls to schedule a first appointment. The surgeon/practitioner/physician can employ a questionnaire to be filled out by the patient at home prior to the office visit or over the internet. The RN can partner with the physician in screening questionnaires and patients for appropriateness. The nurse can ask important but sometimes sensitive historical questions about medication use, medical history, surgical history, allergies, social habits, expectations regarding the procedure and sedation. She/he can discover the patient's previous experiences with anesthesia, sedation, and other procedures. It is important to uncover intolerances to medications, positioning issues, or any history of unexpected events during procedures. The patient will not always know what historical information is important, but the patient may be more likely to confide in the nurse, while telling the physician what he/she thinks the physician wants to hear.

Criteria for selection

Avoid complications and sedation failure by selecting patients who are amenable to easy and safe sedation. Consider scheduling patients with the following characteristics under anesthesia rather than sedation:

- obesity
- difficult airway/significant craniofacial abnormalities
- beards (small chins both predict difficult airways and lead patients to grow beards)
- sleep apnea
- personal or family history of malignant hyperthermia
- coagulopathy/hypercoagulability
- heart or lung disease that is a threat to life
- significant neurological disease
- other organ-system disease that presents a significant hazard, such as diabetes
- history of anesthesia/sedation complications or sedation failure
- intolerance of medications routinely used for sedation
- routine medications or drugs that may react with sedation agents
- chronic pain or anxiety with a baseline need for analgesics or anxiolytics
- pediatric patients who are not consenting individuals and are thus not obligated to cooperate
- extremes of age

Sedation plan

The plan for sedation must be made according to the type and length of the procedure, using rapid-onset and short-acting agents. It is advisable in the outpatient setting to use agents, such as fentanyl and midazolam, which have readily available reversal agents. A relatively short-acting oral benzodiazepine such as alprazolam might be included as premedication. Diphenhydramine and ondansetron are helpful adjuncts for treating side effects of opioids. It is important that the physician and the nurse be familiar with the contraindication, actions, and adverse effects of all medications used, as well as with the proper administration of reversal agents.

Reversal-agent doses (dose and volume needed) for each patient should be known and written down in advance so that they are easy to administer quickly and accurately. A hurried IV push with an incorrect dose may produce an adverse event in itself. It is wise to prepare "cheat sheets" before each case with the doses, volume, onset, and duration written out for each patient's weight before the case is started. This will make administration more efficient and eliminate the effort of performing unfamiliar calculations in the heat of an adverse patient reaction to sedation. Many hospitals have "drug calculators" built into their computer systems for easy use by the staff, and dosing calculators are available on the internet. These are commonly used for pediatric patients, but they are useful for all patients, saving time and preventing errors. If the patient's weight is known in advance, a chart can be prepared prior to the day of the procedure.

Many patients express the desire to be "knocked out" for a procedure. If the patient expresses this, and the procedure is amenable to local anesthesia with minimal or moderate sedation, it is important to address this gently but honestly, rather than misleading the patient. The patient may believe he/she was unconscious during a similar procedure in a similar setting because he/she has no recollection of being awake during the procedure, and this should be explained.

If the plan is for sedation, the patient must be reassured that this is standard practice, and that his/her anxiety and/or pain will be anticipated and managed. If the patient's referring physician (this is particularly common with diagnostic procedures) has told him/her something other than what the staff at the site of the procedure is offering, mistrust may develop. It is important to assure the patient that the physician said what he/she believed to be the truth, but that he/she may not be familiar with the procedural practice. Assure the patient that there is certainly no attempt being made to mislead on either side. The patient needs to be educated about the facts and the process involved from this point, and must be allowed to give full informed consent to whatever plan is chosen.

Sometimes a quick, relatively painless procedure can be done with local anesthetic only. If this produces anxiety, the anxiety may be treated with one dose of oral or intravenous medication, in addition to the local anesthetic. This would be considered minimal sedation. The RN may not be required to assist with or monitor such a case, which may sometimes be done with only the physician and the technologist present. Since it cannot be guaranteed that a patient will tolerate minimal sedation, it is wise to be prepared to assess the patient and prepare for moderate sedation. This leaves options open, since one can always give less medication than anticipated.

Music (with headphones if appropriate), virtual-reality glasses (if appropriate), and pleasant conversation ("verbal valium") are wonderful and safe adjuncts to pharmacologic sedation.

A patient may not even want sedation. In this case, the RN may stand by to offer comfort, conversation, and reassurance that action will be taken if the patient needs something. If a patient is very old or frail, it may be appropriate to initiate the procedure without sedation of any kind. In most cases, a patient too frail for any type of sedation should have his/her procedure in a setting that allows a higher level of care. Most patients will get at least local anesthetic and minimal sedation to start with. A comfortable patient allows a successful procedure. Every attempt should be made to make the patient comfortable enough to easily tolerate the procedure.

If moderate sedation is required to allow cooperation with a longer or more painful procedure, all assessments, monitors, staff, equipment, medications, and capacity to rescue must be present. Deep sedation/monitored anesthesia care (MAC) or general anesthesia should not be administered in the office/outpatient setting in the absence of an anesthesia provider. The RN as guardian needs to understand the continuum of sedation and anesthesia and prepare accordingly.

Recovery and discharge

Recovery

A safe physical environment should be provided during recovery from sedation under the supervision of an RN qualified in sedation and recovery until discharge criteria are met. The recovery area should be quiet and appropriately equipped (standard monitors, oxygen, facemasks, and nasal cannulas, suction, airway devices (masks, oral and nasal airways, laryngeal mask airways/intubation equipment), bag-valve masks, crash cart, emergency medications, reversal agents, fluids, and a malignant hyperthermia (MH) kit if general anesthetics are ever administered in the facility).

The RN may care for two recovering patients or care for one recovering patient while preparing a second patient for a procedure. The RN should not be administering sedation to one patient while recovering or interviewing another patient. A nurse should never be alone in an isolated area with a potentially unstable patient.

Patients should be monitored for at least 60 minutes after the last transmucosal, intramuscular, or intravenous drug administration, or until they have returned to baseline mental status (which should be established and documented prior to initiation of sedation). The patient's status should be assessed and documented on admission to an appropriate recovery area and at least every 15 minutes until the patient reaches defined discharge criteria (minimum of 30 minutes post-procedure). When a reversal agent (flumazenil or naloxone) has been administered, the patient should be monitored for possible re-narcotization or re-sedation for at least 2 hours following administration of the last dose of reversal agent.

Monitoring for all patients should include blood pressure, heart rate, respiratory rate, oxygen saturation, level of sedation, and pain, at least every 15 minutes or as indicated by the patient's condition, and cardiac monitoring when indicated.

It must be stressed that sedation is a continuum. It is never certain which way a patient will go on the sedation scale until he/she has returned to his/her baseline level of consciousness and hemodynamic parameters.

Discharge

When the patient is ready for discharge, he/she should be presented with written discharge instructions. After sedation medication, a patient who seems entirely oriented at discharge may forget what was explained to him/her when he/she arrives home. Discharge instructions should include diet, activity, special care of the procedural wound, and timing, dose, and name of all medications given. This is to ensure that if the patient needs to seek emergency care, the emergency providers can factor in the events/medications associated with the procedure, and render care appropriately. The patient should have a reliable adult with him/her the rest of the day and overnight if appropriate to be alert for any adverse post-procedure events at home. This person should listen to the discharge instructions and escort the patient home. The patient should be informed of all instructions, conditions for seeking emergency care, and follow-up. This form should be signed by the patient and witnessed by a licensed person, physician, or RN. Most often, the nurse will do this.

Contingency plan

There is no substitute for preparation. Even if the outpatient setting is adequately equipped and staffed, adverse events occur. Errors can be made or patients may react in unexpected ways. It is important to recognize a problem immediately, and to recognize when a situation is beyond the capabilities of the team.

In a setting attached to a medical center, the team would deliver immediate care (capability to rescue) while calling the medical center rapid response team, code blue, or airway emergency or appropriate consultant. It is important for all staff to know when and how to contact these teams. Occasional drills and prominently posted numbers can prevent delays in an emergency situation.

In a remote outpatient surgical center or office location, the most prudent plan is to call the emergency ambulance services as rescue measures are initiated. Time is critical to avoid permanent harm to a patient who suffers an adverse event during sedation. Two very common adverse events are hypotension and desaturation, easily treated with stimulation and a bolus of intravenous fluid or jaw-lift, stimulation, and oxygen. It may be necessary to give positive pressure with a bag-valve mask and an oral or nasal airway. Sometimes reversal agents may be needed. The team should be able to function quickly, effectively, and efficiently, and must be able to recognize when the circumstances are beyond the team's capacity to rescue and a higher level of care is needed.

Summary

The chapter covers the individual responsibilities of periprocedural team members and requirements unique to sedation in the office/outpatient setting. Safe sedation includes selection of appropriate procedures and patients and development of a sedation plan which includes the procedure itself, the recovery period and criteria for discharge. Development of a contingency plan is critical in a location distant from immediate aid.

References

1. Gawande A. *The Checklist Manifesto: How to Get Things Right.* New York, NY: Metropolitan Books, 2009.

2. Joint Commission. National patient safety goals. In *Comprehensive Accreditation Manual for Hospitals.* Oakbrook Terrace, IL: Joint Commission, 2011. e-dition.jcrinc.com/frame.aspx (accessed December 2010).

3. AORN position statement on allied health care providers and support personnel in the perioperative practice setting. AORN, 2011. www.aorn.org/PracticeResources/ AORNPositionStatements (accessed June 2011).

4. AORN position statement on creating a practice environment of safety. AORN, 2011. www.aorn.org/PracticeResources/ AORNPositionStatements (accessed June 2011).

5. AORN position statement on one perioperative registered nurse circulator dedicated to every patient undergoing a surgical or other invasive procedure. AORN, 2007. www.aorn.org/ PracticeResources/AORNPositionStatements (accessed June 2011).

6. American Society of Anesthesiologists Task Force on Preanesthesia Evaluation. Practice advisory for preanesthesia evaluation. *Anesthesiology* 2002; **96**: 485–96.

7. University HealthSystem Consortium Consensus Group on Deep Sedation. *Deep Sedation Best Practice Recommendations.* Oak Brook, IL: UHC, 2006.

8. University HealthSystem Consortium Consensus Group on Moderate Sedation. *Moderate Sedation Best Practice Recommendations.* Oak Brook, IL: UHC, 2005.

Further reading

Catchpole K, Mishra A, Handa A, McCulloch P. Teamwork and error in the operating room: analysis of skills and roles. *Ann Surg* 2008; **247**: 699–706.

Frank RL. Procedural sedation in adults. *UpToDate* 2011. www.uptodate.com/ contents/procedural-sedation-in-adults (accessed June 2011).

Nestel D, Kidd J. Nurses' perceptions and experiences of communication in the operating theatre: a focus group interview. *BMC Nursing* 2006; **5**: 1.

www.biomedcentral.com/1472-6955/5/1 (accessed June 2011).

Ogg M, Burlingame B. Clinical issues: recommended practices for moderate sedation/analgesia. *AORN J* 2008; **88**: 275–7.

Reynolds A, Timmons S. The doctor–nurse relationship in the operating theatre. *Br J Perioper Nurs* 2005; **15**: 110–15.

Sedation in dentistry

Benjamin R. Record and Alfredo R. Arribas

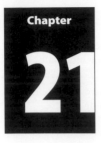

Introduction

Modern dentistry has made much progress in pain control and in providing a patient-friendly service, which has expanded the dentist's ability to perform a wide range of treatments in a pain-free environment. Nevertheless, despite revolutionary new dental techniques, it is well recognized in the dental literature that substantial fear exists concerning seeking dental care. This fear can be so extensive that people from all races and socioeconomic categories can be affected by it in some form. And even though the majority of these "dental phobics" know they must see the dentist twice a year, the fear of walking in the door presents an insurmountable obstacle.

The literature shows that approximately 15% of the US population fears the dentist enough to avoid care completely. Among dental patients who regularly seek care, as many as 50% report some level of fear and anxiety toward their dental experiences and view many of the routine procedures in a dental office as *frightening* [1,2]. These results are supported by the recent survey released by the American Association of Endodontists (AAE) [3]. Not surprisingly, the report from the AAE shows that fear of pain is the root cause, more so than previous experiences.

Fear and anxiety

A major difference between fear and anxiety is the immediacy of the threat to the person. Anxiety is a response to an anticipated event, while fear is a response to an immediate threat. In the dental situation, the term *anxiety* describes reactions that develop in

Moderate and Deep Sedation in Clinical Practice, ed. Richard D. Urman and Alan D. Kaye.
Published by Cambridge University Press. © Cambridge University Press 2012.

Table 21.1. Characteristics of fear and anxiety

Fear	Anxiety
Short-lived phenomenon	Not likely to be dispelled as quickly as fear
Disappears when the external danger or threat passes	The emotional response is usually an internal one and is not readily recognized
A feeling that something terrible is going to happen	Anxiety tends to be a learned response, acquired from personal experience or secondarily through the experiences of others
Physiologic changes • tachycardia • profuse perspiration • hyperventilation • overt behavioral movements, such as becoming jittery or shaking	Anxiety arises from anticipation of an event, the outcome of which is unknown
These clinical manifestations comprise the "fight or flight" response	

anticipation of "the shot," whereas *fear* refers to the reaction to "the shot" itself. If you compare the two responses, you can see appropriate actions a clinician can take to prevent fear and/or anxiety in a dental office setting, as outlined in Table 21.1.

Most persons share basic fears that contribute to fear of dentistry [4]:

(1) Fear of pain
(2) Fear of the unknown
(3) Fear of helplessness and dependency
(4) Fear of bodily change and mutilation
(5) Fear of death

These basic fears can be seen in, or transferred into, a routine dental visit. When you add the stress of a dental appointment, you see a patient who is unable to handle the situation at hand – these are our "dental phobics". The level of phobia will dictate the appropriate level of sedation used to help alleviate and control the patient's responses, from iatrosedation to inhalational sedation, enteral sedation, parenteral sedation and general anesthesia.

Levels of anxiety/phobia in dentistry

The levels of anxiety in the typical dental patient can be classified into severe, moderate, or low to moderate.

Severe dental anxiety – These patients are rare, but create a dual problem for the dentist and the dental team. They delay treatment to the extreme. Now, instead of only treating the physiological concern (pain and/or infection), we must treat a psychological emergency as well. The dental pain is exacerbated by the patient's fear of pain, creating a vicious cycle. If the patient's fear is not addressed, treating the dental problem only creates more stress and increased frustration for the dentist and dental team while furthering the fear and distrust felt by the patient.

Moderate dental anxiety – These patients are the easiest to identify, as they will typically avoid routine care but usually will come to office with problems before they become

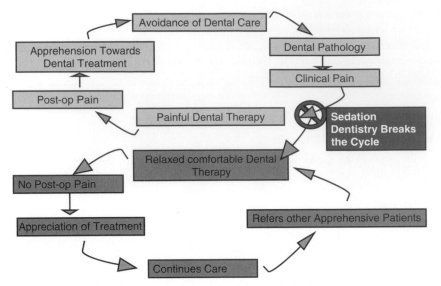

Figure 21.1. Breaking the vicious cycle: the role of sedation in dentistry.

emergencies. Their signs of anxiety and/or fear will be somewhat obvious: rescheduling routine care, signs and symptoms of anxiety in the waiting room and dental chair. These patients may sit in the chair, but they will be hyperresponsive to tactile stimulation and the clinician may require permission to perform even a routine dental examination [4]. **Low to moderate dental anxiety** – Patients with low to moderate dental anxiety are the most common patients seen in the dental office [4]. These are patients who have no irrational fears of dentistry; however, they do feel some form of anxiety as the day approaches. This fear does not prevent them from coming in, because the desire to maintain oral hygiene and health, and/or to obtain relief from pain, overrides any fear of avoidance, because they know the consequences. However, while in the dental office, this patient has some signs of anxiety: sweaty palms, tachycardia – and admittedly would much rather be somewhere else.

The many techniques of behavioral modification, iatrosedation, and pharmacologic intervention can help control fear and anxiety in dental patients [5]. Although a number of behavioral techniques are available for the treatment of dental fear, minimal/moderate sedation and general anesthesia are still major modalities in the provision of dental treatment to phobic patients [1]. Figure 21.1 illustrates how effective sedation techniques can break the vicious cycle of apprehension and fear.

Sedation in dentistry: aims and indications

The following general goals can be achieved with the use of various sedation methods:

(1) To allay anxiety and fear
(2) To provide analgesia
(3) To provide amnesia
(4) To control secretions
(5) To counteract hyperactive gag reflex

(6) To allow for lengthy and difficult dental procedures
(7) To enable treatment of medically compromised patients (unable to tolerate the stress of the dental visit)
(8) To enable treatment of special populations:

    (a) developmentally disabled patients
    (b) children

History of sedation in dentistry

Anxiety and pain control for medical and dental surgery began with two dentists in the nineteenth century. In 1844 Horace Wells discovered the use of nitrous oxide as an anesthetic, and in 1846 William T. G. Morton, was the first to successfully demonstrate anesthesia to the medical establishment, using ether.

In the twentieth century, several dentists, including Allison, Hubbell, and Monheim, advanced the training and practice of general anesthesia in dentistry. Other dentists, including Jorgensen, Driscoll, and Trieger, recognized the potential of combining the ideal sedative and amnesic effects of general anesthetic drugs with the analgesic effects of local anesthetics. They became advocates of moderate (conscious) sedation, which produced an altered state of consciousness, analgesia, and amnesia without producing unconsciousness. By the end of the twentieth century, the dental profession had developed several different anxiety and pain control options, including local anesthesia alone; minimal, moderate, and deep sedation with local anesthesia; and general anesthesia [6].

Guidelines, rules, and regulations

According to the American Dental Association (ADA), the administration of local anesthesia, sedation, and general anesthesia is an integral part of dental practice [7]. A number of organizations, including the ADA, the American Association of Oral and Maxillofacial Surgeons (AAOMS), the American Academy of Pediatric Dentistry (AAPD), the American Academy of Periodontology (AAP), and the American Dental Society of Anesthesiology (ADSA), have developed strict guidelines for the use of anesthesia and sedation in the dental setting. The purpose of these guidelines is to assist dentists in the delivery of safe and effective sedation and anesthesia. These are often referred to as guidelines for controlling "pain or anxiety," although anesthesia and sedation may be used for other reasons. The existing guidelines incorporate definitions, educational requirements and clinical guidelines for the dentist and auxiliary personnel, including patient evaluation, preoperative preparation, personnel and equipment requirements, monitoring and documentation, recovery and discharge, and emergency management, all divided by the level of sedation and anesthesia [7–12].

Dentists providing sedation and anesthesia should also be in compliance with their state rules and regulations. Most state dental boards require dentists to have additional training (postgraduate residency or continuing education) in order to be licensed to provide nitrous oxide sedation, minimal and moderate sedation via enteral (oral) or parenteral routes, and/ or general anesthesia. The legislation by state board typically focuses on the *intent* of sedation by dentists, and also takes into consideration the route of administration. Minimal sedation (anxiolysis) and moderate sedation by the enteral route are the most commonly used methods, followed by moderate/deep sedation via the parenteral route, and then general anesthesia. The ADA has adopted the definitions of the American Society of Anesthesiology [13], and the ADA's definitions of levels of sedation are as set out below [7].

Minimal sedation dentistry (anxiolysis)

Minimal sedation is "a minimally depressed level of consciousness, produced by a pharmacological method, that retains the patient's ability to independently and continuously maintain an airway and respond normally to tactile stimulation and verbal command. Although cognitive function and coordination may be modestly impaired, ventilatory and cardiovascular functions are unaffected ... The drug(s) and/or techniques used should carry a margin of safety wide enough never to render unintended loss of consciousness ... When the intent is minimal sedation for adults, the appropriate initial dose of a single enteral drug is no more than the maximum recommended dose (MRD) of a drug that can be prescribed for unmonitored home use." [7]

Typically, a patient can take a single dose of a drug at home the night before the appointment (optional), and a second dose of the same or a different drug can be administered by the dentist on the morning of the appointment [4].

"The use of preoperative sedatives for children (aged 12 and under) except in extraordinary situations must be avoided due to the risk of unobserved respiratory obstruction during transport by untrained individuals. Children ... can become moderately sedated despite the intended level of minimal sedation; should this occur, the guidelines for moderate sedation apply." [7]

Moderate (conscious) sedation dentistry

Moderate sedation is "a drug-induced depression of consciousness during which patients respond *purposefully* to verbal commands, either alone or accompanied by light tactile stimulation. No interventions are required to maintain a patent airway, and spontaneous ventilation is adequate. Cardiovascular function is usually maintained ... The drug(s) and/or techniques used should carry a margin of safety wide enough to render unintended loss of consciousness unlikely. Repeated dosing of an agent before the effects of previous dosing can be fully appreciated may result in a greater alteration of the state of consciousness than is the intent of the dentist. Further, a patient whose only response is reflex withdrawal from a painful stimulus would not be considered to be in a state of moderate sedation." [7]

Deep sedation

Deep sedation is "a drug-induced depression of consciousness during which patients cannot easily be aroused but respond purposefully following repeated or painful stimulation. The ability to independently maintain ventilatory function may be impaired. Patients may require assistance in maintaining a patent airway, and spontaneous ventilation may be inadequate. Cardiovascular function is usually maintained." [7]

General anesthesia

General anesthesia is "a drug-induced loss of consciousness during which patients are not arousable, even by painful stimulation. The ability to independently maintain ventilatory function is often impaired. Patients often require assistance in maintaining a patent airway, and positive pressure ventilation may be required because of depressed spontaneous ventilation or drug-induced depression of neuromuscular function. Cardiovascular function may be impaired." [7]

Note that "For children 12 years of age and under, the American Dental Association supports the use of the American Academy of Pediatrics/American Academy of Pediatric Dentists *Guidelines for Monitoring and Management of Pediatric Patients During and After Sedation for Diagnostic and Therapeutic Procedures*. Nitrous oxide/oxygen may be used in combination with a single enteral drug in minimal sedation. Nitrous oxide/oxygen when used in combination with sedative agent(s) may produce minimal, moderate, deep sedation or general anesthesia" [7]. See Chapter 19 for additional discussion of pediatric sedation.

Physical and psychological assessment

Dental care can have a profound effect on both the physical and psychological well-being of the patient, and it is extremely important for the person treating the patient to know beforehand the most likely problems to be encountered. Asking pertinent questions and uncovering answers until you are satisfied will help you prepare for any possible situations or emergencies. It has been stated that "when you prepare for an emergency, it ceases to exist" – and in sedation dentistry this is amplified. In developing your sedation plan for your patient, there are specific goals of your assessment. The clinician must remain diligent not only in the physical assessment but also in the psychological exam, because the sedative and hypnotic drugs that will be used may have detrimental affects on someone not mentally stable. The considerations during the physician and psychological assessment are described below.

Goals of the physical and psychological assessment

- To determine the patient's ability to:
  - tolerate physically the stresses involved in the planned dental treatment
  - tolerate psychologically the stresses involved in the planned dental treatment
- To determine whether treatment modification is indicated to enable the patient to better tolerate the stresses of dental treatment
- To determine which technique of sedation is most appropriate for the patient.
- To determine whether contraindications exist to:
  - the planned dental treatment
  - any of the drugs to be used

Physical and psychological evaluation

The physical and psychological evaluation in dentistry consists of the following three components:

- Medical history questionnaire
- Physical examination
- History obtained by dialogue

With this information, the dentist can determine the physical and psychological status of the patient (assign him/her an ASA classification), determine if there is a need for medical consultation, and modify the treatment in any way if indicated.

Patients should be classified according to their medical risk when undergoing a dental/ surgical procedure. Depending on the classification, the sedation level and route of administration can best be determined to avoid complications or emergencies. The system most commonly used is the American Society of Anesthesiologists (ASA) physical status classification system, which has been in use continually since 1962:

ASA 1

- A normal and healthy patient
- Able to carry out normal activity without distress

ASA 2

- A patient with mild systemic disease
- Healthy, but has extreme anxiety and fear toward dentistry, or older (> 60 years), or pregnant
- Able to complete normal activities, but must rest because of distress

ASA 3

- A patient with moderate systemic disease that limits activity but is not incapacitating
- Does not exhibit signs or symptoms of distress while at rest (e.g., in the reception room), but in stressful situations (e.g., dental chair) signs and symptoms may develop

ASA 4

- A patient with severe systemic disease that is a constant threat to life
- Exhibits signs and symptoms of the medical problem(s) at rest, seated in the reception room of the dental or medical office; such patients exhibit undue fatigue, shortness of breath, or chest pain

ASA 5

- A moribund patient not expected to survive 24 hours without the operation
- Almost always a hospitalized patient with an end-stage disease

ASA 6

- A declared brain-dead patient whose organs are being removed for donor purposes.

E

- Emergency operation of any variety (used to modify one of the above classifications: e.g., ASA 3E)

After a thorough assessment, and assignment of ASA classification, a dentist can then proceed with sedation plan. While we accept that every patient responds differently to sedation, this is an important part of the process. The following is a suggested approach according to the patient's ASA physical status:

- ASA 1 patients are candidates for any sedation technique or for outpatient general anesthesia.
- ASA 2 patients are less stress-tolerant than ASA 1 patients. However, they still represent a minimal risk during treatment. Elective treatment is in order, with consideration given to treatment modifications as warranted by the particular condition.
- ASA 3 patients are less able to tolerate stress than those classified as ASA 2. Elective dental care is still appropriate; however, the need for stress-reduction techniques

and other treatment modifications is increased. Outpatient general anesthesia is not usually recommended for these patients, and many of the pharmacosedation techniques may be used with some potential modification as to length of procedure and depth of sedation.

- ASA 4 patients represent a significant risk during treatment, and elective care should be postponed until the patient's medical condition has improved to at least an ASA 3. Management of dental emergencies such as infection and pain should be undertaken as conservatively as possible until the patient's physical condition improves. When possible, emergency care should be noninvasive, consisting of the prescription of drugs such as analgesics for pain and antibiotics for infection. In situations in which it is believed that immediate intervention is required (incision and drainage, extraction, pulpal extirpation), it is recommended that, when possible, the patient receive such care within the confines of an acute care facility (e.g., hospital). Although the risk to the patient is still significant, the chance of survival should an acute medical emergency arise is likely increased.

Sedation techniques for dentistry

In this chapter we focus on enteral (oral) and parenteral (intravenous) sedation techniques for adults, although we recognize that inhalation (nitrous oxide) is one of the more commonly used techniques for sedation in outpatient dental clinics. The combination of nitrous oxide/oxygen administered safely with appropriate armamentarium provides a fast and effective means of sedation that is extremely safe because of its ease of titration and the limited side effects for patients. However, there are limitations to nitrous oxide/oxygen in a dental office, including issues concerning storage, cost, and side effects to dental personnel, and these have limited its use [4]. Many practitioners regularly use nitrous oxide/oxygen in conjunction with both oral and intravenous sedation in the dental office. For the remainder of this chapter, however, we will focus on enteral and parenteral sedation techniques, in each case discussing the indications, advantages, and disadvantages.

Oral (enteral) sedation

Oral sedation dentistry (OSD) provides dentists with an almost ideal form of outpatient surgery sedation technique by allowing the practitioner to manage the patient's anxiety before the appointment. The goal with most oral sedation dentistry is that of *minimal sedation* or in some cases, *moderate sedation* [7]. Oral sedation dentistry has significant advantages for the patient and the dentist, but also a number of disadvantages.

Particular advantages of OSD include the ability to manage anxiety before a dental appointment by prescribing an anxiolytic at home before the appointment. The typical drug/dose would be a long- or medium-acting benzodiazepine at or below the maximum recommended dose (MRD) for unmonitored home use. This can be given the night before and repeated in the dental office before the appointment. Other advantages include the almost universal acceptance (children and special-needs patients being exceptions), ease of administration, and relative safety of orally administered drugs [4]. Unwanted side effects may occur with any drug, but they are less likely and less intense with the oral than the parenteral route, so in general the routine medications used for OSD are safe when used in the correct manner. Another distinct advantage of OSD is that postoperative pain control is well managed, because of the long duration of action of orally administered drugs.

Oral sedation dentistry, however, does possess several significant disadvantages that must also be considered, as they may serve to limit the clinical use of the oral route in the management of pain and anxiety [4]. Some of these include a long latent period, unreliable drug absorption, an inability to easily achieve a desired drug effect (lack of titration), and the prolonged duration of action. If one understands the pharmacology of the chosen sedative, however, its properties can be used for greater success.

The pharmacology of orally administered drugs (absorption, metabolism, distribution, and excretion) presents unique problems in the case of oral sedatives, the clinical effect of which is usually not seen for up to 30 minutes, or longer, depending on a variety of factors. The greatest degree of clinical effectiveness is not seen until a peak plasma concentration is reached, and this is typically at around 60 minutes [4]. The rate-limiting step of OSD is the "time of clinical effect" that arises from this slow onset of action and the delay in reaching maximal effect. Because of this, titration to desired effect is not possible. The clinician must administer a predetermined dose, and many factors alter a patient's response and affect the desired outcome. It is up to the practitioners of oral sedation to properly plan and educate patient and staff, to eliminate the variables that can be controlled.

The duration of action for most orally administered pain-controlling and anxiolytic drugs is prolonged, approximately 3–4 hours. For OSD, this is a problem with the long-acting benzodiazepines and other anxiety-reducing drugs, as the patient will still be under influence after most appointments. The need for post-sedation instructions, postoperative monitoring, and escorts, and the inability to drive or operate machinery, is most critical for orally sedated patients.

Postoperative pain control is well managed by the longer duration of action, and many of the anxiety-reducing drugs help potentiate relief of postoperative discomfort. However, because of the disadvantages, *intraoperative control* of anxiety and pain (unplanned administration) is not highly recommended for an orally sedated patient [4].

A typical oral-sedation visit for a patient constitutes an at-home dosage of a chosen anxiolytic or sedative-hypnotic the night before (optional) and an hour before the dental appointment in the office. If one chooses to sedate the night before, a mild, long-acting anxiolytic is typically prescribed. In the dental office, a shorter-acting, more moderate sedative-hypnotic is chosen, and the dose is usually between $0.5 \times$ and $1 \times$ MRD.

Patients are then monitored for level of sedation by monitoring the levels of *oxygenation*, *ventilation*, and *cardiovascular function*, as required by state dental boards [7]. This usually includes pulse oximetry, noninvasive blood pressure, respiratory rate, and monitoring of CNS depression by communication. It is ill-advised to "titrate" oral medications (continually administering doses until desired effect). However, many dentists will administer a second dose at half the initial dose, but not to exceed $1.5 \times$ MRD. This is referred to as "supplemental dosing" by the ADA [7], and is only done after appropriate monitoring for effect of the first dose (one half-life).

Drugs for oral sedation dentistry

For oral sedation dentistry, benzodiazepines represent the most popular class of drugs available today, ideal for the management of dental fear and anxiety. They are the most effective drugs currently available for the management of anxiety (both preoperatively and postoperatively), and they also possess skeletal-muscle-relaxant and anticonvulsant properties. The use of benzodiazepines continues to grow, due to their effectiveness, variation of effectiveness, and duration of action, combined with a wide margin of safety [4]. However, benzodiazepines do not have any analgesic properties.

Benzodiazepines provide a level of minimal to moderate sedation in most patients, and there are many drugs of this class currently available. Because there are significant differences in the onset of action and the duration of action among these drugs, the choice of a specific drug should be made only after consideration of the needs of both the patient and the dentist during the consult appointment. Diazepam, triazolam, lorazepam, and midazolam (typically for oral use in children) remain popular benzodiazepines for the reduction of dental anxiety, providing minimal to moderate sedation in most patients [4].

For *minimal sedation*, one drug should be used, with or without nitrous oxide/oxygen, to achieve the desired effect. If one chooses to use a combination of anxiolytics and sedative-hypnotics, the intent is *moderate sedation* and therefore appropriate education, training, preparation, equipment for monitoring, and emergency protocols should be established. Clinicians are advised to check with their state board of dentistry to verify requirements.

Anxiolytic drugs are used to manage mild to moderate daytime anxiety and tension. At therapeutic dosages they produce the level defined as minimal sedation without impairing the patient's mental alertness or psychomotor performance. Drugs categorized as anxiolytics that are commonly used in oral sedation dentistry include the benzodiazepines diazepam (Valium), oxazepam (Serax), and alprazolam (Xanax). In the past, benzodiazepines have been known by other names, such as minor tranquilizers, ataractics, anxiolytic sedatives, and psychosedatives. The term *antianxiety drugs* is also widely used for this group of drugs.

Sedative-hypnotics are drugs that produce either sedation or hypnosis, depending on the dosage of the drug administered and the patient's response to it. Lower dosages of these drugs produce a calming effect (sedation), usually associated with a degree of drowsiness and ataxia, while higher dosages produce hypnosis (a state resembling physiologic sleep). The benefit of the use of benzodiazepines and nonbenzodiazepines (vs. barbituates) is reduced "hangover" effect [4]. Drugs of this category typically used for oral sedation dentistry include the benzodiazepines midazolam (Dormicum, Versed, Hypnovel), triazolam (Halcion, Rilamir), and lorazepam (Ativan), and the nonbenzodiazepines zolpidem (Ambien) and zaleplon (Sonata).

A review of the pharmacology of benzodiazepines reveals why they are ideal for oral sedation dentistry. Typical benzodiazepines have sedative (relaxing) and hypnotic properties (inducing sleep and allowing for posthypnotic suggestion). Most benzodiazepines work on the gamma-aminobutyric acid (GABA) receptors in the brain's limbic system and thalamus, which is involved in emotions and behaviour. Because of this interaction, they impair neuronal discharge in the amygdala and amygdala–hippocampus nerve transmission, and they depress the limbic system at smaller doses than those required to depress the reticular activating system (RAS) and cerebral cortex. They therefore do not produce a generalized CNS depression as much as barbiturates [4]. Benzodiazepine receptors have been isolated in spinal cord and brain. They parallel GABA major inhibitory neurotransmitter for brain and glycine (spinal cord). Benzodiazepines act by intensifying the physiologic inhibitory effects of GABA, increasing the affinity of GABA on the Cl^- channels and allowing more Cl^- to enter postsynaptic sites and further depolarizing the membrane, preventing conduction.

Benzodiazepines are classified as short-, intermediate-, or long-acting, with the longer-acting benzodiazepines typically prescribed for treatment of anxiety, and those with short and intermediate duration of action used for insomnia. Dentists are using short- and intermediate-acting benzodiazepines off-label for the treatment of dental anxiety immediately before and during a dental appointment, with the occasional use of a long-acting drug the night before an appointment.

Benzodiazepines have a very wide margin of safety, which provides dentists some comfort zone to properly sedate to desired effect without negative side effects. With dental offices typically isolated from ambulatory surgery centers and/or hospitals, providing effective and safe sedation is paramount when choosing a drug. Some of the other benefits of benzodiazepines are a result of the interactions within the CNS: reduction of hostile and aggressive behavior; attenuation of the behavioral consequences of frustration and fear; skeletal muscle relaxant; anticonvulsant (more effective when given intravenously); potential respiratory depression unlikely (but can occur when used in combination with other medications); and virtually no cardiovascular changes in ASA 1 patients.

Metabolism of benzodiazepines occurs in the liver, and they may or may not have active metabolites; learning which ones do can assist in determining the best choice for a given procedure. Plasma half-life and time for peak plasma concentration vary significantly with class (short-, intermediate-, and long-acting), and because they interact with glycine they may also help potentiate local anesthesia. All benzodiazepines are excreted in the feces and urine, with the percentage of urinary excretion varying from 20% to 80% [4].

There is a potential for psychological and physiologic dependence on benzodiazepines to develop with long-term use; however, the incidence of physiologic dependence is considerably less than that of psychological dependence. For the *pretreatment* of dental anxiety, diazepam and oxazepam are indicated; however, diazepam is most often prescribed, as it can be given early and still have effects on the day of the appointment.

Contraindications to benzodiazepines include allergy to medication, psychoses, and acute narrow-angle glaucoma, but they may be administered to patients with open-angle glaucoma who are receiving appropriate therapy [4]. There are some precautions that must be observed when prescribing these anxiolytics and sedatives:

(1) Patients must be advised against driving a motor vehicle or operating hazardous machinery.
(2) Avoid other CNS depressants, such as alcohol, opioids, and barbiturates.
(3) Avoid pregnant patients as a precaution. There is some evidence of birth defects, and benzodiazepines will cross the placental barrier and be excreted in breast milk.
(4) The use of oral diazepam tablets in children younger than 6 months of age is not recommended.

Drugs commonly used in oral sedation

Below we describe pharmacologic and clinical characteristics of the commonly used oral agents for sedation. The reader is also referred to Chapter 2 for an additional discussion of pharmacology.

Benzodiazepines

Diazepam

- Stimulates GABA receptors
- Produces mild sleep

- Onset approximately 1 hour
- Active metabolites
- Half-life about 50 hours (20–100)
- Duration 6–8 hours
- Mild amnesia
- Supplied in 2, 5, 10 mg
- FDA-approved anxiolytic

Indications

- Preoperative reduction of anxiety

Contraindications

- Pregnancy
- Known hypersensitivity
- Pediatric patients < 6 months
- Acute narrow-angle glaucoma

Dental use

- 2.5–10 mg the night before and/or the morning of appointment

Triazolam

- Sedative-hypnotic, benzodiazepine
- Stimulates GABA receptors
- No long-term active metabolites
- Plasma half-life 2–3 hours
- Duration of action 1.5–5.5 hours
- Very little hangover effect
- Wide effective dose range (minimum effective concentration varies with patients)
- Peak plasma levels seen in little as 1.3 hours
- Anticonvulsant
- Respiratory depressant in high doses
- Relaxation adequate for pain control (difficult anesthesia patients)
- No nausea
- LD50 is 5 g/kg in rats

Indications

- Preoperative sedation
- Night-time sleep

Cautions

- Overdose may occur at $4 \times$ MRD of 0.5 mg (2.0 mg, or eight 0.25 mg tablets)
- Hallucinations, paranoia and depression (several reports with extended medication time)
- Anterograde amnesia
- Reduce dose in elderly or debilitated patients
- Dry mouth

Contraindications

- Acute narrow-angle glaucoma (can dry up eyes and increase ocular pressure)
- Known hypersensitivity
- Psychosis (absolute contraindication in schizophrenia)
- Pregnancy and breastfeeding: excreted in milk
- Concurrent use of alcohol can lead to severe respiratory depression

Dental use

- 0.125–0.5 mg/day; 1 hour before dental appointment in office; MRD 0.5 mg
- Elderly: maximum 0.25 mg/day
- Always use lowest effective dose
- Typically given 1 hour before appointment (0.125–0.5 mg)
- Supplemental dose of half initial dose after one half-life has been observed, not to exceed 1.5 × MRD, is appropriate in some patients to achieve minimal sedation in a dental office setting

Lorazepam

- Benzodiazepine; works on GABA receptors
- Produces mild/moderate sleep
- Onset 1 hour
- No active metabolites
- Half-life 12–14 hours
- Duration 6–8 hours
- Moderate amnesia
- Dosage forms 0.5, 1, 2 mg tablets
- Metabolized by glucuronidation

Indications

- Preoperative sedation
- Night-time sleep

Contraindications

- Known hypersensitivity
- Pregnancy
- Children less than 12 years old
- Acute narrow-angle glaucoma

Dental use

- 1–5 mg adult (ASA 1, 2); ASA 3 or elderly: half the normal dose
- Taken 1 hour before appointment in the office
- Onset is slightly slower than other benzodiazepines, and possible to have patient take earlier
- Usually used in patients needing longer procedures (> 2 hours), patients with hepatic dysfunction, patients where triazolam was ineffective

Midazolam

- Oral dosage form in USA is 2mg/mL syrup
- Absorption and onset of clinical action faster than comparable benzodiazepines (mainly diazepam)
- Peak action within 30 minutes
- No active metabolites
- Half life 1–3 hours
- Anterograde amnesia very good
- Mostly used for pediatric sedation; not as effective in adults

Nonbenzodiazepine sedative-hypnotics

Zaleplon (a pyrazolopyrimidine) and zolpidem (an imidazopyridine) are used for the short-term management of insomnia. Although unrelated structurally to benzodiazepines, they interact with a GABA–benzodiazepine receptor complex and share some of the pharmacologic properties of benzodiazepines.

They are strong sedatives with only mild anxiolytic, myorelaxant, and anticonvulsant properties. Both have been shown to be effective in inducing and maintaining sleep in adults. They are rapidly absorbed from the gastrointestinal tract and are metabolized in the liver. They are converted into inactive metabolites and eliminated primarily through renal clearance.

Precautions include respiratory depression, but this is not usually seen in healthy patients receiving average doses. If they are used in patients with compromised respiratory function, however, the likelihood of depressed respiratory drive is increased.

Zaleplon (Sonata) and Zolpidem (Ambien)

- Nonbenzodiazepine sedative-hypnotics: pyrazolopyrimidine (zaleplon); imidazopyridine (zolpidem)
- Used for short term insomnia
- Work on benzodiazepine–GABA receptor sites
- Produce high sleep
- Onset 45 minutes (zaleplon); 30 minutes (zolpidem)
- Time to peak concentration 1 hour (zaleplon); 1.5 hours (zolpidem)
- No active metabolites
- Elimination half-life 1 hour (zaleplon); 2.5 hours (zolpidem)
- Duration of action 1–2 hours (zaleplon); 2–4 hours (zolpidem)
- Moderate amnesia
- Not an FDA-approved anxiolytic but similar to midazolam in efficacy
- Zaleplon is absorbed and eliminated more quickly, and is used for short appointments

Contraindications

- Children < 18 years
- Severely depressed patients

Warnings

- CYP450 inhibitors
- Aldehyde oxidase inhibitors (diphenhydramine)
- Elderly patients

Dental use

- Dose 5–15 mg for zaleplon; 5–10 mg for zolpidem
- Administered 30 minutes to 1 hour before appointment and used in short appointments
- Onset of sedation is rapid and, because of short half-life, recovery is quick

Histamine (H$_1$) blockers (antihistamines)

CNS depression (sedation and hypnosis) is a known side effect of some drugs used primarily for other purposes. Such effects occur with many of the histamine blockers, drugs used primarily in the management of allergies, motion sickness, and parkinsonism.

Several histamine blockers demonstrate this property and are marketed primarily as sedative-hypnotics. These drugs include methapyrilene, pyrilamine, diphenhydramine, promethazine, and hydroxyzine. The two histamine blockers most frequently used for their sedative/anxiolytic properties are promethazine and hydroxyzine.

In dentistry, these drugs have proven to be quite useful, especially in pediatric dentistry. Hydroxyzine is the most common form used in oral sedation dentistry, used alone or most commonly in addition to a benzodiazepine or opioid. The sedative actions of hydroxyzine are not produced by cortical depression; it is thought to suppress some hypothalamic nuclei and extend its actions peripherally into the sympathetic portion of the autonomic nervous system.

The oral liquid form of hydroxyzine hydrochloride is more pleasant-tasting to most patients than the liquid form of hydroxyzine pamoate. This fact is of particular importance in pediatric dentistry.

When these drugs are administered in combination with benzodiazepines or opioids, their dosage should be decreased by 50%, because the depressant actions of opioids are potentiated by hydroxyzine. In dental practice, the use of hydroxyzine as a sole drug is almost always limited to the management of children with mild to moderate fear, and it is often used in combination with meperidine for the management of more fearful pediatric patients.

The incidence of side effects is quite low, with transient drowsiness observed most commonly. Fatal overdose with hydroxyzine is extremely uncommon, and withdrawal reactions after long-term therapy have never been reported.

Hydroxyzine

- Moderate sleep
- Anxiolytic, antihistaminic, and antiemetic actions
- Onset 1 hour
- Metabolized in liver/excreted via kidneys
  - No active metabolites (cetirizine has minimal sedation activity)
- Half-life 3–7 hours
- Duration 3 hours
- No amnesia
- No specific antidote
- Helps those patients with increased nausea and vomiting, increased gag reflex, hypersalivation; useful in smokers

Indications

- Preoperative management of anxiety
- Potentiation of sedative effects of anxiolytics

Contraindications

- Early pregnancy
- Known hypersensitivity
- Nursing mothers
- Children <1 year
- Acute narrow-angle glaucoma

Dental use

- 10–50 mg dose for adults
- Typically 1.1–2.2 mg/kg (reduced by 50% in combination) in children
- Taken at same time as other CNS depressants in the office

Opioids ("narcotics")

Opioids are classified as strong analgesics, and their primary indication is for the relief of moderate to severe pain. Mainly, opioids alter a patient's *psychological response* to pain and suppress anxiety and apprehension.

In dentistry, many opioids are used *parenterally* as preanesthetic drugs because of their sedative, anxiolytic, and analgesic properties. Meperidine has lost favor with many because of its adverse side effects at the higher doses that are often required (because it is not as effective as newer opioid derivatives), and we only discuss it here because it is still occasionally used, especially in pediatric oral sedation.

In the absence of pain, opioids administered alone frequently produce dysphoria instead of sedation. To achieve anxiolytic and sedative effects, opioids should not be administered via the oral route in adults. Absorption following oral administration is not as consistent as it is with parenteral administration, and the incidence of unwanted side effects (postural hypotension, nausea, and vomiting) is considerably greater. For adults, it is recommended that opioids should generally be avoided for oral sedation dentistry, given their lack of effect and the increased risk of complications, especially in medically compromised patients. Opioids are included for the sake of completeness, and because they are used in pediatric dentistry in combination with histamine blockers and/or benzodiazepines.

Oral sedation protocols

As a guideline in the use of oral sedation in an outpatient setting, the following protocols are provided. Note, however, that they are only a guide, and that the practitioner must be trained in advanced airway techniques and at a level of sedation above their intent for "rescue" purposes.

Minimal sedation

The following sample protocols are typically used in dental offices where the intent is minimal to moderate sedation (depending on the response of the patient). The addition of diazepam the night before or the morning of the appointment is optional, and is not recommended on the first sedation visit.

Sample protocol #1

Approximately 45 minutes to 1 hour of treatment in adults (18 years and older)

- Diazepam 2.5–10 mg PO night before appointment
- Zaleplon 5–15 mg PO in office 30–45 minutes before appointment
- Nitrous oxide/oxygen during administration of local anesthesia, and at end of appointment if need to extend procedure

Sample protocol #2

Approximately 1–2 hours of treatment in adults (18 years and older)

- Diazepam 2.5–10 mg PO night before appointment
- Triazolam 0.125–0.5 mg PO in office1 hour before appointment. Typical protocol for ASA 1 or 2 minimally to moderately anxious patient:
  - 0.25 mg in office 1 hour before "doctor" time
  - 45 minutes later evaluate for signs of sedation and move to dental chair
  - at 60–90 minutes, may administer a supplemental dose, no more than half initial dose and given only after clinical half-life has been exceeded. Should not exceed $1.5 \times$ MRD
- Nitrous oxide/oxygen during administration of local anesthesia and at end of appointment if need to extend procedure

This is a first-line attempt for minimal-sedation dentistry on a majority of dental patients using oral sedation dentistry. The reader should note the following:

- It is often used for a target appointment in patients where your desire is to perform examination, obtain radiographs, and attempt prophylaxis on moderate to severe dental-phobic patients.
- In mild to moderate dental-phobic patients, one can get more profound anesthesia.
- In special-needs or medically compromised patients, dosages are often decreased.
- It is a great starting point for most new patients who are severely anxious and not sure if they want to proceed with deeper sedation.

Sample protocol #3

Approximately 1–3 hours of treatment

- Diazepam 2.5–10 mg night before appointment
- Lorazepam 1–5 mg PO in office 1–1.5 hours before appointment
  - Supplemental dosing not recommended due to long half-life and slow onset
- Nitrous oxide/oxygen during admininstration of local anesthesia and at end of appointment if need to extend procedure

Moderate sedation

The following protocols are intended to provide a deeper level of sedation, where the patient's responses will be "purposeful" to verbal or light tactile stimulation and respiratory depression will be unlikely. Clinicians and patients should see more profound amnesia and more relaxation with the following protocols.

Sample protocol #1

Approximately 2 hours of treatment (varies)

- Diazepam 2.5–10 mg PO night before appointment
- Triazolam 0.125–0.5 mg (up to 0.75 mg) PO in office 1 hour before appointment

- Hydroxyzine 50–100 mg PO in office 1 hour before appointment
- Nitrous oxide/oxygen during administration of local anesthesia and at the end of the appointment, if there is a need to extend the procedure
- Hydroxyzine is great for "gaggers" and smokers
- Combination helps with more profound amnesia and deeper sedation, but patients will recover more quickly

Sample protocol #2

Approximately 3–4 hours of treatment, depending on patient

- Diazepam 2.5–10 mg night before; morning of appointment
- Lorazepam 1–5 mg PO in office 1 hour before appointment
- Hydroxyzine 10–50 mg PO in office 1 hour before appointment
- Nitrous oxide/oxygen during admininstration of local anesthesia and at end of appointment if need to extend procedure
- Alteration would be to substitute meperidine for hydroxyzine

When learning oral sedation dentistry, it is advised that the clinician should learn two to three protocols and the drugs used. One should also remember that there are other benzodiazepines and nonbenzodiazepines that vary in chemical structure and half-life, and that if a protocol is no longer working on a patient, the possible causes should be considered: the patient may be taking new medications that interfere with the metabolism of benzodiazepines, or the patient may have developed a tolerance. In either case, a different benzodiazepine may produce the desired effect. Learning to use appropriate drug reference resources will assist the clinician in making an informed decision.

Meperidine is still used by some clinicians for oral sedation dentistry, especially in the sedation of children and special-needs patients. Some practitioners occasionally use orally administered meperidine in conjunction with a benzodiazepine if there is a contraindication to hydroxyzine; they may use it with both drugs if the intent is moderate sedation in a patient who has not responded to normal protocols and intravenous sedation/general anesthesia is absolutely contraindicated. In these cases, it is wise to administer sedation in a setting with full ACLS capabilities, advanced airway and anesthesia support. If it is decided that meperidine is safe, it would replace hydroxyzine or the benzodiazepine in the above protocols at a dose of 50–100 mg by mouth.

Emerging techniques

There has been some clinical use of clonidine as a premedication to supplement oral and intravenous sedation in dentistry. Especially in procedures that are expected to be longer in duration [14], or in patients who have not responded to the typical "recipe," there has been some evidence that preloading with 0.1–0.2 mg of clonidine has an additive effect for benzodiazepines, histamine blockers, and/or opioids without significant decrease in respiratory or cardiovascular function. This is not indicated in patients currently on clonidine or with low blood pressure, but it has proven effectiveness. Clonidine is an alpha-2-adrenergic agonist hypotensive medication that may decrease heart rate and vascular resistance, allowing smoother flow of blood. This is a direct counteraction of the effects that "fear" (which leads to catecholamine release) and epinephrine (injected with local anesthetic) have on the body, especially during a time of anxiety. Specifically, clonidine prevents the "fight of flight" response produced by stimulation of the sympathetic nervous system (tachycardia, hypertension), especially during high-anxiety events such as a dental visit. Clonidine has many uses as a presedation adjunct prior to surgery [15–18].

The techniques described above will allow a clinician to achieve minimal or moderate sedation in a low to moderately anxious dental patient, and to do so with relative predictability. However, oral sedation still has its limitations, chief among which are the inability to titrate and the prolonged sedation time. Parenteral (intravenous) sedation techniques will eliminate those issues.

Intravenous (parenteral) sedation

The intravenous (IV) route of drug administration is a parenteral technique that represents the most effective method of ensuring predictable and adequate sedation at all levels (mild, moderate, and deep) in virtually all patients [4]. Table 21.2 describes some advantages and disadvantages of intravenous sedation.

Armamentarium for intravenous sedation

The following supplies and monitoring equipment are generally necessary for the safe and effective administration of intravenous sedation. Additional equipment may be necessary.

- Intravenous fluids
- Delivery tubing and drug pump
- Intravenous catheters
- Drugs
- Monitors
  - electrocardiography
  - blood pressure
  - pulse oximetry
  - respiration
  - exhaled CO_2
  - temperature

Table 21.2. Advantages and disadvantages of intravenous sedation

Advantages	Disadvantages
Rapid onset of action	Venipuncture is necessary
Can titrate drug to desired effect	Complications in the site of venipuncture
Can easily accomplish any level of sedation	Requires more intensive monitoring
Shorter recovery time	Need for an escort after discharge
Can reverse drugs or have access for emergency drugs	Some drugs cannot be reversed
Fewer side effects (nausea and vomiting)	Need for extra and extensive training of staff
Control of secretions	Bigger investment for practitioner (equipment, drugs, personnel, insurance)
Diminished gag reflex	

Fluid management and intravenous access

Most office-based intravenous sedation procedures are of short duration and involve minimal blood loss. The need for fluid resuscitation perioperatively is not a major concern in everyday practice. The intent of fluid management in office-based surgery is primarily to rehydrate a patient, as opposed to replacing intraoperative fluid losses. Normally patients who undergo sedation will be required to be NPO for at least 6 hours. An 8-hour fast will create a 750 mL fluid deficit in a 70 kg healthy patient.

For a short-duration dental IV procedure, the choice of fluids, between normal saline (0.9 NaCl), half normal saline (0.45 NaCl), lactated Ringer's (LR), and 5% dextrose in water (D5W), depends on convenience. To administer drugs and fluids, constant intravenous access is required. The armamentarium, anatomy, and access techniques are discussed in greater detail in Chapter 5.

Pharmacology

Several different anesthetic drugs and techniques are used in IV sedation in dentistry to facilitate procedures and patient comfort. The ideal properties of IV sedation drugs in the dental setting include the following:

- amnesia
- analgesia
- suppression of stress response
- hemodynamic stability
- sedation/immobilization
- hypnosis
- rapid onset and short duration of action

The most commonly used drugs for IV sedation in the dental setting are benzodiazepines, opioids, ultra-short-acting anesthetic agents (e.g., propofol or methohexital), and ketamine. These drugs are administered in various combinations, and in combination with nitrous oxide/oxygen and local anesthetics, and are normally administered by incremental boluses [19]. The pharmacology of these drugs is extensively covered in Chapter 2; therefore this chapter will cover only the drugs most commonly used in IV sedation in the dental setting, and their relevant properties.

Benzodiazepines

Benzodiazepines are the most effective drugs in the management of anxiety. They have muscle-relaxant and anticonvulsant properties, and anterograde amnesic properties.

- **Midazolam (Versed)** is water-soluble, and therefore causes no irritation or phlebitis when applied, and no second peak effect. Beta half-life: 1.7–2.4 hours; alpha half-life: 4–18 minutes. It has anterograde amnesic properties. It is more amnesic but less sedating than diazepam, and it is known to cause dizziness. It is contraindicated in acute pulmonary insufficiency, secondary to its respiratory-depressant properties, and in patients allergic to midazolam. Dosage: start with 1–2.5 mg, then titrate to effect. Titrate with 2 mg increments. Average sedative dose: 2.5–7.5 mg.
- **Diazepam (Valium)** is lipid-soluble, creating local irritation of the vein, phlebitis, and even thrombosis when applied. It may have rebound effect or second peak effect.

Peak blood level: 1–2 minutes. Beta half-life: 30 hours; alpha half-life: 45–60 minutes. It provides 45–60 minutes of sedation, and can cause respiratory depression, can elevate seizure threshold, and has anterograde amnesic properties. Contraindicated in patients with glaucoma and hypersensitivity to valium. Other adverse reactions include hyperactivity, confusion, nausea, changes in libido, decreased salivation, and emergence delirium. Dosage: 5–20 mg titrated slowly, usually in 5 mg increments.

Opioids

Opioids are administered primarily for their analgesic properties. Opioids may be classified as natural or synthetically derived. Reliable sedation cannot be achieved without producing some level of respiratory depression. Respiratory depression is worsened by the concomitant administration of benzodiazepines or ultra-short-acting anesthetics.

- **Fentanyl (Sublimaze)** is a synthetic opioid. It is 100 times more potent than morphine. Has rapid onset and is short-acting. Onset in less than 1 minute with blood and brain equilibration time of 6.4 minutes. Its effects are usually gone in about 30–60 minutes. It may cause muscular rigidity of thoracic and abdominal muscles, related to fast administration, and its respiratory-depressant effects outlast its analgesic effects. Contraindicated in patients allergic to fentanyl, patients with chronic obstructive pulmonary disease (COPD), and patients with advanced respiratory disease. This drug has a very narrow therapeutic index and should be used with extreme caution. Dosage: start with 25–50 µg, then titrate to effect. Titrate in 25 µg increments. Average sedative dose: 100 µg.
- **Meperidine (Demerol)** is a synthetic opioid. Historically, meperidine was the most commonly used opioid by dentists for IV sedation, falling out of favor because of side effects and cleaner alternatives such as fentanyl. It is one-tenth as potent as morphine. Onset of action 2–4 minutes; duration of action 30–45 minutes. It has vagolytic properties, increases heart rate, and decreases salivary secretions. It also triggers histamine release at the site of injection (resolves spontaneously), and it is known to cause seizures, secondary to its metabolite normeperidine. It is contraindicated in patients allergic to meperidine and patients with COPD and decreased respiratory reserve. Average sedative dose: 37.5–50 mg. Maximum single dose: 50 mg. Titrate to effect in doses of 25 mg.

Reversal agents

- **Naloxone (Narcan)** is an opioid antagonist. Its onset of action is 2 minutes and its duration is 30 minutes. Contraindicated in patients allergic to naloxone and in patients with opioid dependency. Dosage: 0.1–0.2 mg every 2–3 minutes. Maximum dose: 1.2 mg.
- **Flumazenil (Romazicon)** is a benzodiazepine antagonist. It has a short onset of action of 3–5 minutes and duration of approximately 60 minutes. Contraindicated in patients allergic to flumazenil and in patients who have been given benzodiazepines for status epilepticus or increased intracranial pressure. Dosage: 0.2 mg every minute up to maximum dose of 1.0 mg.

It is important to note that patients who are reversed from sedation with any of these reversal agents will need to be monitored for approximately 2 hours. Reversal agents most of the time have shorter duration of action than the sedative drugs, creating the risk of re-sedation.

Barbiturates

Barbiturates are sedative-hypnotic drugs, anticonvulsants (except for methohexital), and CNS and respiratory depressants. They have no analgesic properties. They are known to cause "hangover" effects, secondary to their redistribution to fat. Barbiturates are also known to cause idiosyncratic reactions such as excitement and lower pain threshold, and to increase rates of laryngospasm.

- **Methohexital (Brevital)** is used IV to induce general anesthesia. Can also be used to maintain unconsciousness as the hypnotic component of a balanced anesthetic technique or a total intravenous anesthetic technique. It is known to cause seizures in high doses and to increase heart rate. It has no reversal agent. It is contraindicated in use with other CNS depressants such as alcohol, monoamine oxidase (MAO) inhibitors, antihistamines, etc. Its onset of action is 1 minute and its duration of action is 5–8 minutes. Induction dose: 1.5 mg/kg with bolus dosage of 10–20 mg and infusion rate of 20–60 µg/kg/min.

Propofol

Propofol (Diprivan) is a general anesthetic drug used for induction and maintenance of anesthesia as well as for sedation. It is not water-soluble, but is available in aqueous solution. The solution contains soybean oil, glycerol, and egg lecithin (egg yolks, not whites); therefore it is recommended to be used within 6 hours of opening the bottle. It causes pain with IV administration that can be lessened by pretreatment with IV lidocaine. Propofol has high lipid solubility that results in rapid onset of action and short duration. It is available in 10 mg/mL concentration. The typical recommended dose for sedation is 50–100 µg/kg/min until appropriate level of sedation is obtained, followed by a maintenance infusion of 25–75 µg/kg/min. Its onset of action is 90–100 seconds and its duration of action is 2–8 minutes. However, prolonged administration can result in drug accumulation and prolonged wake-up time.

Ketamine

Ketamine (Ketalar) is a dissociative anesthetic that dissociates the thalamus from the limbic cortex. The patient appears conscious (e.g., eye opening, swallowing, muscle contracture), but is unable to process or respond to sensory input. It can be administered through an IV or IM route. It can increase blood pressure, heart rate, and cardiac output; therefore, it should be avoided in patients with coronary artery disease, congestive heart failure, arterial aneurysms, and uncontrolled hypertension. It is a potent bronchodilator, useful in patients with asthma, but it also increases salivation. Lithium may prolong duration of action and diazepam attenuates its cardiostimulatory effects and prolongs half-life. Ketamine is known to cause the so-called "emergence phenomenon," for which its use in combination with benzodiazepines is recommended. Maximum doses: 2mg/kg IV or 4mg/kg IM.

Anticholinergics

These drugs are competitive antagonists to acetylcholine in the parasympathetic nervous system, effective in dryness of the mouth and upper respiratory tract.

- **Glycopyrrolate (Robinul)** does not cross lipid membranes (blood–brain barrier), with no CNS depression or delirium-type reactions. Its time of onset is 1 minute and its duration of action is 2–3 hours for its vagal effects and up to 7 hours as an antisialagogue. It is contraindicated in patients with glaucoma, adhesions between the iris and the lens, prostate disease, myasthenia gravis, contact lenses, and asthma. Its usual therapeutic dose is 0.1 mg, and it may be repeated every 2–3 minutes. Maximum dose: 0.3 mg.

Techniques of administration

There are as many techniques for administering and combining drugs for IV sedation in the dental setting as there are practitioners administering IV sedation. In order to simplify the techniques, it may be helpful to classify the drugs in the following categories:

Premedication

- **Nitrous oxide/oxygen.** Widely available to the dental practitioner. It can be used to reduce anxiety, even before venipuncture, and as a support drug during IV sedation.
- **Steroids** (dexamethasone, methylprednisolone). Can be administered to decrease postoperative edema in traumatic procedures. Also can be given to decrease histamine release reactions created by some of the sedative drugs.
- **Antihistamines** (diphenhydramine). Used to decrease histamine release reactions created by some of the sedative drugs. Some antihistamines provide added sedative properties.
- **Anticholinergics** (glycopyrrolate, scopolamine, atropine). Used for control of secretions.

Anxiolysis/analgesia

- **Nitrous oxide/oxygen.** Support drug during IV sedation to reduce amounts of sedative drugs used and to provide oxygen supplementation.
- **Benzodiazepines** (diazepam, midazolam). Most effective drugs in the management of anxiety. Most commonly used in combination with opioids in IV sedation.
- **Opioids** (fentanyl, meperidine). Administered primarily for analgesia. In combination with benzodiazepines accomplish ideal levels for moderate IV sedation.

Deep sedation

- **Anesthetic drugs** (ketamine, propofol, barbiturates). Administered to increase level of sedation during particularly painful or difficult portions of the procedure (e.g., local anesthesia injections), or when ideal level of sedation cannot be accomplished with anxiolytic/analgesic drug combination.

Day of procedure

On the day of the procedure, certain preoperative, documentation and discharge planning requirements must be met. Below is a rough guide to help the practitioner improve patient confort and safety, and to ensure proper documentation and monitoring during and after the procedure.

Preoperative requirements

(1) Current medical history
(2) Pre-procedure diagnosis, appropriateness of procedure, rationale for sedation and sedation plan, i.e., medications to be administered

(3) Verify NPO status for at least 4 hours following oral intake of clear fluids and at least 6 hours following oral intake of nonclear fluids or food

(4) A physical examination, to include at least the patient's vital signs, airway, and blood oxygenation

(5) Signature on appropriate consent form for the procedure and for the administration of parenteral sedation/analgesia

(6) Verification of the presence of a patient escort, a responsible adult who will stay in the waiting area during the procedure and take the patient home upon completion of the procedure

(7) Loose-fitting garments

(8) Morning appointments

(9) Short waiting-room time

(10) Restroom

(11) Monitors

(12) Oxygen/nitrous oxide

(13) Intravenous (IV) line placement

Documentation

(1) Respiratory rate (documented every 5 minutes and preoperatively, intraoperatively, and postoperatively)

(2) Level of consciousness (documented every 5 minutes); can be assessed by different scales (e.g., AVPU scale)

(3) Heart rate (documented every 5 minutes and preoperatively, intraoperatively, and postoperatively)

(4) Blood pressure (documented every 5 minutes and preoperatively, intraoperatively, and postoperatively)

(5) Pulse oximetry with continuous auditory and visual display of oxygen saturation (documented every 5 minutes and preoperatively, intraoperatively, and postoperatively)

(6) ECG monitoring (3–5 lead ECG): constant, with printing capabilities (not required for oral sedation dentistry)

Recovery and discharge

- Never leave patient unattended
- Adjust dental chair position slowly
- Vital signs must return close to normal
- Never discharge alone after sedation
- Written and verbal instructions to patient and escort
- Discharge on wheelchair and with escort
- Continue to document until patient is discharged

Discharge criteria

- Patient has stable vital signs
- Patient easily arousable and with intact protective reflexes
- Adequately patent airway
- Adequately hydrated

- Patient can talk, and can sit unaided
- Patient can walk with minimal assistance
- Can use a scoring systems to document adequacy of discharge (e.g., modified Aldrete or PADSS)

Complications associated with intravenous sedation for dental treatment

The literature shows that the administration of IV sedation and general anesthesia during dental treatment is a safe and effective modality, and the overall complication rate is similar to or less than the rates reported in hospital-based anesthesia practices [20–25]. Boynes and colleagues showed that the overall complication rate for IV sedation during dental treatment is 24.7%, with *airway obstruction* (5.8%) and *nausea and vomiting* (4.7%) as the primary complications [20]. Airway obstruction is the complication reported more frequently in the dental setting when compared with hospital-based practices (2–4%). This could be explained by the nature of the procedures, in which the airway is shared by both the dentist and anesthesia provider working in the same area. Other complications were not reported to be very different than in the hospital-based practices, and these are discussed at length in Chapter 11.

Summary

Every dental visit must begin with the recognition that dental phobia exists, and a clinician will begin to "sedate" his or her patients the moment they enter the dental office. By relying solely on the use of drugs, in enteral or parenteral sedation, you invite the occasional failure and expose yourself to risk of oversedation and/or adverse drug reaction. Remember that, regardless of the severity of the phobia and the level of sedation chosen, a clinician must always utilize iatrosedation as the foundation of every visit.

Minimal, moderate, and deep sedation are major modalities of pharmacological intervention and behavior modification that assist the dental profession in providing dental treatment to patients with different levels of dental anxiety and fear, and they have become an integral part of dental practice.

There are many safe and effective medications available to the dental practitioner for sedation, all possessing slightly different clinical characteristics and various degrees of risk. Careful consideration needs to be given to the objectives of the sedation when deciding which pharmacologic agents and route of administration to use. The appropriateness of the procedure, the rationale for sedation, and the sedation plan should be reviewed to ensure that the sedation procedure is as safe as possible.

Careful attention also needs to be given to physical and psychological assessment of the patient, to determine his or her ability to tolerate (both physically and psychologically) the stresses involved with the planned dental treatment and to determine whether treatment modifications, including modification of sedation protocols, are indicated to enable the patient to better tolerate these stresses.

The dental practitioner should have a complete understanding of, and should be in compliance with, the national and/or state regulations that define moderate and deep sedation, including the educational requirements, clinical guidelines, and licensure.

Finally, even though the administration of moderate and deep sedation during dental treatment is a safe and effective modality, basic preparation for all emergency situations is critical for the successful management of any unexpected sedation-related emergencies that may arise.

References

1. Slovin M, Falagario-Wasserman J. Special needs of anxious and phobic dental patients. *Dent Clin North Am* 2009; **53**: 207–19.

2. Gale E. Fears of the dental situation. *J Dent Res* 1972; **51**: 964–6.

3. American Association of Endodontists. How to ease fear of the dentist. www.aae. org/uploadedFiles/News_Room/ Press_Releases/RCAW09_MAT.pdf (accessed June 2011).

4. Malamed, SF. *Sedation: a Guide to Patient Management*, 5th edn. St Louis, MO: Mosby, 2009.

5. Rubin J, Slovin M, Kaplan A. Assessing patients' fears: recognizing and reacting to signs of anxiety. *Dent Clin North Am* 1986; **1**: 14–18.

6. Weaver JM. Two notable pioneers in conscious sedation pass their gifts of pain-free dentistry to another generation. *Anesth Prog* 2000; **47**: 27–8.

7. American Dental Association (ADA). *Guidelines for the Use of Sedation and General Anesthesia by Dentists*. Chicago, IL: ADA, 2007. www.ada.org/sections/about/ pdfs/anesthesia_guidelines.pdf (accessed June 2011).

8. Glassman P, Caputo A, Dougherty N, *et al.* Special Care Dentistry Association consensus statement on sedation, anesthesia, and alternative techniques for people with special needs. *Spec Care Dentist* 2009; **29**: 2–8.

9. American Dental Association (ADA). *Guidelines for Teaching Pain Control and Sedation to Dentists and Dental Students*. Chicago, IL: ADA, 2007. www.ada.org/ sections/about/pdfs/anxiety_guidelines.pdf (accessed June 2011).

10. American Academy of Pediatrics; American Academy of Pediatric Dentistry, Coté CJ, Wilson S; Work Group on Sedation. Guidelines for monitoring and management of pediatric patients during and after sedation for diagnostic and therapeutic procedures: an update. *Pediatrics* 2006; **118**: 2587–602. www.aapd.org/media/Policies_Guidelines/ G_Sedation.pdf (accessed June 2011).

11. American Association of Oral and Maxillofacial Surgeons (AAOMS). Statement by the American Association of Oral and Maxillofacial Surgeons concerning the management of selected clinical conditions and associated clinical procedures: the control of pain and anxiety. Rosemont, IL: AAOMS, 2010. www.aaoms. org/docs/practice_mgmt/condition_ statements/control_of_pain_and_anxiety. pdf (accessed June 2011).

12. American Association of Oral and Maxillofacial Surgeons (AAOMS). Anesthesia in outpatient facilities. In *AAOMS Parameters of Care: Clinical Practice Guidelines*, 4th edn (AAOMS ParCare 07). 55.PC07-CD. Rosemont, IL: AAOMS, 2007.

13. Continuum of depth of sedation: definition of general anesthesia and levels of sedation/ analgesia. Committee of origin: Quality Management and Departmental Administration (approved by the ASA House of Delegates on October 27, 2004, and amended on October 21, 2009). Available online at www.asahq.org/ For-Healthcare-Professionals/Standards- Guidelines-and-Statements.aspx.

14. Hall DL, Tatakis DN, Walters JD, Rezvan E. Oral clonidine pre-treatment and diazepam/meperidine sedation. *J Dent Res* 2006; **85**: 854–58.

15. Fazi L. A comparison of oral clonidine and oral midazolam as preanesthetic medications in the pediatric tonsillectomy patient. *Anesth Analg* 2001; **92**: 56–61.

16. Wright PMC, Carabine UA, McClune S, Orr DA, Moore J. Preanesthetic medication with clonidine. *Br J Anaesth* 1990; **65**: 628–32.

17. Carabine UA, Wright PMC, Moore J. Preanesthetic medication with clonidine: a dose–response study. *Br J Anaesth* 1991; **67**: 79–83.

18. Segal IS, Jarvis DJ, Duncan SR, White PF, Maze M. Clinical efficacy of oral transdermal clonidine combinations during the perioperative period. *Anesthesiaology* 1991; **74**: 220–5.

19. Treasure T, Bennett J. Office-based anesthesia. *Oral Maxillofac Surg Clin N Am* 2007; **19**: 45–57.

20. Boynes SG, Lewis CL, Moore PA, Zovko J, Close J. Complications associated with anesthesia administered for dental treatment. *Gen Dent* 2010; **58**: e20–5.

21. D'Eramo EM. Mortality and morbidity with outpatient anesthesia: the Massachusetts experience. *J Oral Maxillofac Surg* 1999; **57**: 531–6.

22. Nkansah PJ, Haas DA, Saso MA. Mortality incidence in outpatient anesthesia for dentistry in Ontario. *Oral Surg Oral Med Oral Pathol Oral Radiol Endod* 1997; **83**: 646–51.

23. Hines R, Barash PG, Watrous G, O'Connor T. Complications occurring in the postanesthesia care unit: a survey. *Anesth Analg* 1992; **74**: 503–9.

24. Lunn JN, Hunter AR, Scott DB. Anaesthesia related surgical mortality. *Anaesthesia* 1983; **83**: 1090–6.

25. Tarrac SE. A description of intraoperative and post anesthesia complication rates. *J Perianesth Nurs* 2006; **21**: 88–96.

Sedation for assisted reproductive technologies

Patricia M. Sequeira

Introduction

Assisted reproductive technologies (ART) refers to a set of techniques used to help couples conceive by artificial or partly artificial means. ART has been made possible, and has developed to its current state, by advances in endocrine assays, controlled ovarian stimulation, hormonal manipulation, cryopreservation, ultrasonography, and a range of procedures on eggs, sperm, and embryos. An ART physician is a gynecologist specially trained in reproductive endocrinology. In vitro fertilization (IVF) is a term used to describe the process of obtaining an ovum and uniting it with sperm in a laboratory, and later placing the fertilized egg in the uterus. Transvaginal ultrasound-guided (TVUG) oocyte retrieval (OR) has replaced laparoscopic methods. Egg retrieval is the most painful part of an IVF cycle and therefore requires sedation and analgesia. Sedation for oocyte retrieval and related ART procedures is described in this chapter.

A man and woman of reproductive age who are unable to conceive for a given period of time, usually 1 year, are considered to be infertile. Infertility may be due to tubal (fallopian) factors, ovulatory dysfunction, diminished ovarian reserve, endometriosis, uterine factors, male factors (very low sperm count or abnormal sperm motility), other factors (not treatable by current available methods), or unknown factors. Approximately one-third of infertility is traced to female factors, one-third to male factors, and the remaining third are due to a mixture of female and male problems or unknown factors.

The IVF cycle and ART procedures

A woman starts with an IVF cycle, which consists of a series of treatments in several steps over a period of approximately 2 weeks. The cycle starts when the woman begins taking

Moderate and Deep Sedation in Clinical Practice, ed. Richard D. Urman and Alan D. Kaye.
Published by Cambridge University Press. © Cambridge University Press 2012.

hormonal drugs to stimulate oocyte production, or starts ovarian monitoring, with the intention of having embryos transferred. An IVF cycle starts either naturally or with medication, followed by the production of eggs. Egg retrieval follows. If fertilization is successful, then the next step is embryo transfer. The IVF cycle may require discontinuation due to the absence of egg production, excessive ovarian hyperstimulation, or other medical reasons.

Controlled ovarian hyperstimulation

Controlled ovarian hyperstimulation (COH) is an ART hormonal process through which the ovaries are purposely stimulated to develop more than one dominant follicle (Figure 22.1). This is the start of an IVF cycle. Multiple dominant follicles with eggs will increase the number of eggs retrieved and the likelihood of pregnancy. COH is used to promote the development of a relatively synchronous cohort of ovarian follicles and thus assist in the timing of egg retrieval. COH also helps with the development of the proper endometrial environment for embryo transfer. A typical protocol uses a combination of a gonadotropin-releasing-hormone agonist (GnRH-a), human menopausal gonadotropin (hMG), and human chorionic gonadotropin (hCG). Ovarian suppression and follicular variation are achieved with GnRH-a. Ovarian stimulation is begun with hMG. Oocyte retrieval is usually 36 hours after the start of hCG. The hormonal protocols differ from clinic to clinic, endocrinologist to endocrinologist, patient to patient, as well as according to individual patient hormonal response. COH is carefully monitored throughout with serial ultrasound examination to evaluate the follicle size and progression of hormonal blood levels.

Ovarian hyperstimulation syndrome

Controlled ovarian hyperstimulation can have adverse effects. Ovarian hyperstimulation syndrome (OHSS) is an iatrogenic consequence of COH. OHSS at its most severe stage can have life-threatening physiologic complications. The patient with moderate to severe OHSS may have signs of rapid weight gain, oliguria, hemoconcentration, leukocytosis, hypovolemia, electrolyte imbalance, ascites, pleural and pericardial effusions, acute respiratory

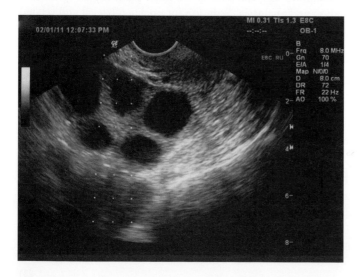

Figure 22.1. Ultrasound view of a hyperstimulated ovary with five follicles.

distress syndrome, hypercoagulability and thromboembolic events, and multiorgan failure. OHSS should be self-limiting, and regression takes place as long as prompt and appropriate supportive medical care is provided. Exogenous and endogenous hCG will worsen OHSS.

Oocyte retrieval

The reproductive medicine physician selectively retrieves eggs from the individual ovarian follicles that have been stimulated via COH. There is a window of time in which the eggs can be retrieved. Oocyte retrieval is a specially scheduled and timed procedure. Retrievals may be performed seven days a week in a busy ART center.

Embryo transfer

Embryo transfer is an ultra-short ART procedure. The process consists of transferring embryos from the laboratory to the patient's uterus. Patients with difficult, or abnormal, cervical or uterine anatomy and those who are extremely anxious may require sedation.

Dilatation and curettage

The ART patient is at a higher risk for increased miscarriage. The dilatation and curettage (D&C) procedure in a setting outside the operating room, such as an ART center, should be done only on selected patients. A patient should be healthy and of normal weight, with normal coagulation, no excessive bleeding, and less than 12 weeks pregnant. Morbidly obese patients, those with a full stomach, and pregnancies greater than 12 weeks should be reserved for the operating room with anesthesia.

Sperm retrieval

Microscopic epididymal sperm aspiration (MESA), percutaneous epididymal sperm aspiration (PESA), and testicular sperm extraction (TESE) are sperm retrieval procedures that take place at an infertility center. For certain cases of male infertility the urologist performs these procedures. MESA uses microsurgical techniques to obtain sperm from the epididymis. The TESE technique removes a small sample of testis tissue for extraction of sperm by the andrology lab. PESA uses a needle to draw sperm from the epididymis.

The patient is in the supine position with the scrotum sterilely prepped and draped. The urologist administers local anesthesia and may use an operating microscope for the sperm retrieval, which usually lasts less than 1 hour. The patient and/or urologist may request sedation.

Patient demographics

The patients are usually healthy adult women. Overweight and obese women are occasionally encountered. Very few well-controlled asthmatics and hypertensive patients are found. Anxiety, depression, and stress due to infertility status may arise. The age range for the ART patient is late twenties to mid-forties.

Procedural risks

Procedure risks for transvaginal ultrasound-guided oocyte retrieval may include bleeding, infection, and injury to pelvic or abdominal organs. These complications may require hospitalization, and possibly surgery. Oskowitz *et al.* reported on a series of 6776 procedures performed in a freestanding surgical facility dedicated to ART [1]. They recorded the number of patients who required hospital admission during the first 24 hours after surgery. Following 4199 vaginal oocyte retrieval procedures, seven patients were admitted. Two patients had serious morbidity, defined as requiring major intervention such as surgery. Nausea and vomiting, syncope, hemoperitoneum, and ovarian hematoma were included in the admitting diagnoses.

ART facilities and personnel

According to a postal questionnaire conducted in 2004, 69% of ART centers in the United Kingdom perform oocyte retrieval outside of the general operating room environment [2]. A typical ART procedure room may be located within a university-based or freestanding fertility clinic. The embryology and andrology laboratories are adjacent to the procedure room, for immediate processing of the oocytes and sperm.

Another postal questionnaire of ART centers in the UK revealed significant variations in personnel present during oocyte retrievals, the use of drugs, degree of monitoring, and the availability of emergency drugs [3]. Eighty-four percent of the ART centers used intravenous sedation and 16% used general anesthesia for transvaginal oocyte retrieval.

Results from a telephone survey of 278 ART programs in the United States revealed that 91 private (68%) and 41 academic (56%) programs used personnel from the department of anesthesiology [4]. A large number of ART programs used their own trained personnel to provide sedation. Ninety-five percent of the transvaginal oocyte retrieval and transcervical embryo transfer were performed under sedation. For the remaining 5%, general, regional, or local anesthesia was used. The majority of the ART personnel typically used meperidine and midazolam, while 90% of the anesthesiology personnel used midazolam and/or propofol with fentanyl.

Sedation for ART procedures

The procedure that most commonly requires sedation during an IVF cycle is oocyte retrieval. Occasionally, an embryo transfer procedure will be scheduled with sedation. The dilatation and curettage procedure is infrequently encountered. On very rare occasions the urologist incorporates MESA and TESE procedures in the ART sedation schedule.

Sedation goals

The sedation goals for oocyte retrieval and related procedures are effective pain relief and sedation with minimal postoperative nausea and vomiting. The procedure should be executed in a safe manner, and the goals also include ease of administering intravenous medications and patient monitoring. The medications should be short-acting and easily reversible. The drugs should minimally affect the oocytes, embryos, and the endocrine and immune systems. ART procedures are costly, and economic factors should be considered.

Sedation considerations

The principal consideration for the ART patient in the pre-procedural period is the management of patient anxiety. The patients may have stress, anxiety, and depression due to their infertile status. They may arrive with anxiety from the expectant wait of the oocyte count. Empathy from all those involved in their care, including the nursing staff, the procedure-room staff, the embryologist, the reproductive medicine physician, and the sedation provider, is invaluable.

Pre-procedural sedation concerns are typically minor, because of the general good health of the ART patient. Airway issues can arise from patients who have a history of loud snoring, sleep apnea, or obesity. The patient with a history of asthma or hypertension is usually medically compliant and well controlled. The hyperstimulated patient may feel bloated and nauseated prior to the ART procedure. A history of postoperative nausea and vomiting (PONV), or motion sickness, should be obtained and reduction of baseline risks initiated. Pain management should be discussed with the patient.

Airway issues should be communicated to the ART physician, since the sedation level may be different than the usual. Care should be taken in the placement of the patient in the dorsal lithotomy position. Positioning while awake and not sedated ensures proper padding and positioning of the patient. Adequate sedation should ensure a cooperative patient and avoid injury to pelvic vessels or organs.

Sedation risks

Apnea is a risk when administering intravenous (IV) sedation agents, especially when mixing two or more. Reducing the IV agents and providing a greater stimulus (chin-lift or a painful jaw-thrust) may help overcome the apnea. Control of the airway with a bag-valve mask may be necessary. Opioid or benzodiazepine reversal should be available, but not routinely used. The desired sedation level should be achieved by careful titration of the IV agents.

Patients at risk for aspiration should be identified. Suctioning equipment should be readily available. Laryngospasm is a risk in the oversedated and obtunded patient. Successful laryngospasm management includes early recognition followed by positive-pressure ventilation and waking the patient. Hypotension from sedation agents is treated with generous fluid hydration and the reduction of IV sedation. Vasopressors are rarely needed. PONV can be seen in this patient population, and those at risk should be identified.

Selection of sedation and analgesia

The selection for sedation and analgesia will depend on the ART center and the physician's preference. The sedation provider should be familiar with the ART procedures, the fertility center's choice of sedation/analgesia, the individual physician's needs, and those of the ART patient. There is variation in the sedation provider personnel and drugs used. Patient preference has a limited impact, since most ART centers usually have set sedation protocols.

Sedation for oocyte retrieval

Transvaginal ultrasound-guided oocyte retrieval can be performed under a paracervical block, moderate sedation, deep sedation, or general anesthesia. The literature concerning effective sedation and analgesia should be interpreted with caution. There are insufficient data to support any one method as superior to others in terms of pregnancy outcomes, pain relief, and patient satisfaction. Specific anesthetic drugs and techniques should be evaluated for their compatibility. Animal data may not reflect the human experience.

Intravenous moderate sedation for TVUG-OR is reportedly the most used anesthetic strategy. The personnel may include nursing staff and/or an ART physician who is trained and experienced in sedation for ART procedures.

The patient's chart is reviewed; medications and allergies, height and weight, as well as baseline vital signs are noted. The patient interview includes the nothing by mouth (NPO) status, medical, surgical, and sedation/anesthesia history, as well as history of PONV or motion sickness. The discussion of the sedation plan and the expectations of the peri-procedure period are explained to the patient. This explanation helps alleviate some of the anxiety associated with the procedure. The discussion should include the information that the patient will be sleepy yet responsive to touch or voice for the evaluation of pain or discomfort. Reassure the patient that comfort and pain control are the goals of sedation.

The readiness of the ART procedure team is checked so that the patient can be brought into the procedure room. This is necessary because the embryology laboratory also partici-pates in this procedure by accepting the collected eggs and reporting the egg count. Once in the procedure room, the ART staff will identify the patient, and the embryologist also follows a similar patient identification process.

The patient is positioned supine on the operating-room table. The routine monitors that are placed include a continuous electrocardiogram, pulse oximetry, and noninvasive blood pressure. CO_2 analysis is encouraged, especially for deep sedation. An intravenous catheter is placed. Oxygen is usually provided via a nasal cannula. The patient is repositioned in the dorsal lithotomy position with the perineum at the edge of the table, just as for a vaginal examination.

The opioid is usually the first agent given, since the primary goal of sedation is pain management during the oocyte retrieval. The opioid most frequently used is fentanyl. The usual dose of fentanyl is in the range of 50–100 µg, intravenously. Once fentanyl titration is begun then the anxiolytic is administered. The most common agent is a benzodiazepine, such as midazolam or diazepam. Usually 2–4 mg of midazolam IV is given, titrated so the patient is relaxed and sleepy yet responsive to light touch and voice.

When the desired sedation level is achieved, the surgeon places the vaginal ultrasound into the vagina. Both ovaries are examined, and the physician reports to the sedation provider a gross estimate of eggs to be retrieved. This helps gauge the length of time that the procedure is expected to take. Generally younger patients have more eggs than older patients. The placement of the vaginal probe can be very stimulating when the ovaries are difficult to visualize and maximal pressure is applied into the posterior vaginal wall. The next stimulus is the puncture through the vaginal wall into the ovary. A 16-gauge needle is used alongside the vaginal probe. The follicles are aspirated. This process is then repeated on the contralateral ovary. Once the retrieval is complete, the probe is used to evaluate the ovaries for possible bleeding, or surrounding vessel and tissue injury. The probe is withdrawn and a vaginal speculum is then placed to evaluate for bleeding or vaginal wall injury. Pressure is typically held at the vaginal wall puncture sites. Additional medication is not needed at this point because the inspection of the vagina may not be uncomfortable or painful. If the physician needs to place a suture, or hold extensive vaginal pressure, additional opioids may be needed as well as further verbal reassurance. Once there is no reported bleeding, the patient is transferred to the recovery area. Table 22.1 summar-izes the steps involved in sedation for oocyte retrieval.

Sedation for embryo transfer

Embryo transfer usually does not require sedation. The ART center will administer an oral benzodiazepine for those with mild to moderate anxiety, for the patient is kept "awake."

Table 22.1. Sedation for transvaginal ultrasound-guided oocyte retrieval: a summary

Preparation in the procedure room
Check availability of emergency equipment
Pre-procedure interview and documentation
Confirm patient identification in the room
Place routine monitors
Peripheral IV
Give oxygen via nasal cannula
Position patient in dorsal lithotomy position
Start sedation with fentanyl 50 µg IV
Give midazolam 2 mg IV
Titrate IV fentanyl and midazolam
Keep communicating with the patient
Give reassurance throughout the retrieval
Treat pain with fentanyl
Follow the progression by talking to the ART physician

On occasion, the extremely anxious patient is going to request sedation for the embryo transfer. The main reason is to alleviate the procedural anxiety and discomfort of the vaginal speculum and cervical stimulation. The reproductive medicine physician may also request moderate sedation for a patient with a difficult cervical or uterine anatomy. Having the patient under moderate sedation will facilitate maneuvering the small plastic catheter containing the embryos into the uterus. This ultra-short procedure is not very stimulating or painful.

The patient chart is reviewed and the history and physical exam are obtained. The goal of the anesthetic is discussed with the patient. Patient safety, comfort, and anxiolysis are emphasized. Describing the sedation/ART procedure helps ease any pre-procedural anxiety.

In the procedure room, the patient identification is verified by the ART staff, and again by the embryologist. The patient is positioned supine on the table. The routine monitors and an intravenous catheter are placed. Then the patient is repositioned into the dorsal lithotomy position. Pressure points are padded and checked. The sedation is started during the vaginal wash, which also includes the placement of a vaginal speculum by the procedure technician. Moderate sedation can be accomplished with a combination of fentanyl and midazolam. Approximately 50 µg of fentanyl is titrated along with 2–4 mg of midazolam. Verbal reassurance is used when administering moderate sedation.

Sedation for dilatation and curettage

The sedation provider will from time to time be scheduled to administer moderate to deep sedation for a missed abortion. This is not unusual, since the ART patient has a higher risk for a missed abortion. The patient for a D&C in the ART center should be a healthy patient.

The reproductive physicians who elect to do the D&C in the ART facility may facilitate moderate sedation with a paracervical block.

The patient's chart is reviewed and the approximate gestational age is noted. The laboratory work is reviewed for the hematocrit, platelet count, and blood type. When a rhesus-negative woman carries a rhesus-positive pregnancy, Rhogam is given to prevent the woman's immune system from reacting to Rh-positive blood of any subsequent pregnancy.

The goals of ART sedation are reviewed with the patient. Safety and comfort are emphasized. Empathy and reassurance helps with pre-procedural anxiety.

The procedural risks include uterine bleeding and perforation. The reproductive medicine physician will request a dose of antibiotic to prevent pelvic infection. The most stimulating part of the D&C is the serial dilatation of the cervical os and canal.

In the procedure room, the nursing staff verifies the patient identification. The patient is positioned supine on the operating-room table. The routine monitors are placed. An IV catheter (minimum 20-gauge) is placed. The patient is then repositioned in the dorsal lithotomy position, with the perineum at the lateral edge of the table. Pressure points are checked. Oxygen is administered via a nasal cannula. Midazolam 2–4 mg is given for anxiolysis and amnesia. A few minutes later fentanyl is titrated in doses of 25 μg. The usual required doses of fentanyl range from 50 to 100 μg, with the most common total being a 100 μg dose. Titrating the sedation agents carefully will ensure that the patient breathes spontaneously with minimal airway assistance.

Post-sedation considerations

Patient care is transferred to the recovery-room nurse. The patient care transfer begins with proper patient identification, followed by a description of the procedure, the sedation agents used, drug allergies, antiemetics, antibiotics, and fluids that were administered. Sedation or procedure complications encountered are communicated. Pertinent patient details such as history of PONV, extreme pre-procedural anxiety, large amounts of sedation medications given, retrieval of no eggs, few eggs, or many eggs should be communicated. A young patient or egg donor with many eggs retrieved will most probably require additional analgesics in the recovery period.

Upon arrival to the recovery area, attention is focused on oxygenation, ventilation, and circulation by monitoring pulse oximetry, breathing frequency, airway patency, systemic blood pressure, and heart rate. Supplemental oxygen and suction should be readily available. The vitals signs are recorded every 15 minutes. On occasion, care may be directed toward the need for airway support for a sleepy patient. This is treated by patient stimulation and a chin-lift. Hypotension is usually secondary to the sedation and is typically self-limiting. Continuing the IV fluids and waking the patient usually resolves the hypotension. Moderate to severe pain on admission should be immediately treated with IV fentanyl 25–35 μg. Proactively addressing pain management should aid in the prompt discharge of the patient, and in avoidance of PONV.

ART patients usually stay in the recovery area for 90–120 minutes. Typical causes for a delay in the discharge from the recovery room are abdominal cramping or pain, PONV, a vasovagal event, or delay in urination.

Moderate to severe pelvic pain is treated with IV opioids, whereas mild pain is treated with nonopioids such as acetaminophen and/or nonsteroidal anti-inflammatory agents. Verbal reassurance also helps. The reproductive medicine physician should evaluate unrelenting pain. A full bladder may also be responsible for ongoing abdominal pain. The patient is encouraged to urinate. Rarely is catheterization of the bladder needed.

PONV considerations should start during the pre-procedure period, recognizing that the ART population is at risk. According to Apfel and colleagues, the four primary risk factors for PONV are female gender, nonsmoking status, a history of PONV, and opioid use [5]. The typical ART patient has at least three of the four risk factors. A history of PONV and motion sickness can be specifically determined during the patient interview. Strategies to reduce baseline PONV risk factors should be deployed. These include reduction in pre-procedural anxiolysis, aggressive intravenous hydration, supplemental oxygen, and minimizing opioids. PONV antiemetic prophylaxis coupled with these strategies is known as a multimodal approach.

When PONV occurs in the recovery area and the patient has not received prophylaxis, a 5-hydroxytryptamine (serotonin) receptor 3 (5-HT$_3$) antagonist such as ondansetron should be administered. In the event that PONV prophylaxis with a 5-HT$_3$ antagonist is inadequate, an additional dose of 5-HT$_3$ antagonist should not be used as a rescue agent since it does not give additional benefit when used within the first 6 hours after surgery [6]. Compazine, droperidol, dexamethasone, or metoclopramide have been used for PONV rescue.

On occasion, a patient may experience lightheadedness and nausea as a result of a vasovagal event. This patient is nauseated as well as bradycardic and hypotensive. The patient is placed in the supine position and a bolus of crystalloid fluid is administered. Symptoms usually resolve quickly. If bradycardia and hypotension persist, a dose of atropine 0.5 mg IV should be administered. Crampy pain may be responsible for the vasovagal event, and this should be treated.

Very rarely, brisk vaginal bleeding is observed in the recovery area. The reproductive medicine physician should evaluate the patient. The patient may be brought back to the procedure room for a thorough vaginal/pelvic examination.

The ART nursing staff documents the patient recovery course. Once the criteria for discharge are met, the patient and the adult escort are given written discharge instructions. A post-procedure follow-up telephone call is made the following morning by the ART staff.

Summary

Oocyte retrieval is a very important part of the IVF cycle. Transvaginal ultrasound-guided oocyte retrieval remains the most painful part of an IVF cycle. Moderate/deep sedation is commonly used for egg retrieval and its related procedures in the United States and the United Kingdom. There is variability in personnel and medications used. A significant number of ART centers are providing their own sedation teams. The best sedation and anesthetic practice for pain relief and pregnancy rates has yet to be determined.

References

1. Oskowitz SP, Berger MJ, Mullen L, et al. Safety of a freestanding surgical unit for the assisted reproductive technologies. Fertil Steril 1995; 63: 874–9.

2. Yasmin E, Dresner M, Balen A. Sedation and anaesthesia for transvaginal oocyte collection: an evaluation of practice in the UK. Hum Reprod 2004; 19: 2942–5.

3. Elkington NM, Kehoe J, Acharya U. Intravenous sedation in assisted conception units: a UK survey. Hum Fertil (Camb) 2003; 6: 74–6.

4. Ditkoff EC, Plumb J, Selick A, Sauer MV. Anesthesia practices in the United States

common to in vitro fertilization (ART) centers. *J Assist Reprod Genet* 1997; **14**: 145–7.

5. Apfel CC, Läärä E, Koivuranta M, Greim CA, Roewer N. A simplified risk score for predicting postoperative nausea and vomiting: conclusions from cross-validations between two centers. *Anesthesiology* 1999; **91**: 693–700.

6. Kovac AL, O'Connor TA, Pearman MH, *et al.* Efficacy of repeat intravenous dosing of ondansetron in controlling postoperative nausea and vomiting: a randomized, double-blind, placebo-controlled multicenter trial. *J Clin Anesth* 1999; **11**: 453–9.

Further reading

Bokhari A, Pollard BJ. Anaesthesia for assisted conception. *Eur J Anaesthesiol* 1998; **15**: 391–6.

Elkington M, Kehoe J, Acharya U. Policy and Practice Committee of the British Fertility Society. Recommendations for good practice for sedation in assisted conception. *Hum Fertil (Camb)* 2003; **6**: 77–80.

Gan TJ, Meyer T, Apfel CC, *et al.* Consensus guidelines for managing postoperative nausea and vomiting. *Anesth Analg* 2003; **97**: 62–71.

Kwan I, Bhattacharya S, Knox F, McNeil A. Conscious sedation and analgesia for oocyte retrieval procedures: a Cochrane review. *Hum Reprod* 2006; **21**: 1672–9.

Schenker JG, Ezra Y. Complications of assisted reproductive techniques. *Fertil Steril* 1994; **61**: 411–22.

Toledano RD, Kodali BS, Camann WR. Anesthesia drugs in the obstetric and gynecologic practice. *Rev Obstet Gynecol* 2009; **2**: 93–100.

Trout SW, Vallerand AH, Kemmann E. Conscious sedation for in vitro fertilization. *Fertil Steril* 1998; **69**: 799–808.

Tsen LC. From Darwin to desflurane? Anesthesia for assisted reproductive technologies. *Anesth Analg* 2002; **94** (Suppl): 109–14.

Wallach EE, Zacur HA. *Reproductive Medicine and Surgery*. St Louis, MO: Mosby, 1995; 849.

Chapter

23

Sedation for interventional pain management procedures

Ron Banister, Rahul Mishra, and Alan D. Kaye

Locations

The administration of anesthetics for moderate and deep sedation during pain management procedures is a challenge to any provider. While minor and interventional procedures are routinely performed in operating theaters, it is increasingly common for these same procedures to be performed in a variety of other settings and even without sedation at all. These sites include remote locations within the hospital, outpatient pain management centers, diagnostic centers, and physician offices.

Practitioners must be aware of the specific characteristics of their location to ensure patient safety. This includes, for example, logistics for contacting medical assistance or obtaining equipment for medical emergencies. It is equally prudent to realize that standards of care are unchanged regardless of practice setting. As mandated by various organizations, such as The Joint Commission (TJC), the American Society of Anesthesiologists (ASA), and the Occupational Safety and Health Administration (OSHA), the requirements for intravenous conscious sedation in any given location may be legally enforced. All practitioners and assisting personnel must survey the site prior to the commencement of a procedure to ensure that adequate care is delivered in a controlled and routine manner.

Established standards of care

The ASA has established several guidelines including the requirements for anesthesia delivery in an office-based setting and for interventional pain procedures. The concept of anesthesia delivery in the office, referred to as office-based anesthesia (OBA), is considered a subset of ambulatory anesthesia. ASA policies mandate that a licensed physician be in

Moderate and Deep Sedation in Clinical Practice, ed. Richard D. Urman and Alan D. Kaye.
Published by Cambridge University Press. © Cambridge University Press 2012.

attendance at the facility and at least available by telephone in the event of overnight patient care until discharge criteria are met. Resuscitation equipment and emergency transfer should be immediately available to the facility. Additionally, minimal care standards such as appropriate written consent, patient education regarding follow-up, and discharge instructions apply to all patients undergoing procedures. OBA is unique in that, unlike a hospital or licensed ambulatory surgical facility, physician offices have minimal regulatory control or oversight by government agencies. However, this underscores the importance of meeting requirements for delivering sedation for pain procedures. The practitioner must be confident that all issues are addressed in order to reduce risk and liability.

The ASA's statement on anesthesia delivered for interventional pain procedures outlines that, unless unique circumstances are present, patients should only need local anesthesia. Any procedures that are prolonged and/or painful should follow the guidelines for sedation or monitored anesthesia care (MAC) discussed further below. Procedures performed with sedation, MAC or local anesthesia must balance the risk of possible harm to the patient, especially those undergoing elective cervical spine procedures. Patients must be alert enough during a pain procedure to be able to communicate with the pain practitioner if they are experiencing pain when a needle is misplaced intraneurally, within the spine itself, or in another aberrant location.

OSHA also sets specific standards for the care of patients in settings outside of the operating suite. OSHA guidelines cover safety items such as radiation exposure, high sound levels, and heavy mechanical equipment, which can all be applicable to the practice of pain management.

TJC outlines several standards for the anesthetic care of patients, from environmental guidelines and emergency management to leadership structure and infection control. There are aspects of office-based surgery outlined in TJC's *Accreditation Handbook for Office-Based Surgery* specific to the delivery of sedation and anesthesia. For example, the permission given to a practitioner to administer sedation stipulates that he or she must be able to rescue the patient from any depth of anesthesia (e.g., "when the patient slips from moderate into deep sedation or from deep sedation into full anesthesia"). It is further clarified that the availability of a cardiorespiratory rescue team is not acceptable in lieu of a practitioner who is qualified to administer sedation, and thus also qualified to rescue a patient from any depth of anesthesia.

Facilities and equipment

There are basic characteristics of non-operating-room sites that need to be met for adequate delivery of anesthesia care to patients. The ASA, OSHA, and TJC outline the standards that each remote location should fulfill prior to administration of sedation for pain management procedures. At the conclusion of procedures, travel distances to recovery areas vary, and therefore it is vital to have an adequate supply of supplemental oxygen with fully functional backup, monitoring equipment, and immediate access with keys to elevators or corridors. In the event of an emergency, there should be efficient access to oxygen, suction, emergency drugs, monitors, and defibrillator. The crash cart should be stocked and within reasonable distance from the patient area along with instruments for intravenous access (gloves, tourniquets, alcohol wipes, catheters, tubing, syringes). Furthermore, reliable transfer to an outside facility should also be in place for emergent situations requiring a higher level of care.

Additionally, the practitioner and staff should be familiar with the exact location of the nearest defibrillator, fire extinguisher, and exit. Pain procedures often require fluoroscopy, and radiation safety is therefore of the utmost importance. Advanced preparation should be made for proper storage and handling of machines, lead aprons or glass shields, and thyroid shields. Dosimetry data should comply with state and federal regulations. The remote locations where pain procedures are performed should also have adequate illumination, power outlets, and fault circuit breakers. There should be ample provision of physical space for equipment and all participating personnel.

Personnel and staffing

An anesthesiologist is not always involved in the care of the patient, and sedation/analgesia is frequently administered by non-anesthesiologists or other non-anesthesia professionals. Delivery of anesthesia requires the understanding that sedation and general anesthesia are on a continuum. But not all those who are administering medications may be able to appreciate the importance of this concept, based on their background and training. The ASA has established standards for granting privileges for administering moderate sedation to practitioners who are not anesthesia professionals. Only physicians, dentists, or podiatrists who are qualified by education, training, and licensure should supervise the administration of moderate sedation. The non-anesthesiologist should not only be able to pre-assess patient comorbidities and be competent in the use of routine sedation medications, but also be trained and skilled in the use of airway equipment and emergency resuscitative care (e.g., oral airway, laryngoscope, endotracheal tubes, and resuscitation bag-mask). These qualifications are needed in order to provide complete care for patients undergoing routine pain procedures in remote locations where emergent situations may arise.

There are numerous people involved in the care of a patient before, during, and after the procedure, including nurses, radiology technicians, and surgical technicians. Open communication between parties is essential for adequate anesthetic delivery to the patient in an environment where staff members are skilled in different areas. This is extremely important in a situation where skilled anesthesia care may not be in the immediate vicinity. It may also be prudent to ensure that staff members are able to assist in patient resuscitation, if needed (Basic Life Support, Advanced Cardiac Life Support).

Patient evaluation

Appropriate pre-procedural evaluation of each patient is recommended by the ASA. The pre-assessment allows for reduction in risk of adverse outcomes and in turn leads to improved patient outcomes. Qualified practitioners should familiarize themselves with and document major organ-system abnormalities, previous exposure to sedation anesthesia, and noted complications, current medical history and medications, allergies, and social history including tobacco, alcohol, and substance abuse. The subpopulation of patients undergoing interventional pain management procedures requires that the provider have a detailed understanding of not only routine medications, but additionally of various analgesics, muscle relaxants, sedatives, and other adjunct medications, to avoid oversedation and other adverse events perioperatively. This includes knowing how many of these drugs were taken in recent days, including on the day of the pain procedure, and a good understanding of the baseline level of sedation.

Complete physical examination assessing the heart, lungs, and airway should be completed. Many pain procedures are performed with the patient in the prone position, and a thorough evaluation for airway limitations is prudent for a successful outcome. Extra precaution should be taken for patients with increased body habitus, short neck, limited range of motion of head and neck, dysmorphic features of the head and neck, small mouth, trismus, or history of sleep apnea, because these factors increase the likelihood of airway obstruction during spontaneous ventilation and difficult airway management. Additional laboratory workup is indicated for underlying medical conditions which have the potential to affect the delivery of anesthetic care.

Obtaining consent for anesthetic care is required in most situations. Since many of these procedures are performed with moderate sedation only, it is important that patients have a good understanding that they may feel a portion of the procedure, in particular a local anesthesia wheal at the surface of the injection site. They need to understand that it is against local, regional, and national standards to render a pain patient unconscious for typical interventional pain procedures. For example, if the injection is placed directly into the spine, the patient will not be able to communicate effectively that the injectable is being placed into the wrong area.

Further, the patient must be informed that routine measures are taken to ensure safe delivery of medical care, but more invasive techniques may need to be employed if sedation fails to provide adequate analgesia and the patient and surgeon wishes to proceed with the procedure. In this regard, there is always a rare chance for an unanticipated procedural complication or an acute reaction to medications, which can include the potential for catastrophic allergic response with loss of the airway, cardiovascular instability, and even death. The risks and benefits of all types of anesthetic care should be explained and questions answered, to ensure that the patient clearly understands the plan of action. It is recommended that procedures not be performed if a responsible adult is not available to accompany the patient home after the procedure.

Monitoring

A primary cause of morbidity associated with sedation cited by the ASA is drug-induced respiratory depression. Adequate monitoring of ventilatory function via observation of chest rise and auscultation is recommended to avoid adverse outcomes. Additional monitors should be employed to ensure proper oxygenation and circulation with pulse oximetry and ECG. Blood pressure, end-tidal CO_2, and temperature monitoring are standard ASA monitors and should be employed. The healthcare practitioner providing sedation for pain procedures will be ill-equipped to ascertain the cause of symptoms such as sudden onset of lightheadedness, shortness of breath, oversedation, nausea, or changes in mental status, without appropriate monitors.

As cited earlier, the depth of anesthesia, from sedation to general anesthesia, is a continuum (see Table 1.2). The adequate delivery of anesthesia requires the practitioner to understand the difference between conscious sedation and monitored anesthesia care (MAC), because the level of care can change from moment to moment based on the titration of a given drug. The essential component of MAC is the assessment and management of anticipated physiologic changes during the case, with the provider of the anesthetic prepared and qualified to convert to general anesthesia if necessary. For practitioners administering moderate or deep sedation, there should not be such an expectation, meaning

Table 23.1. The Ramsay scale for monitoring of sedation level

Sedation level	Description
1	Anxious and agitated
2	Cooperative, tranquil, oriented
3	Responds only to verbal commands
4	Asleep with brisk response to light stimulation
5	Asleep without response to light stimulation
6	Nonresponsive

Modified from: Ramsay MAE, Savege TM, Simpson BRJ, Goodwin R. Controlled sedation with alphaxalone–alphadolone. *Br Med J* 1974; **2**: 656–9.

that the integrity of the patient's physiologic status and airway should remain intact for the entirety of the procedure. The patient should also respond purposefully to verbal command and tactile stimulation. In this regard, the degree of postoperative care required for patients after MAC is higher (e.g., assessment for return to baseline mental status, relief of pain).

In addition to physiologic monitoring, assessment of level of sedation and pain is vital for adequate sedation for pain procedures. Some facilities use brain-wave monitors such as the Bispectral Index (BIS) and Sedline to help the clinician assess the depth of anesthesia of pain patients under sedation. Common additional tools include the Ramsay Sedation Scale (RSS; Table 23.1) and the Richmond Agitation–Sedation Scale (RASS; see Tables 4.1 and 8.1). RSS is scaled 1 (anxious and agitated) to 6 (nonresponsive), while RASS is from +4 (combative) to –5 (unarousable) The visual analog scale (VAS) and the Faces scale (see Figure 3.1) are most commonly used to assess and document a patient's comfort level.

Drugs

Various sedatives, opioids, and dissociative agents are used in the management of patients undergoing pain procedures. Here we present a brief review of the effects of these drugs; see Chapter 2 for fuller details of the pharmacology of sedative agents. Obviously, it is imperative for the practitioner to have immediate access to airway equipment when administering any of these medications.

Midazolam (Versed) and diazepam (Valium) are common benzodiazepines used in the premedication of pain patients prior to their pain procedure. These drugs interact with discrete benzodiazepine receptors in the cerebral cortex, and while they have no direct analgesic properties they do have anxiolytic, amnesic, sedative, and muscle-relaxant properties. Benzodiazepines cause minimal cardiovascular depression, which can be seen as a decrease in blood pressure or decreased heart rate mediated via decreased vagal tone. These medicines also cause respiratory depression from a decreased response to CO_2, especially when administered intravenously. The relatively high potency of midazolam necessitates careful titration to avoid overdose and resulting apnea. The use of opioids with benzodiazepines has a synergistic effect on cardiovascular depression, which can be especially pronounced in patients with ischemic heart disease. Careful review of a patient's chart is also warranted, to avoid drug interactions. Cimetidine reduces the metabolism of diazepam, erythromycin inhibits metabolism of midazolam, and heparin increases the free drug concentration of diazepam in blood twofold.

The commonly used opioids, fentanyl and alfentanil, are used for pain control. These drugs inhibit postsynaptic responses to noxious stimulus in nociceptive neurons. The high lipid solubility of these two drugs is reflected in the rapid onset of action, but the duration of action is considerably shorter. If multiple doses are administered then plasma concentrations do not decrease rapidly, and this may prolong duration of analgesia and suppression of ventilation. Alfentanil is one-fifth to one-tenth as potent as fentanyl and has about one-third the duration of action, which provides many clinical advantages over fentanyl for analgesia. Side effects are similar to those of morphine (e.g., reduced peristalsis leading to constipation) without the accompanying histamine release and hypotension. Opioids do not depress cardiac function, but high doses may cause vagus-mediated bradycardia. However, opioid-mediated respiratory depression is subject to close titration. In addition to blunting a patient's response to CO_2, these drugs also induce chest wall rigidity, which may impair adequate ventilation.

Propofol is an induction agent used for general anesthesia that can also be used for deep sedation in a variety of settings. Combined with active hypnotic and antiemetic properties, its short duration of action makes it an ideal anesthetic adjuvant for deep sedation for certain complex and lengthy interventional pain procedures, as well as resulting in a prompt recovery. Physiologic changes result in decreased arterial blood pressure, in which large changes occur with large intravenous doses, rapid injection, and advanced age. Careful titration and adequate monitoring of patient vital signs during administration is critical, because profound respiratory depression can be seen, which may lead to apnea with multiple or larger doses.

Ketamine is a highly lipid-soluble dissociative anesthetic that renders patients unable to process sensory information while appearing to be conscious. Uniquely, the cardiovascular effects are increased blood pressure and heart rate, which typically needs to be avoided in patients with coronary artery disease. Respiratory drive is minimally affected and, in fact, it is a bronchodilator, which is an advantage for asthmatic patients (although the drug also increases secretions in a dose-dependent manner). Although this drug is not considered a first-line sedation drug for interventional pain procedures, it can be a useful agent for difficult patients and/or challenging pain procedures. Patients should be educated about the undesirable psychotomimetic effects (e.g., illusions, disturbing dreams, delirium). Drug interaction with diazepam prolongs ketamine's elimination half-time.

Dexmedetomidine is a selective alpha-2 agonist with sedative properties and some analgesic effects. There is no significant depression of respiratory drive, but excessive sedation may cause airway obstruction. Other side effects include bradycardia, heart block, hypotension, and nausea. Therefore, dexmedetomidine should be used with caution in patients taking vasodilators, beta-blockers, or drugs that decrease heart rate.

Competitive antagonists (reversal agents) should also be available to the practitioner, such as naloxone and flumenzail. Naloxone is an opioid reversal agent that can rescue patients from the effects of opioid overdose. But reversal of opioid overdose (e.g., respiratory depression) can also reverse opioid analgesia and result in sympathetic stimulation from sudden increased perception of pain. Flumenazil is a benzodiazepine reversal agent that antagonizes the hypnotic effects more effectively than the amnesic properties. Side effects include anxiety reactions and nausea and vomiting. Both reversal agents can also cause withdrawal symptoms if patients are tolerant or have long-standing treatment with the given opioid or benzodiazepine.

Emergency rescue drugs, including epinephrine, diphenhydramine (Benadryl), and dexamethasone (Decadron), should always be available in a crash cart that is easily accessible to the site of procedure. The practitioner and staff should be prepared for situations such as sudden loss of consciousness, seizure, allergic reaction, and adverse procedural outcomes.

Procedures

Typical procedures in pain management are varied, and the clinician providing sedation should have an understanding so that appropriate sedation can be delivered effectively and efficiently (Table 23.2). It is critical to perform a time-out before the interventional pain

Table 23.2. Overview of pain procedures for the non-anesthesiologist

Short-duration procedures (15–30 minutes)
1. Diagnostic blocks and infusions
2. Trigger-point/myofascial injections (e.g., injections directly into muscle beds)
3. Cryoablation injections
4. Facet joint injections
5. Epidural steroid injections, including cervical, thoracic, and lumbar
6. Transforaminal nerve root injections
7. Caudal injections
8. Sacroiliac joint injections
9. Hip injections
10. Radiofrequency thermocoagulation (RFTC)
11. Pulsed electromagnet field injections (PEMF)
12. Knee injections
13. Most sympathetic/ganglion blocks, including sphenopallantine ganglion, stellate ganglion, dorsal root ganglion, splanchnic nerve, celiac plexus block, thoracic and lumbar sympathetic, hypogastric plexus, and ganglion of Impar
14. Intercostal nerve blocks
15. Suprascapular nerve blocks
Longer-duration procedures (30–60 minutes)
1. Discograms: cervical, thoracic, lumbar
2. Epidurolysis/epiduroscopy
3. Augmentation techniques, including spinal cord stimulation (dorsal column stimulation testing and permanent implantation) of the occipital nerve, cervical, thoracic, lumbar, or sacral spinal cord
4. Intrathecal implantation
5. Neurolytic and neurolysis blocks, including ethyl alcohol, phenol, hypotonic, hypertonic, and glycerol injections
6. Decompressive neuroplasty (Racz procedure)
7. Vertebroplasty

Table 23.3. Key anesthetic considerations for the non-anesthesiologist

1. Ensure supplemental oxygen supply
2. Ensure that tools for intravenous access and airway equipment are functional and available
3. Develop skills for early recognition in oversedation
4. Document vital signs before, during, and after procedure
5. Ensure personnel are on standby for emergency
6. Be vigilant!

physician starts his/her procedure, to ensure that the correct procedure on the correct side is being performed. Many busy pain practitioners perform 10–20 procedures in a day, and confusion must be minimized. Fairly straightforward interventional pain procedures, which are typically between 30 and 60 minutes in duration and can be managed effectively with moderate sedation, include diagnostic blocks and infusions, trigger-point injections, cryoablation injections, ganglion injections, facet injections, epidural steroid injections, transforaminal nerve root injections, caudal injections, sacroiliac joint injections, hip injections, pulsed radiofrequency and pulsed electromagnet field injections, knee injections, discograms, epidurolysis, and most sympathetic blocks. There are many other types of injections and most of them can be performed successfully with moderate sedation. In most cases, experience with the pain practitioner, appropriate monitoring, careful titration of drugs, and effective communication will ensure success for these patients. Key anesthetic considerations are outlined in Table 23.3.

Patient recovery

Immediately following a pain procedure, the patient should be transported with the practitioner providing the sedation to a recovery area. Supplemental oxygen and monitors for transport may be required if a long distance to recovery care is expected. Upon arrival, vital signs, level of sedation, and degree of pain should be immediately reassessed. The patient's general condition should be noted, and staff should be available to accept the transfer of care. Because stimulation from the procedure is no longer present, prolonged effects of the sedatives or decreased metabolism may contribute to cardiorespiratory suppression. Prior to release from the facility, appropriate discharge criteria should be met such as return to baseline mental status, stable vital signs, and a sufficient time elapsed since last documented dose of medication. Discharge from the facility should only be done when the patient is accompanied by a responsible adult. Finally, it is imperative that discharge instructions are provided to the patient, indicating appropriate diet, medications, acceptable activities, and contact information in case of emergency.

Summary

Providing safe and effective sedation for pain patients can be challenging and rewarding. Even for longtime anesthesia providers, interventional pain procedures require careful planning and prudent decision making. Many interventional pain practitioners perform procedures without sedation, which can be both terrifying and painful for the patient in need of these treatments. Regardless of the location, e.g. an office, a radiology suite, an ambulatory facility, or a hospital operating room, sedation can be a critical component of an interventional pain procedure. However, in ill-equipped hands, pain patients can potentially have morbidity and mortality when sedation is utilized. Competence and defined standards of experience and expertise are not only warranted but essential for successful sedation of the pain patient.

Further reading

ASA guidelines:

Continuum of depth of sedation: definition of general anesthesia and levels of sedation/analgesia. Committee of origin: Quality Management and Departmental Administration (approved by the ASA House of Delegates on October 27, 2004, and amended on October 21, 2009).

Distinguishing monitored anesthesia care ("MAC") from moderate sedation/analgesia (conscious sedation). Committee of origin: Economics (approved by the ASA House of Delegates on October 27, 2004 and last amended on October 21, 2009).

Guidelines for ambulatory anesthesia and surgery. Committee of origin: Ambulatory Surgical Care (approved by the ASA House of Delegates on October 15, 2003, and last amended on October 22, 2008).

Guidelines for office-based anesthesia. Committee of origin: Ambulatory Surgical Care (approved by the ASA House of Delegates on October 13, 1999, and last affirmed on October 21, 2009).

Practice guidelines for sedation and analgesia by non-anesthesiologists. *Anesthesiology* 2002; **96**: 1004–17.

Statement on anesthetic care during interventional pain procedures for adults. Committee of origin: Pain Medicine (approved by the ASA House of Delegates on October 22, 2005 and last amended on October 20, 2010).

Statement on granting privileges for administration of moderate sedation to practitioners who are not anesthesia professionals. Committee of origin: Ad Hoc Committee on Credentialing (approved by the ASA House of Delegates on October 25, 2005, and amended on October 18, 2006).

Statement on nonoperating room anesthetizing locations. Committee of origin: Standards and Practice Parameters (approved by the ASA House of Delegates on October 15, 2003 and amended on October 22, 2008).

Statement on qualifications of anesthesia providers in the office-based setting. Committee of origin: Ambulatory Surgical Care (approved by the ASA House of Delegates on October 13, 1999, and last amended on October 21, 2009).

Miller RD, ed. *Anesthesia*, 7th edn. Philadelphia, PA: Churchill Livingstone, 2009.

Raj PP, Lou L, Erdine S, *et al. Interventional Pain Management: Image-Guided Procedures*, 2nd edn. Philadelphia, PA: Elsevier, 2008.

Ramsay MAE, Savege TM, Simpson BRJ, Goodwin R. Controlled sedation with alphaxalone–alphadolone. *Br Med J* 1974; **2**: 656–9.

Sessler CN, Gosnell MS, Grap MJ, *et al.* The Richmond Agitation–Sedation Scale: validity and reliability in adult intensive care patients. *Am J Respir Crit Care Med* 2002; **166**: 1338–44.

Stoelting RK, Miller RD. *Basics of Anesthesia*, 5th edn. Philadelphia, PA: Churchill Livingstone, 2007.

The Joint Commission. *Accreditation Handbook for Office-Based Surgery: What You Need to Know About Obtaining Accreditation.* www.jointcommission.org/assets/1/18/2011_OBS_Hdbk.pdf (accessed June 2011).

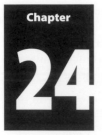

Chapter 24

Emergency resuscitation algorithms: adults

Eunhea Kim and Richard D. Urman

Introduction

Moderate and deep sedation occurs in numerous settings, and healthcare providers may unexpectedly find themselves in situations where emergency resuscitation of patients will be required. A discussion of key concepts found in the latest AHA guidelines follows, to prepare the provider for these potential emergencies. For more detailed information, the reader is referred to the 2010 American Heart Association (AHA) guidelines for cardiopulmonary resuscitation and emergency cardiovascular care [1].

Basic life support (BLS)

Basic life support (BLS) skills for the healthcare provider include immediate recognition of sudden cardiac arrest (SCA), early cardiopulmonary resuscitation (CPR), and rapid defibrillation with an automated external defibrillator (AED) (Table 24.1) [2].

The first step is to check for the patient's responsiveness. The healthcare provider can check for the absence of breathing or normal breathing, as well as try to appreciate a response to stimulus (e.g., voice). Immediate activation of the emergency response system should follow if the patient is unresponsive, and an AED should be obtained if it is nearby and easily accessible.

It is important to note, however, that the 2010 AHA guidelines "deemphasize" checking for breathing, as well as checking for a pulse, because healthcare providers may not always be able to accurately do so or may take too long and delay prompt intervention. As a result, the provider should take no longer than 10 seconds to check for a pulse, and if no pulse is appreciated in that time, chest compressions should be initiated without further delay. However, if the patient suddenly collapses or is not breathing, pulse checks should not even be attempted and the provider should assume that SCA has occurred and begin chest compressions.

Moderate and Deep Sedation in Clinical Practice, ed. Richard D. Urman and Alan D. Kaye.
Published by Cambridge University Press. © Cambridge University Press 2012.

Table 24.1. Key steps in BLS

1. Check patient's responsiveness
2. Activate emergency response system
3. Obtain AED/defibrillator, if nearby

4. Begin CPR
   • 30 : 2 compression/ventilation ratio
   • "Push hard and fast"

5. After AED arrives, check rhythm
6. SHOCKABLE rhythm → shock and immediately follow with CPR for 2 minutes NOT SHOCKABLE rhythm → CPR for 2 minutes
7. Check rhythm every 2 minutes, then go back to step 6

An important change in the latest guidelines is this emphasis on early chest compressions. Chest compressions should be initiated before ventilation ("CAB" rather than "ABC"), and this priority shift is a result of growing evidence on the importance of chest compressions to ensure oxygen delivery to the heart and brain.

However, if a definite pulse is palpable, then the healthcare provider should not initiate chest compressions, but give one mouth-to-mouth breath every 5–6 seconds and recheck the patient's pulse every 2 minutes. The patient should also be placed in a recovery position on his/her side with the lower arm in front of the body.

To start chest compressions, the patient should be placed on a firm surface, or a backboard should be placed under the patient if he/she is in a hospital bed. The heel of one hand should be placed on the center of the patient's chest, with the heel of the other hand on top of the first. The chest wall should be allowed to completely recoil after each compression to prevent higher intrathoracic pressure, which can lead to decreased hemodynamics. Chest compression rate should be at least 100 compressions per minute, and the sternum should be depressed 2 inches (5 cm) ("push hard and fast"). If two or more providers are present, they should alternate every 2 minutes to prevent fatigue and poor compression quality. It is also important to note that chest compressions should be minimally interrupted to check for a pulse, analyze rhythm, or other activities. If an interruption occurs, it should be limited to less than 10 seconds, except when placing an advanced airway or defibrillating. CPR should continue until an AED arrives, the patient wakes up, or advanced life support personnel arrive.

After the initiation of chest compressions, ventilation should be attempted. The compression/ventilation ratio is 30:2 if there is no advanced airway, such as an endotracheal tube. Ventilation can be performed using the head-tilt/chin-lift maneuver if there is no evidence of head or neck trauma. Each mouth-to-mouth breath is delivered by opening the airway, pinching the patient's nose, and creating an airtight seal with each breath given over 1 second to produce visible chest rise. Each breath should be a "regular" breath and not a deep breath. Mouth-to-barrier device, mouth-to-nose, mouth-to-stoma breathing are other alternatives, depending on the patient-specific situation. Bag-valve-mask ventilation with room air or oxygen can also be performed when available. A tight seal should be obtained between the face and mask, and the bag should be squeezed two-thirds of its volume for a 1 L bag and one-third its volume for a 2 L bag. In all of the ventilation methods, the compression/ventilation ratio is still 30 : 2. Once an advanced airway (endotracheal tube, Combitube, or laryngeal mask airway [LMA]) is placed, one breath should be delivered every 6–8 seconds, or 8–10 breaths per minute, with no interruption of chest compressions. These recommendations are given to prevent excessive ventilation, which can lead to gastric inflation and complications such as regurgitation and aspiration.

Early defibrillation with an AED is the next key step in the adult BLS sequence and is the treatment of choice for ventricular fibrillation (VF) of short duration. Defibrillation is performed after a 2-minute cycle of CPR in the BLS sequence. However, there is not enough evidence to recommend delaying defibrillation until a cycle of CPR has been done. For in-hospital settings where an AED is available, the defibrillator should be used as soon as possible. If more than one healthcare provider is present, one provider should initiate compressions while the other activates the emergency response system and obtains an AED. Once the AED has been obtained, the defibrillation sequence is as follows: power AED on, follow AED prompts to check rhythm and give one shock if the rhythm is "shockable," and resume CPR immediately after shocking. If the rhythm is "not shockable," CPR should resume immediately, and the rhythm should be checked every 2 minutes.

Lastly, there are special situations that warrant discussion, especially because the healthcare provider can have a significant impact on patient outcome if they are properly recognized. Two of those situations will be discussed here.

Acute coronary syndrome (ACS) is commonly manifested by chest pain, radiation of pain to the upper body, shortness of breath, sweating, nausea, and lightheadedness. Immediate activation of the emergency medical service (EMS) system should follow when these symptoms are present. When appropriate, EMS providers are trained to administer chewable, nonenteric aspirin 160–325 mg, obtain a 12-lead ECG, administer oxygen to keep oxygen saturation ≥ 94%, administer nitroglycerin in select patients, and administer analgesics such as morphine. Additionally, if an ECG demonstrates ST-segment elevation myocardial infarction (STEMI), the patient must then be rapidly transported to a percutaneous coronary intervention (PCI) facility. Prompt PCI has been associated with improved outcomes in STEMI.

Acute ischemic stroke is another situation in which proper recognition and immediate activation of the EMS system can have a significant impact on the patient's outcome. Commonly manifested symptoms of stroke are acute in onset and can include the following: numbness and weakness of the face, upper or lower extremities, confusion, difficulty speaking or understanding, difficulty walking, dizziness, loss of balance or coordination, and severe headache. If fibrinolytic therapy is given within the first hours of symptom onset, neurologic injury is reduced and patients can have improved outcomes. Patients should be transported directly to a stroke center when possible.

As with any other situation, if the patient is unresponsive, then the BLS sequence, as well as the following advanced cardiac life support (ACLS) components, are critical and should not be delayed, regardless of whether or not the root cause is an ACS or acute ischemic stroke.

Advanced cardiac life support (ACLS)

ACLS builds on the BLS sequence and includes airway management and ventilation support, management of cardiac arrest, and treatment of bradyarrhythmias and tachyarrhythmias [3].

Advanced airway placement and ventilation support allow for oxygenation and elimination of carbon dioxide. There are not sufficient data to recommend when to place an advanced airway in relation to other interventions during resuscitation. However, airway placement should not delay initial CPR and defibrillation, and it is important to note that airway placement can be achieved without interruption of chest compressions. Additionally, only those healthcare providers who have been trained in airway placement should do this, and the guidelines suggest frequent training for skill maintenance. If advanced airway placement cannot be achieved, bag-valve-mask ventilation can be used as a backup. Cricoid pressure, oropharyngeal airways, and nasopharyngeal airways can all be used as adjuncts until an advanced airway is placed.

Once an endotracheal tube or supraglottic airway (e.g., Combitube or LMA) is placed, an immediate assessment for proper placement should follow. Physical examination should reveal bilateral chest rise, bilateral breath sounds, and no breath sounds over the epigastrum. For endotracheal tubes, exhaled CO_2 detectors can also be used to confirm correct placement. Additionally, continuous waveform capnography is now recommended, as it is the most reliable method to confirm and monitor for correct placement of an endotracheal tube. Continuous waveform capnography also has the advantage of reflecting poor-quality CPR if partial-pressure end-tidal CO_2 ($PETCO_2$) decreases below 10 mmHg, and reflecting the return of spontaneous circulation (ROSC) if there is an abrupt and sustained increase in $PETCO_2$ (> 40 mmHg).

After successful placement of an advanced airway, the rate of chest compressions is 100 per minute with no interruptions for ventilation. Ventilation should be given as one breath every 6–8 seconds, or 8–10 breaths per minute. Providers should switch roles every 2 minutes to prevent fatigue. There are not sufficient data to suggest the goal tidal volume, respiratory rate, and inspired oxygen concentration, but 100% inspired oxygen is often empirically used.

In addition to CPR and ventilation support, management of cardiac arrest involves rhythm-based management with an AED. The adhesive pads or paddles of an AED should be placed in an anterior-lateral position. Other positions are anterior-posterior, anterior-left infrascapular and anterior-right infrascapular. VF, pulseless ventricular tachycardia (VT), pulseless electrical activity (PEA), and asystole are heart rhythms that can lead to cardiac arrest. VF and VT are "shockable" rhythms, whereas PEA and asystole are "not shockable" rhythms. If a rhythm check with an AED reveals VF or VT, the initial shock should be delivered at 120–200 J for a biphasic defibrillator and 360 J for a monophasic defibrillator (Table 24.2). After shocking, CPR should resume immediately for 2 minutes, followed by another rhythm check. If VF or VT is revealed again, then another shock is delivered, immediately followed by CPR. Additionally, during this 2-minute cycle of CPR, epinephrine 1 mg IV/IO can be given and repeated every 3–5 minutes. Again, if in 2 minutes VF or VT is revealed, another shock is delivered, immediately followed by CPR. During this cycle of CPR, a bolus dose of amiodarone 300 mg IV/IO can be given. Subsequent to this initial round of cycles, medications given should alternate between epinephrine 1 mg IV/IO and amiodarone 150 mg IV/IO. Alternatively, vasopressin 40 units IV/IO can replace the first or second dose of epinephrine, but should only be given once. If a rhythm check at any time reveals PEA or asystole, which are not shockable rhythms, the sequence outlined below is initiated.

For PEA or asystole, CPR (and not defibrillation) should continue for 2 minutes, followed by another rhythm check (Table 24.3). Epinephrine 1 mg IV/IO every 3–5 minutes can be given during this cycle of CPR. If PEA or asystole is revealed again, CPR resumes for 2 minutes. If a rhythm check at any time reveals VF or VT, the preceding sequence for

Table 24.2. VF/VT management in ACLS

1. Initial shock at 120–200 J (biphasic defibrillator) or 360 J (monophasic defibrillator)

2. CPR for 2 minutes, followed by rhythm check

3. If VF/VT, shock again (at same energy dose or higher)

4. CPR for 2 minutes, followed by rhythm check
   - Epinephrine 1 mg IV/IO every 3–5 minutes
   - Vasopressin 40 u IV/IO can replace first or second dose of epinephrine

5. If VF/VT, shock again (at same energy dose or higher)

6. CPR for 2 minutes, followed by rhythm check
   - Amiodarone 300 mg IV/IO bolus
   - Amiodarone 150 mg IV/IO for second dose

7. If VF/VT, go back to step 4 and follow with steps 5–6 if appropriate

Table 24.3. PEA/asystole management in ACLS

1. CPR for 2 minutes, followed by rhythm check
   - Epinephrine 1 mg IV/IO every 3–5 minutes
   - Vasopressin 40 u IV/IO can replace first or second dose of epinephrine

2. If PEA/asystole, CPR for 2 minutes, followed by rhythm check

3. If PEA/asystole, go back to step 1 and follow with step 2 if appropriate

shockable rhythms is initiated. For the treatment of PEA or asystole, atropine is no longer recommended for routine use, because of a lack of supporting evidence.

Medications given during cardiac arrest have the primary goal of facilitating ROSC. Epinephrine hydrochloride is a vasopressor whose alpha-adrenergic agonist properties include increasing coronary perfusion pressure and cerebral perfusion pressure. The benefits of epinephrine's beta-adrenergic agonist properties are less clear, and it may increase myocardial work and reduce subendocardial perfusion. Vasopressin is a peripheral vasopressor that causes coronary and renal vasoconstriction and has not been shown to be superior to epinephrine in cardiac arrest. There is evidence that vasopressors may be associated with an increased rate of ROSC, although not necessarily an increase in rate of neurologically intact survival to hospital discharge. Amiodarone is an antiarrhythmic drug and is preferred for treatment of VF and pulseless VT. It acts at sodium, potassium, and calcium channels, as well as alpha- and beta-adrenergic receptors as an antagonist. There is evidence that amiodarone increases short-term survival to hospital admission compared to lidocaine or placebo, but there has been no evidence suggesting increased survival to discharge.

It is important to note that other ACLS interventions, such as obtaining vascular access, administering drugs, placing an advanced airway, and monitoring continuous waveform capnography, are recommendations in the AHA guidelines and should not interrupt CPR or defibrillation. Additionally, timely identification and treatment of the underlying cause of cardiac arrest is essential. "The Hs and Ts" are identified in the guidelines as potentially reversible causes of cardiac arrest and are as follows: hypovolemia, hypoxia, hydrogen ion excess (acidosis), hypoglycemia, hypo-/hyperkalemia, hypothermia, tension pneumothorax, tamponade (cardiac), toxins, thrombosis (pulmonary), and thrombosis (coronary). Examples of interventions that may be critical for effective resuscitation include crystalloid administration for hypovolemia due to sepsis, empiric fibrinolytic therapy for suspected pulmonary embolism, and needle decompression for tension pneumothorax.

Another integral component of ACLS is the timely identification and treatment of unstable bradyarrhythmias and tachyarrhythmias. "Unstable" is defined by the AHA guidelines as "a condition in which vital organ function is acutely impaired or cardiac arrest is ongoing or imminent," and it can be manifested as acute mental status changes, chest pain, acute heart failure, shock, and hypotension. Hypoxemia is a common cause of unstable bradycardia and tachycardia, and as a result each ACLS treatment algorithm begins with an evaluation of the patient's breathing by physical examination and monitors such as pulse oximetry. Patients often require supplemental oxygen and assistance with breathing.

Bradycardia is a heart rate less than 60 beats per minute and should be immediately treated if it is the cause of the patient's instability. The first-line treatment is atropine 0.5 mg IV, which can be repeated every 3–5 minutes up to a maximum dose of 3 mg. If unresponsive to atropine, a dopamine infusion at 2–10 µg/kg per minute, epinephrine at 2–10 µg per minute, or temporary transcutaneous pacing may be utilized. Expert consultation and/or transvenous pacing may also be required.

There are many types of tachycardia, and they can be classified according to whether they are narrow-complex versus wide-complex or regular versus irregular. Additionally, they may or may not require treatment. However, for an unstable tachyarrhythmia, immediate synchronized cardioversion should follow. Intravenous access and patient sedation should be established prior to cardioversion when possible, but should not delay cardioversion if the patient is too unstable.

Cardioversion is synchronized with the QRS complex, and the energy dose is adjusted depending on the nature of the rhythm. For unstable atrial fibrillation, the initial biphasic energy dose is 120–200 J. For unstable atrial flutter, the initial energy dose is 50–100 J. For unstable monomorphic/regular VT, the initial energy dose is 100 J. If synchronization is not possible, if the QRS complex has a polymorphic appearance, or if the appearance of the QRS complex cannot be determined, then the energy dose should be set as high-energy unsynchronized shocks (i.e., energy doses used for defibrillation). It is important to note that with a heart rate less than 150 beats per minute and the absence of ventricular dysfunction, the tachyarrhythmia is more likely a secondary manifestation of the underlying condition, rather than the root cause of the patient's instability. If the patient is not hypotensive, the AHA guidelines suggest a trial of adenosine 6 mg IV with a 12 mg second dose if needed.

In a stable patient with a tachyarrhythmia, further evaluation and intervention can be considered depending upon the nature of the QRS complex. If the QRS complex is wide ($\geq$ 0.12 seconds), the following can be considered: IV access, 12-lead ECG, adenosine if monomorphic, antiarrhythmic infusion, and cardiology consultation. The following antiarrhythmic infusions can be given: procainamide, amiodarone, or sotalol. If heart failure or QT prolongation is absent, procainamide should be administered at 20–50 mg per minute until arrhythmia resolves, hypotension occurs, or QRS increases to greater than 0.18 seconds (50% increase). After this initial dose, the maintenance dose of procainamide is 1–4 mg per minute. Alternatively, amiodarone can be given as 150 mg over 10 minutes and repeated as necessary, followed by a maintenance dose of 1 mg/min for the first 6 hours. If QT prolongation is absent, sotalol can also be considered and given as 100 mg (1.5 mg/kg) over 5 minutes.

If the QRS complex is narrow ($\leq$ 0.12 seconds) in a stable patient with a tachyarrhythmia, the following can be considered: IV access, 12-lead ECG, vagal maneuvers (i.e., Valsalva maneuver, carotid sinus massage), adenosine if monomorphic, beta-blocker or calcium channel blocker, and cardiology consultation.

There are many pharmacologic treatment options for the various types of tachyarrhythmias, and a discussion of each is beyond the scope of this book. However, the current AHA guidelines provide drug tables that explain indications for use, dosing, common side effects, and contraindications for use.

Once ROSC has been achieved, the guidelines emphasize the need for prompt transition to post-cardiac-arrest care. For patients in an outpatient setting, transport to a hospital that can provide coronary intervention, neurologic care, critical care, and hypothermia is the first step. For inpatients who are in a hospital setting, transfer to a critical care unit is the next step. What the best care is for patients after an SCA is an ongoing area of research, but a timely initiation of a multidisciplinary, multisystem approach to patient care is vital, as most deaths occur in the first 24 hours.

References

1. American Heart Association. 2010 American Heart Association Guidelines for Cardiopulmonary Resuscitation and Emergency Cardiovascular Care. *Circulation* 2010; **122** (18 Suppl 3): S639–933.

2. Berg RA, Hemphill R, Abella BS, *et al.* Part 5: adult basic life support: 2010 American Heart Association Guidelines for Cardiopulmonary Resuscitation and Emergency Cardiovascular Care. *Circulation* 2010; **122** (18 Suppl 3): S685–705.

3. Neumar RW, Otto CW, Link MS, *et al.* Part 8: adult advanced cardiovascular life support: 2010 American Heart Association Guidelines for Cardiopulmonary Resuscitation and Emergency Cardiovascular Care. *Circulation* 2010; **122** (18 Suppl 3): S729–67.

Chapter

25

Emergency resuscitation algorithms: infants and children

Joyce C. Lo and Richard D. Urman

Introduction

Healthcare practitioners must always be prepared for an emergency situation in which they are responsible for the initial resuscitation of their patient. While the principles behind the emergency resuscitation of adults can be broadly applied to pediatric patients, there are many important differences to be noted. In infants and children, cardiac arrest most commonly occurs as the end result of progressive respiratory failure – hypoxemia, hypercapnea, and acidosis leading to bradycardia and hypotension, and, ultimately, cardiac arrest. This is in contrast to adults, in whom cardiac arrest is most often due to a primary cardiac cause. Pulseless ventricular tachycardia (VT) and ventricular fibrillation (VF) is found as the initial cardiac rhythm in approximately 5–15% of pediatric patients, with its incidence increasing with age. This chapter outlines an approach towards the resuscitation of pediatric patients adapted from the 2010 American Heart Association (AHA) guidelines for cardiopulmonary resuscitation and emergency cardiovascular care [1].

Pediatric basic life support (BLS)

Pediatric basic life support (BLS) encompasses prevention, early cardiopulmonary resuscitation (CPR), and prompt access to the emergency response system, and these latter two components pertain to the practitioner providing sedation (Table 25.1) [2]. It is valuable to first note a key change in the 2010 AHA guidelines as compared to prior editions. Instead of beginning with BLS with "look, listen, and feel for breathing" followed by the Initiation of CPR with rescue breaths (traditional "ABC"), there is now a clear emphasis on early chest compressions ("CAB"). It was controversial that pediatric BLS should begin with compressions as opposed to ventilations, since most pediatric cardiac arrests are due to asphyxia.

Moderate and Deep Sedation in Clinical Practice, ed. Richard D. Urman and Alan D. Kaye.
Published by Cambridge University Press. © Cambridge University Press 2012.

Table 25.1. Key steps in pediatric basic life support

1. Check for patient responsiveness and breathing
2. Activate emergency response system *and* obtain AED, if available If lone rescuer: a. Deliver 2 minutes of CPR prior to activating emergency response system/obtaining AED b. After returning, begin CPR with chest compressions prior to using AED
3. Check for definite pulse (up to 10 seconds) DEFINITE PULSE → Give 1 breath every 3 seconds → Add compressions if pulse remains < 60/min with signs of poor perfusion → Recheck pulse every 2 minutes NO PULSE → Continue to step 4
4. Begin CPR if no pulse with compressions ("push fast, push hard") 1 rescuer: cycles of 30 : 2 compression/ventilation ratio 2 rescuers: cycles of 15 : 2 compression/ventilation ratio
5. Use AED to check rhythm when available
6. SHOCKABLE rhythm (e.g., VF or rapid VT) → Give 1 shock, resume CPR immediately for 2 minutes starting with compressions NOT SHOCKABLE rhythm (e.g., asystole or PEA) → Continue CPR for 2 minutes, recheck rhythm every 2 minutes

However, because most pediatric cardiac arrest patients do not receive bystander CPR, due to rescuer uncertainty or confusion, the CAB approach aims to improve the likelihood of bystander intervention and CPR. This new sequence would delay rescue breaths by only approximately 18 seconds (the time to deliver 30 chest compressions). It is reasonable, of course, for the healthcare practitioner to tailor the sequence of rescue actions in a witnessed arrest to treat the most likely inciting event.

If a child is found unresponsive and not breathing (or only gasping), the healthcare provider should immediately send someone to activate the emergency response system and obtain an automated external defibrillator (AED) or other defibrillator. CPR should begin (with chest compressions) after 10 seconds of searching for a pulse. Any prolonged search for a pulse may be unreliable and time-consuming, delaying the onset of CPR. In infants, one should check for a brachial pulse, and in children, a femoral or carotid pulse. In the event that there is a lone rescuer, CPR should begin immediately with chest compressions for 2 minutes prior to activating the emergency response system and obtaining a defibrillator.

If a child is found with a palpable pulse of 60 per minute or more but inadequate breathing, a rescue breath should be given every 3–5 seconds with pulse checks (lasting up to 10 seconds) every 2 minutes. If the pulse is less than 60 per minute and there are signs of poor perfusion despite support via oxygenation and ventilation, chest compressions should be initiated, as cardiac output in children is heavily dependent on heart rate.

CPR should be initiated with 30 chest compressions. For a *child*, healthcare providers should "push fast, push hard," using the heel of one or two hands to provide at least 100 compressions per minute with enough force to depress the lower half of the sternum at

Table 25.2. Characteristics of high-quality CPR

Rate > 100/min ("push fast")

At least 1/3 the anterior-posterior diameter of the chest ("push hard") compressed: ~1½ inches (4 cm) in infants, ~2 inches (5 cm) in children

Complete recoil between compressions

Minimize interruption between compressions

Avoid excessive ventilation

Deliver chest compressions on a firm surface

least one-third of the anterior-posterior dimension of the chest (approximately 2 inches, or 5 cm). One should take care to avoid the xiphoid and ribs. After each compression, the chest should be allowed to completely recoil so that the heart can refill with blood. Interruptions between compressions should be minimized, but to avoid rescuer fatigue, the compressor role should be rotated every 2 minutes. High-quality chest compressions (Table 25.2) are required to provide adequate blood flow to vital organs and achieve return of spontaneous circulation (ROSC).

In *infants*, the two-finger chest compression technique should be used when there is a lone healthcare provider, and the two-thumb-encircling hands technique should be used when there are two rescuers. In the two-finger technique, the two fingers are placed below the intermammary line, avoiding the xiphoid and ribs. In the two-thumb-encircling hands technique, the infant's chest is encircled with both hands – fingers around the thorax and thumbs together over the lower third of the sternum – and the sternum is compressed by the thumbs. This latter technique is thought to provide improved coronary artery and systemic perfusion. The depth of compression should be at least one-third the anterior-posterior diameter of the chest (approximately 1.5 inches, or 4 cm).

In a scenario with a single rescuer, after 30 compressions, two breaths should be given with a jaw-thrust or head-tilt/chin-lift maneuver. For two-rescuer CPR, one provider is responsible for chest compressions and the other provider maintains an open airway and delivers ventilations at a 15 : 2 ratio. Ventilation is either given mouth-to-mouth or by bag-valve-mask ventilation, but given that bag-mask ventilation is more complex, it is reserved for two-rescuer CPR. When a bag-valve-mask is used, the patient's airway should be opened with a chin-lift and a tight seal must be maintained between the mask and the patient's face. When additional healthcare practitioners are present, a two-person bag-valve-mask technique may provide for more efficient ventilation. A small self-inflating bag with a volume of at least 450–500 mL should be used for infants and small children and an adult-sized bag (1000 mL) should be used for older children. When a self-inflating bag is connected to supplementary oxygen at 10 L/min, the inspired oxygen concentration varies between 30% and 80%. If an oxygen reservoir is attached to the bag, oxygen concentrations can increase to 60–95%.

AEDs can detect shockable rhythms and attenuate the delivered energy to an appropriate dose for children under 8 years old. For infants, a manual defibrillator is preferred over an AED. Defibrillation should begin at a dose of 2 J/kg, followed by at least 4 J/kg for second and subsequent doses, up to and not exceeding 10 J/kg or the adult dose. At this time, there is still limited evidence regarding effective or maximum energy doses in the pediatric patient. Shocks should be delivered immediately following compressions, and CPR, beginning with compressions, should resume immediately after the shock. An AED will prompt the rescuer to reanalyze the rhythm every 2 minutes.

Pediatric advanced life support (PALS)

Pediatric advanced life support (PALS) builds upon BLS and relies on a team of organized healthcare providers working effectively, rapidly, and simultaneously to resuscitate a patient [3]. While chest compressions begin, other providers must provide ventilations, obtain a defibrillator, connect monitors, establish vascular access (peripheral venous or intraosseous access), and determine which medications are to be administered. Also, extracorporeal life support (ECLS) should always be considered early, if available, when cardiac arrest is refractory to standard resuscitation and there is a potentially reversible cause.

Emergency drugs can be administered intravenously (IV) or intraosseously (IO). Given the general difficulty in obtaining central venous access, this should be deferred until the patient has been stabilized. Initial resuscitation medications should be dosed based on actual body weight (not exceeding the standard adult dose) or determined with the use of a body-length tape with precalculated doses.

Beyond standard monitoring (electrocardiography, pulse oximetry, noninvasive blood pressure measurement), arterial catheterization and end-tidal CO_2 monitoring can be helpful in PALS resuscitation. An arterial waveform can be used to provide important information on adequacy of hand position and depth during chest compressions, as well as to indicate ROSC. In addition to confirmation of endotracheal tube position, capnography may help to assess quality of compressions during CPR. With partial-pressure end-tidal CO_2 ($PETCO_2$) < 10–15 mmHg, one must be aware of the possibility of excessive ventilation or inefficient chest compressions. On the other hand, an abrupt and sustained increase in $PETCO_2$ may herald ROSC and may be able to prevent stopping compressions for an additional pulse check.

The PALS cardiac arrest algorithm organizes care around 2-minute periods of uninterrupted CPR. Based on a trained healthcare provider's interpretation of the ECG, or by AED analysis, the rhythm will either be "shockable" (e.g., VF or rapid VT) or "not shockable" (e.g., PEA or asystole). For shockable rhythms (Table 25.3), defibrillation is necessary and could be curative. Ideally, there should be minimal time between the last compression and shock delivery, after which compressions should immediately begin again. Compressions can continue while the defibrillator is charging, and, as described above, the initial shock can be given at a dose of 2 J/kg. If the rhythm is still shockable after 2 minutes of CPR, a shock should be given at 4 J/kg and can increase with subsequent shocks to a maximum dose of 10 J/kg (not to exceed the adult dose). During CPR, epinephrine 0.1 mg/kg IV (maximum of 1 mg) should be administered every 3–5 minutes with chest compressions. If epinephrine has been dosed, amiodarone (5 mg/kg IV bolus) can also be given repeated up to two times. In the absence of amiodarone, lidocaine 1 mg/kg IV can be given. Attempts should be made to treat reversible causes of cardiac arrest (Table 25.4).

If defibrillation is successful, a pulse must be verified and, if present, post-cardiac-arrest care should commence. If VF or pulseless VT recurs, CPR should be restarted, amiodarone should be administered, and a shock should be delivered at a dose at least equal to the previous successful dose. If at any time the rhythm becomes "nonshockable," management switches to the PEA/asystole algorithm (Table 25.5). In nonshockable rhythms, CPR is the

Table 25.3. Management of pediatric VF/VT

1. Shock at 2 J/kg
2. Resume CPR immediately for 2 minutes, recheck rhythm   Obtain IV/IO access
3. If VF/VT, shock again at 4 J/kg

4. Resume CPR for 2 minutes, recheck rhythm
   Administer epinephrine 0.01 mg/kg IV every 3–5 minutes (maximum 1 mg)
   Consider advanced airway

5. If VF/VT, shock again at 4 J/kg or higher dose up to 10 J/kg (not to exceed adult dose)

6. Resume CPR for 2 minutes, recheck rhythm
   Administer amiodarone (5 mg/kg IV bolus), repeat up to two times
   Treat reversible causes
   Return to step 3 if rhythm continues to be shockable

* If rhythm becomes "nonshockable" at any point, proceed to the PEA/asystole algorithm (Table 25.5).
* If defibrillation is successful, verify a pulse is present. If so, begin post-cardiac-arrest care.
* If defibrillation is successful but VF recurs, resume CPR and administer amiodarone before shocking again at previously successful dose.

Table 25.4. Reversible causes of cardiac arrest

Hypovolemia	Tension pneumothorax
Hypoxia	Tamponade (cardiac)
Hydrogen ion excess (acidosis)	Toxins
Hypoglycemia	Thrombosis (coronary, pulmonary)
Hypo /hyperkalemia	
Hypothermia	

mainstay of therapy. Epinephrine should be administered as described above, and the rhythm should be rechecked every 2 minutes for either an organized or shockable rhythm. Reversible causes should be explored and treated.

Since ventilation is key, various airway devices may aid in ventilating the patient. Oropharyngeal and nasopharyngeal airways may help to maintain a patent airway. It is important to select an appropriate size in order to maintain an open airway but avoid obstruction. A laryngeal mask airway (LMA) can be considered when ventilation is unsuccessful and endotracheal intubation is not possible. Endotracheal intubation requires a trained provider, as the pediatric airway poses challenges given the different airway anatomy in children. When appropriate, endotracheal intubation should be facilitated with rapid sequence induction and confirmed with condensation on endotracheal tube, bilateral chest rise and equal breath sounds, exhaled CO_2 on capnometry or capnography, and chest x-ray. When an advanced airway is in place, a breath is given every 6–8 seconds (or 8–10 breaths/minute). If a patient's condition worsens, consider dislocation or obstruction of the tube, pneumothorax, or equipment errors.

Table 25.5. Management of pediatric PEA/asystole

1. CPR for 2 minutes, recheck rhythm
   - Obtain IV/IO access
   - Administer epinephrine 0.01 mg/kg IV every 3 to 5 minutes (maximum 1 mg)
   - Consider advanced airway

2. If SHOCKABLE
   → refer to VF/VT management algorithm

   If NOT SHOCKABLE
   → resume CPR for 2 minutes
   → treat reversible causes

3. Recheck rhythm. If organized rhythm is present, check for pulse and begin post-cardiac-arrest care.

When circulation has been restored and arterial oxyhemoglobin saturation monitoring is possible, begin titrating down the inspired oxygen concentration (if appropriate equipment is available). Given the risk of harm from hyperoxemia, there is a recommendation to titrate down inspired oxygen to maintain an arterial oxyhemoglobin concentration $< 100\%$ and $\geq 94\%$. Note that adequate oxygen delivery to end organs is determined by arterial oxyhemoglobin saturation, as well as cardiac output and hemoglobin concentration.

In a child with bradycardia (heart rate < 60), supplemental oxygen should be provided, IV access should be obtained, and an ECG monitor/defibrillator should be attached. No further action needs to be taken if ventilation and perfusion are adequate. However, if there are signs of cardiorespiratory symptoms such as poor perfusion in a patient with bradycardia, CPR should be initiated and the patient should be reevaluated after 2 minutes. Epinephrine 0.01 mg/kg IV should be given for persistent bradycardia. Atropine 0.02 mg/kg IV should be given for bradycardia due to increased vagal tone or AV block. Transcutaneous pacing should be used for complete heart block or sinus node dysfunction.

In a child with tachycardia, one should first check for pulses and assess perfusion. If the patient has poor perfusion or is pulseless, immediately begin the PALS algorithm as described above. Otherwise, place monitors, provide supplemental oxygen, obtain vascular access and a 12-lead ECG. Once the ECG is available, determine QRS duration. A narrow-complex tachycardia (QRS ≤ 0.09 s) may be either sinus tachycardia (for which reversible causes should be explored and treated) or a supraventricular tachycardia. In a hemodynamically stable patient, begin with vagal stimulation by carotid sinus massage, Valsalva maneuver, or, in infants and young children, apply ice to the face. If this is unsuccessful, chemical cardioversion with adenosine 0.1 mg/kg IV given rapidly followed by an immediate saline flush should be attempted. Verapamil 0.1–0.3 mg/kg IV can also be used in older children. If this is ineffective, electric synchronized cardioversion is recommended, preferably with sedation, starting at a dose of 0.5–1 J/kg. If unsuccessful, the dose should be increased to 2 J/kg. Prior to a third shock, amiodarone 5 mg/kg IV (infused over 20–60 min) or procainamide 15 mg/kg IV (infused over 30–60 min) should be given. Expert consultation should be obtained prior to this if the patient is hemodynamically stable.

In a stable child with wide-complex tachycardia (QRS > 0.09 s), expert consultation is strongly recommended, because all treatments have serious potential adverse effects. Pharmacologic and electric cardioversion are both part of treatment that should be guided by an expert in pediatric arrhythmias. In hemodynamically unstable patients, electric cardioversion with 0.5–1 J/kg is recommended, and, if unsuccessful, the dose should be increased to 2 J/kg.

The resuscitation of infants and children with congenital heart disease will not be described in this chapter. However, the 2010 AHA guidelines for CPR and ECC do contain recommendations for the emergency management of these patients and should be reviewed as necessary.

Despite improvement in CPR outcomes, the majority of children with cardiac arrest either do not survive or survive but with significant impairment. Studies have shown that the inclusion of family members during resuscitation has helped family members cope with long-term grief and trauma following such an event.

Summary

Most recent AHA guidelines emphasize the role for early compressions ("CAB") rather than beginning BLS with rescue breaths (traditional "ABC").

High-quality chest compressions (at least 100 compressions a minute with enough force to depress the sternum approximately 5 cm and adequate time for complete recoil between compressions) are required to provide adequate blood flow to vital organs and achieve return of spontaneous circulation.

Two rescue breaths should be given after 30 compressions if there is a single rescuer or after 15 compressions if there are two rescuers. In a patient with an advanced airway in place, a breath should be given every 6–8 seconds (or 8–10 breaths/minute).

In a child who is unresponsive or not breathing, the healthcare provider should delegate someone to activate the emergency response system and obtain a defibrillator, while the healthcare provider starts CPR with chest compressions. If there is a lone rescuer, 2 minutes of chest compressions should be initiated prior to activating the emergency response system and obtaining a defibrillator.

The PALS cardiac arrest algorithm organizes care around 2-minute periods of uninterrupted CPR. If a patient's ECG rhythm is "shockable," defibrillation should occur immediately after the last compression and CPR should begin again with chest compressions immediately following delivery of the shock.

References

1. American Heart Association. 2010 American Heart Association Guidelines for Cardiopulmonary Resuscitation and Emergency Cardiovascular Care. *Circulation* 2010; **122** (18 Suppl 3): S639–933.

2. Berg MD, Schexnayder SM, Chameides L, *et al.* Part 13: pediatric basic life support: 2010 American Heart Association Guidelines for Cardiopulmonary Resuscitation and Emergency Cardiovascular Care. *Circulation* 2010; **122** (19 Suppl 3): S862–75.

3. Kleinman ME, Chameides L, Schexnayder SM, *et al.* Part 14: pediatric advanced life support: 2010 American Heart Association Guidelines for Cardiopulmonary Resuscitation and Emergency Cardiovascular Care. *Circulation* 2010; **122** (18 Suppl 3): S876–908.

Index